The Business of Medical Practice

Advanced Profit Maximization Techniques for Savvy Doctors

2nd Edition

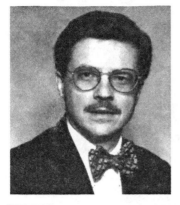 **Dr. David Edward Marcinko, MBA, CFP©, CMP©,** is a health care economist, adjunctive clinical professor, and former private practitioner from Temple University in Philadelphia. He has edited two practice-management textbooks, three medical texts, and four personal financial planning books for physicians and health care professionals. His clinical publications are archived in the Library of Congress and the Library of Medicine at the National Institutes of Health. His economic thought leadership essays have been referenced by *Investment Advisor Magazine,* Medical Group Management Association (MGMA), American College of Medical Practice Executives (ACMPE), American College of Physician Executives (ACPE), JAMA.ama-assn.org, Health Care Management Associates (HMA), CFP© Biz *(Journal of Financial Planning),* and the Financial Planner's Online Library with CD-ROM, among others. A favorite on the lecture circuit, Dr. Marcinko speaks frequently to medical societies and financial institutions throughout the country in an entertaining and witty fashion.

Professor Marcinko received his undergraduate degree from Loyola College (Baltimore), his business degree from the Keller Graduate School of Management (Chicago), and his financial planning diploma from Oglethorpe University (Atlanta). He is a licensee of the Certified Financial Planner© Board of Standards (Denver) and holds the Certified Medical Planner© designation. He earned Series #7 (general securities), Series #63 (uniform securities state law), and Series #65 (investment advisory) licenses from the National Association of Securities Dealers (NASD) and a life, health, disability, variable annuity, and property-casualty license from the State of Georgia. He is also a board-certified surgical fellow.

Dr. Marcinko was cofounder of an ambulatory surgery center that was sold to a publicly-traded company and is a Certified Professional in Health Care Quality (CPHQ); a certified American Board of Quality Assurance and Utilization Review Physician (ABQAURP); a medical-staff vice president of a general hospital; an assistant residency director; a founder of a computer-based testing firm for doctors; and president of a regional physician practice-management corporation in the Midwest.

Currently, Dr. Marcinko is chief executive officer of the *Institute of Medical Business Advisors, Inc.,* a national resource center and referral alliance providing financial stability and managerial peace-of-mind to struggling physician clients.

The **Business** of **Medical Practice**

Advanced Profit Maximization Techniques for Savvy Doctors

2nd Edition

David Edward Marcinko, MBA, CFP, CMP
Editor

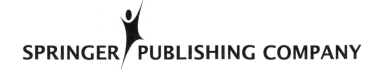

SPRINGER PUBLISHING COMPANY

Springer Publishing Company, Inc.
11 West 42nd Street
New York, NY 10036

Acquisitions Editor: Sheri W. Sussman
Production Editor: Jeanne W. Libby
Cover design by Joanne Honigman

06 07/5 4 3 2

Library of Congress Cataloging-in-Publication Data

The business of medical practice, 2nd ed : advanced profit maximization techniques for savvy doctors / [edited by] David Edward Marcinko.
    p. ; cm.
  Includes bibliographical references and index.
  ISBN 0-8261-2375-9
  1. Medicine—Practice—Finance. 2. Medical offices—Management. [DNLM: 1. Practice Management, Medical—economics. W 80 B9787 2004] I. Marcinko, David E. (David Edward)
R728.B8755 2004
610'.68—dc22   2004008895

Printed in the United States of America by Integrated Book Technology.

Disclaimer:
The information presented in this textbook is not intended to constitute financial, business, insurance, technology, legal, accounting, or management advice. Prior to engaging in the type of activity described, you should receive independent counsel from a qualified professional. Examples are generally descriptive and do not purport to be accurate in every regard. The practice-management and health care industry is evolving rapidly, and all information should be considered time-sensitive.

Dedication

It is an incredible privilege to edit the second edition of *The Business Of Medical Practice: Advanced Profit Maximization Techniques for Savvy Doctors.* One of the most rewarding aspects of my career has been the personal and professional growth acquired from interacting with business, accounting, technology, legal, and financial professionals of all stripes. The mutual sharing and exchange of practice-management ideas stimulates the mind and fosters advancement at many levels.

Creating this text was a significant effort that involved all members of our firm. Over the past year, we interfaced with numerous outside private and public companies to discuss its contents. Although it is impossible to list every person or company that played a role in its production, there are several people we wish to thank for their extraordinary assistance: Robert J. Cimasi, CMP©, and Timothy Alexander, MLS, of Health Capital Consultants, LLC, St. Louis, Missouri; Dr. Richard J. Mata, MS-MI, MS-CIS, health care informaticist from San Antonio, Texas; Dr. Peter R. Kongstvedt, FACP, Partner-Health and Managed Care Consulting Division, Cap Gemini Ernst & Young, LLC; Richard D. Helppie, founder and CEO of the Superior Consultant Corporation (NASD-SUPC); Mike Jensen and Ruth Given, PhD, of Deloitte Health Care Consulting; Dave Pickhardt, vice president for managed health care at Aventis Pharmaceuticals, underwriters of the Managed Care Digest Series™ (which was developed and produced by Forte Information Resources, with data provided by the SMG Marketing Group, Inc.), the Medical Group Management Association (MGMA); and Sheri W. Sussman, editorial director at Springer Publishing Company.

Of course, this second edition would not have been possible without the support of my wife Hope and daughter Mackenzie, whose daily advocacy encouraged me to completion.

It is also dedicated to the contributing authors who crashed the development life cycle in order to produce time-sensitive material in an expedient manner. The satisfaction I enjoyed from working with them is immeasurable.

Dr. David Edward Marcinko, MBA, CFP©, CMP©
Editor-in-Chief
Norcross, Georgia

Contents

SECTION THREE: CONTEMPORARY ASPECTS OF MEDICAL PRACTICE

Contributors

Kriss Barlow, RN, MBA
Corporate Health Group
7 Brayton Meadow,
East Greenwich, RI 02818-1334
715-381-1171 (voicemail)
401-886-5588 (fax)
www.CorporateHealthGroup.com

Kriss Barlow has more than 20 years of health care experience. Her clinical framework is complemented by physician strategy, marketing, and network development success. She holds a bachelor's degree in nursing from Augustana College and an MBA from the University of Nebraska.

Dr. Gary L. Bode, MSA, CMP©
Creative Practice Accounting
2999 Single Tree Court
Leland, NC 28451
800-839-4763 (voicemail)
910-371-5923 (voicemail)
910-520-4670 (mobile)
www.MedicalBusinessAdvisors.com

Gary L. Bode, a former clinician, was managing partner of a multioffice medical practice for a decade before earning his master of science degree in accounting from the University of North Carolina. He is a nationally known financial author, educator, and speaker. Currently, he is managing principal of Comprehensive Practice Accounting (CPA), in Wilmington, North Carolina. He is also chief accounting officer for the Institute of Medical Business Advisors, Inc. Areas of expertise include producing customized managerial accounting reports, appraisals, and valuations, restructurings, and standard financial accounting, as well as proactive tax positioning and tax return preparation for small- to medium-sized businesses.

Daniel J. Buba, JD
Counsel: Law Offices of Liberty Mutual Group
Indianapolis Legal Department
11611 N. Meridian Street, Suite 410
Carmel, IN 46032
317-582-0438-286 (voicemail)
317-582-1281 (fax)
Daniel.Buba@LibertyMutual.com

Dan Buba received his undergraduate degree from Siena Heights University in Michigan and graduated cum laude from the Chicago-Kent College of Law. His practice emphasis is on health care law and on medical insurance and medical malpractice litigation. He writes and lectures extensively for physicians and the bar. He is a member of the Indiana Bar Association (IBA), the Indiana Hospital Association (IHA), and the American Academy of Health Care Attorneys (AAHA).

Render S. Davis, MHA, CHE
3317 Breton Circle
Atlanta, GA 30319
404-256-0264 (voicemail)
rendavis@bellsouth.net

Render S. Davis is a certified health care executive. He served as assistant administrator for general services, policy development, and regulatory affairs at Crawford Long Hospital of Emory University from 1977 to 1995. He is currently an administrator for special projects and cochair of the ethics committee of Crawford Long Hospital and an independent health care consultant in the areas of policy and ethics. He is a founding board member of the Health Care Ethics Consortium of Georgia and has served on the consortium's executive committee, advisory board, futility task force, and strategic planning committee and has chaired the annual conference planning committee since 1995.

DeeVee Devarakonda, MBA
Founder: Filigree, Inc.
4745 Le Beau Ct.
Fremont, California 94555
510-894 0134 (voicemail)
www.filigree-inc.com
deevee@attbi.com

Prior to founding Filigree, DeeVee was chief marketing officer at Quaero—a CRM services company. In her role, she was responsible for building the brand, developing new markets and channels, and establishing the CRM infrastructure. Prior to Quaero, DeeVee worked at Infosys Technologies—an IT services company—where she headed the global marketing group. She designed, developed, and executed marketing programs for Infosys and was responsible for patient attraction and retention initiatives. Prior to Infosys, she worked with Ammiratti Puris Lintas, now a part of Interpublic Group of health care organizations, the second largest advertising group in the world, where she led the media program for Unilever brands. DeeVee has a bachelor's in mechanical engineering from the Indian Institute of Technology, Madras, and earned a master's in management from the Indian Institute of Management, Ahmedabad. She is an author and frequent speaker on multichannel CRM strategies at industry forums such as IQPC and the Direct Marketing Association.

Dr. Charles F. Fenton III, JD
Law Offices
1145 Cockrell Court
Suite # 101
Kennesaw, Georgia, 30152-4760,
404-233-4350 (voice)
404-231-0853 (fax)
www.MedicalBusinessAdvisors.com

Dr. Charles F. Fenton, a board-certified private practitioner from Temple University, received his law degree from and was class valedictorian at Georgia State University. His clients include physicians involved in audits or recoupment actions, as well as disputes with insurance companies and related vendors. He has authored numerous professional and managerial publications for physicians and the bar. In addition to his health-law practice, he is chief legal officer for the Institute of Medical and Business Advisors, Inc.

Eric Galtress
2086 Covington Avenue
Simi Valley, CA 93065
805-522-7207 (voicemail)
805-522-3111 (fax)
Ericteam101@yahoo.com

Eric Galtress held executive level positions in the Professional Employer Organization (PEO) Industry with specialization in both service and manufacturing sectors, as well as other niche markets. He developed and provided instruction in client needs analysis and the proposal process in the field of human resource management and is active in the implementation of tailored services and client retention. Mr. Galtress has written chapters in textbooks and authored many articles for the World Trade Association and for the aerospace, medical, business, and garment industries. With expertise in government compliance, contract management, and business development, he most recently served as senior vice president, chief operating officer, and board member of a training, education, and media company.

Dr. Daniel L. Gee, MBA
Principal: Creative Health Care USA
8467 E. Aster Dr.
Scottsdale, Arizona 85260
480-473-2525 (voicemail)
480-473-1646 (fax)
DNLGee1@cox.net

Dr. Gee is an expert in operating suite dynamics and logistics, having helped establish two hospital-based obstetrical anesthesiology programs in Phoenix, Arizona. Formerly, he was managing partner for a multispecialty anesthesiology practice in the Southwest and chief of anesthesiology at John C. Lincoln Hospital in Phoenix. Dr. Gee designed pharmaceutical protocols for clinical practice, was a speaker for Glaxo Pharmaceuticals, and served on formulary committees and as an investigator for clinical trial programs. He received a BS degree with honors from the University of Southern California, an MBA from Arizona State University, and a medical degree from the University of Arizona. He is a diplomate of the American Board of Anesthesiology and an active medical practitioner.

Allan Gordon
Principal: Phoenix Health Care Consulting, LLC
111 N. Sepulveda Blvd., Suite # 220
Manhattan Beach, CA 90266
888-PHC-6252 (voicemail)
310-379-0916 (fax)

Allan Gordon specializes in managed-care consulting to providers and health plans, including managed-care contracting and network development, market and competitive analysis, physician-network review, and contract negotiations. A graduate of the University of California, Los Angeles, Mr. Gordon has more than 18 years of experience in health plan operations, including provider relations, department integration, provider network development, market and competitor analysis, and strategic planning. His clients include medical groups, IPAs, health plans, and public sector health initiatives.

Angela Herron, CPA
Founder: Phoenix Health Care Consulting, LLC
Phoenix Health Care Consulting
111 N. Sepulveda Blvd., Suite # 220
Manhattan Beach, CA 90266
888-PHC-6252 (voicemail)
310-379-0916 (fax)

Angela Herron's professional experience includes financial management and advisory services to health care clients, including business planning and advisory services on transactions for health care companies and business ventures. She specializes in financial analysis, providing ongoing financial management to numerous medical groups. She also works with physicians to prepare for managed-care contracts and with PHOs to structure and implement integrated managed-care delivery systems. Ms. Heron is a graduate of the University of Northern Iowa, with a bachelor's degree in accounting, and she is a certified public accountant.

Hope Rachel Hetico, RN, MHA, CMP© candidate
Institute of Medical Business Advisors, Inc.
Peachtree Plantation–West
Suite # 5901 Wilbanks Drive
Norcross, Georgia 30092-1141
770-448-0769 (voicemail)
775-361-8831 (fax)
www.MedicalBusinessAdvisors.com

Hope Rachel Hetico received her nursing degree from Valpariso University and her master's degree in Health Care Administration from the College of St. Francis, in Joliet, Illinois. She is author's editor of a dozen major textbooks and is a nationally known expert in reimbursement, case management, utilization review, National Association and Committee for Quality Assurance (NACQA), Health Plan Employer Data and Information Set (HEDIS), and Joint Commission on Accreditation of Healthcare Organization (JCAHO) rules and regulations. Prior to joining the Institute of Medical Business Advisors as president, she was a financial advisor, licensed insurance agent, and Certified Professional in Health Care Quality (CPHQ). She was also Eastern regional director for medical quality improvement at Apria Health Care, in Costa Mesa, California.

Frederick William LaCava, PhD, JD
LaCava & Buba Law Firm
5146 East 75th Street
Indianapolis, IN 46250
317-577-2249 (voice)
317-577-1320 (fax)
LaCavaLaw@aol.com

Dr. Frederick William LaCava (also known as "Duffy"), earned his BA from Emory University, Atlanta, a doctorate in English from The University of North Carolina, Chapel Hill, and a JD from Indiana University School of Law, Bloomington, Indiana. He practices health law at the LaCava & Buba Law Firm, in Indianapolis, Indiana.

Allison McCarthy, MBA
Consultant: Corporate Health Group
P.O. Box 563
West Dennis, MA 02670
508-394-8098 (voicemail)
508-760-6911 (fax)
amccarthy@corporatehealthgroup.com

Nancy McCarthy is a consultant for the Corporate Health Group (CHG), with 15 years experience in physician relations, recruitment, tertiary outreach, and network development. Prior to joining CHG, she was the director of physician relations at Beth Israel Deaconess Medical Center in Boston and vice president of Physician Services at North Suburban Health System/The Malden Hospital, in Malden, Massachusetts. She also held a position in regional council management for the Massachusetts Hospital Association (MHA). Ms. McCarthy earned her MBA, with a concentration in health care management, from Boston University and her undergraduate degree in management from Northeastern University. She is a certified member of the American College of Medical Practice Executives (ACMPE).

Dr. Brent A. Metfessel, MS
Corporate Clinical Research Coordinator
Anthem Blue Cross Blue Shield
Corporate Medical Policy, B3F4
370 Bassett Rd.
North Haven, CT
203.985.7752 (voice)
Brent.Metfessel@anthem.com
www.Anthem.com

In his prior position as senior medical informaticist for Crossroads Technology Solutions, Dr. Metfessel created and enhanced client reporting and analytic technologies using episode of care methodologies. He designs custom-built primary care and specialist provider profiling systems. He is a visionary in the application of the industry-leading clinical episode of care methodology to health care databases, with a decade of experience in general computer science, statistical analysis, artificial intelligence, and computational biology. Now at Anthem, he is a senior clinical research coordinator for health care IT. Dr. Metfessel received his master of science degree, in health informatics, from the University of Minnesota and his medical doctorate from the University of California, San Diego. He also holds a professional certificate in management for physicians from the University of St. Thomas.

Carolyn Merriman
President: Corporate Health Group
7 Brayton Meadow
East Greenwich, RI 02818-1334
888-334-2500 (voicemail)
401-886-5588 (fax)
www.CorporateHealthGroup.com

Carolyn Merriman is founder and president of the Corporate Health Group, providing consultation for strategic planning, occupational health, physician relations, call centers, marketing, and sales efforts. She has been involved in the development and roll-out of a variety of service line strategies. A noted speaker and contributing author for health care periodicals, Merriman is coauthor of *A Comprehensive Guide to Occupational Health Sales and Marketing.* Merriman was recently named for a 3-year term to the board of directors for the Society for Health Care Strategy and Market Development (SHSMD).

Rachel Pentin-Maki, RN, MHA, CMP© cand.
Institute of Medical Business Advisors, Inc.
Peachtree Plantation–West
Suite # 5901 Wilbanks Drive
Norcross, Georgia 30092-1141
770-448-0769 (voicemail)
775-361-8831 (fax)
www.MedicalBusinessAdvisors.com

Rachel Pentin-Maki received her nursing degree from the Community College of Springfield, Ohio, and her master's degree in health care administration from Lewis University, in Evanston, Illinois. Formerly, she helped edit several medical and business textbooks and is a nationally known expert in business staffing and human resource management. Prior to joining the Institute of Medical Business Advisors as chief operating officer, she was the administrator and director of human resources at the Finnish Rest Home, Lantana, Florida. Currently, she is on the board of directors at Finlandia University (Suomi College) in Hancock, Michigan, and is leading the *i*MBA initiative into Helsinki.

Carol S. Miller, MBA, BSN
Senior Principal, Mitretek Systems
3150 Fairview Park Drive South
Falls Church, Virginia 22042-4519
703-610-2458 (corporate voicemail)
703-610-2453 (corporate fax)
carol.miller@mitretek.org

Carol S. Miller is a senior principal at Mitretek Systems, based in Falls Church, Virginia. Her health care career spans 25 years and includes expertise in physician/hospital communications systems, telecommunications strategies, and hospital operations. She has served in executive positions for hospitals, management organizations, and billing services. Ms. Miller holds a master of business administration degree as well as a bachelor of science degree in nursing. She has been published in numerous industry journals and is a member of such organizations as the Health Care Financial Management Association, American College of Health Care Executives, and the Medical Group Management Association.

Patricia A. Trites, MPA, CHBC, CPC, CHCC, CHCO
Health Care Compliance Resources
507 W. Jefferson
Augusta, MI 49012
info@complianceresources.com
616-731-2561 (voicemail)
800-973-1081 (toll free)
616-731-2490 (fax)

Patricia Trites is CEO of Health Care Compliance Resources and holds a master's degree in public administration, specializing in health care, from Western Michigan University. She is a college instructor in health care administration, with intensive coding- and reimbursement-training protocols. She is also a noted speaker for national health care industry conventions. She conducts compliance guidance in the areas of billing and reimbursement, OSHA, Clinical Laboratory Improvement Act (CLIA), and employment law. Her professional memberships and affiliations include The American Compliance Institute, Medical Group Management Association (MGMA), Independent Accountants Association of Michigan, National Association of Health Care Consultants, Institute of Certified Professional Health Care Consultants, American Academy of Professional Coders and Trustees, and the Institute of Certified Health Care Business Consultants.

Foreword

It's never been easy to be a physician, and in many ways the pressures on practitioners are only getting worse. This is why I've been a longtime admirer of what David Edward Marcinko does with his writing and knowledge of medicine and medical practice. Dr. Marcinko's books provide guidance for physicians, helping them to survive organizationally, administratively, and financially so that they can continue to serve their patients.

Helping fellow physicians in one way or another often figures into the motivations of those who have left the joys of a medical practice to pursue health care from a different vector. Some are called into research, giving up the rewards of helping individuals with the hope that they might contribute insights that can lead to the helping of many.

After medical school, my own path took me to the University of Pittsburgh and a doctorate in medical informatics, with visions of helping physicians help their patients through better management of data. Fortunately, I see that vision coming true, especially as I work with my colleagues at Microsoft to create a secure informational infrastructure that gives physicians the information they need at any time, and at any place—including over a wireless device as they attend to a patient at bedside. We call this initiative to provide seamless, yet secure, access to data on an anytime, anywhere, basis Health Care Without Boundaries.

Though we are proud of our work, the greatest wonders come from what we see after we release our products, as physicians do things with our software that we never envisioned. Physicians, by nature—or through selection and training—have scientific minds and a driving curiosity. Over and again, my colleagues and I are dazzled by what physicians are creating by using our technology in unexpected ways. And it is often the work done by private practitioners looking for ways to create their own solutions, because they either couldn't afford a prepackaged one or couldn't find a solution that answered their creative visions.

Physicians, especially those in private or small group practice, are under great stress today. But they are buoyed by a passion for their work and dedication to their patients, and they are extremely resourceful with the brilliance and ingenuity that comes from the curiosity of the scientific mind.

Medical Economics magazine recently ran a story about Robert Novich, a New Rochelle, New York, internist who needed an electronic medical-records system for his solo practice. Suffering from sticker shock and the inflexibility of the commercial EMRs he looked at, he decided to create his own, using Microsoft® Word and a fax machine. Lab reports and other documents received by fax are directly imported into the computer for digital storage. Working with his son Jeff, who was a college student at the time, Dr. Novich created a system that uses Word templates to simplify creation of medical records and Explorer to provide instant file access, slashing time from pulling information out of file cabinets. The system also creates and manages electronic prescriptions.

The results? Dr. Novich said, "I feel like a brand new doctor." This book is filled with a wealth of information on how to survive the financial, administrative, and regulatory pressures that could otherwise draw down on the time you want to spend with your patients. Dr. Marcinko and his contributors cover the spectrum, from developing a medical-office business plan for the new practitioner to placing a value on a practice for the retiring physician preparing to sell. A sampling of topics includes human-resource management and physician recruitment, marketing, insurance coding and health-law compliance, process improvement and medical-care outcomes tracking, cash-flow analysis, office-expense modeling, cost accounting, practice benchmarking, financial and ratio analysis, ROI calculations, CRM, six sigma initiatives, concierge medicine, and medical ethics.

Throughout this book, a common denominator is the need for acquiring and managing information. Fortunately, we live in a time when information technology is providing ever more benefits with an ever lower threshold—both financially and technically.

For less than $500, you can buy a computer today that has a more powerful central processing unit and more memory than the multimillion-dollar mainframes and super computers that were enshrined in regional banks and university research centers in the 1980s. And the advent of point-and-click interfaces and drag-and-drop development environments mean that everyday doctors can do extraordinary things.

Microsoft recently sponsored a contest looking for innovative ways in which our office suite of applications had been used by health care workers. The response was overwhelming—not because of the technology, but because of the innovative ways it was being deployed to solve real-world problems.

Cecil Lynch, an MD and medical informaticist who teaches at the University of California at Davis, is using Microsoft Access to help the U.S. Centers for Disease Control (CDC) enhance the efficiency of its disease surveillance system.

Dr. Duke Cameron of the Division of Cardiac Surgery, Johns Hopkins Hospital, came up with the idea of using the Outlook® Calendar to schedule operating rooms, to help assure the operating room is properly set up with specific implant devices and other special equipment or supplies before the surgical team arrives.

Nick Hoda, a psychologist-in-training at Mississippi State University, uses Microsoft Excel charts and graphs to show his elementary school clients coping with learning and behavioral problems that their behavior really is getting better. He uses the same charts with teachers and administrators to win his young clients another chance at the classroom.

My favorite story, though, came from Dr. Thomas Schwieterman, a fourth-generation physician working in the same medical office his great grandfather established in 1896 in the town of Mariastein, Ohio. From those same historic environs, Schwieterman has used Microsoft Access to create his own physician assistant application. The Schwieterman Family Physicians practice kept him so busy that he was wondering how he could keep up with his patient caseload. Schwieterman wanted a faster way to handle prescriptions, provide medical information, and record data for his patient records. He walked into a McDonald's restaurant one day and had an idea. "I ordered a cheeseburger and fries and watched the person at the counter touch the screen of the cash register a few times, and realized the order was getting transferred back to the food preparation area, and that by the time I paid, my order was ready," he said. "I thought to myself: 'That's what I need!' "

He searched for commercially available solutions, but when he couldn't find an exact match for his needs, and when he found prices steep for a small private practice, he decided to create his own—using Access. He also called upon a friend with a master's degree in electrical engineering to help on the coding. His creation boosted his income by 20%—"Which was important, because we pay more than $60,000 a year for malpractice insurance, even though our clinic has never been sued since it was founded, 107 years ago."

What my friends at Microsoft especially like about this story is that when Dr. Schwieterman's colleagues tried his program, liked it, and suggested he try to sell it, he put together a PowerPoint® presentation and landed a partnership agreement with a major health care supply and services corporation to market his ChartScribe solution.

So, the pressures facing physicians are great, but so are their resources. Information technology is one resource, this book is another, but the greatest resource of all is the innate curiosity and drive to discover and create, which seems to be so much a part of those who are drawn to this noble profession.

Ahmad Hashem, MD, PhD
Global Health Care Productivity Manager
Microsoft's Health Care Industry Solutions Group
Microsoft Corporation
Redmond, Washington

Preface

In the current managed care milieu, *The Business of Medical Practice: Advanced Profit Maximization Techniques for Savvy Doctors* is a textbook of specific value to all medical professionals, as declining payments, increasing expenses, onerous federal regulations, and the shenanigans of Wall Street raise havoc with physician autonomy, income, and patient care. Contrary to conventional wisdom, we do not believe draconian free-market competition in the present guise of managed care will dramatically reduce health care costs, for seven reasons:

- First, it is difficult to define medical quality.
- Second, a perfectly competitive marketplace does not exist.
- Third, the consumer has a voracious appetite for medical care, regardless of accountability or self-restraint.
- Fourth, the demographic economics are against it.
- Fifth, the push for continuous research and development is in the DNA of human beings.
- Sixth, abandoning nonprofitable specialty lines or cutting edge treatments is anathema to medical practitioners.
- Seventh, above all else, medicine is a uniquely personal experience, and American society is not ready for the brutal and rational efficiencies of the business world.

Nevertheless, one in three physicians declined to offer patients useful medical services because they were not covered under health-insurance benefits, according to a 2003 study published in *Health Affairs*. This means some physicians may be violating ethical codes that discourage doctors from withholding information because of coverage restrictions. Furthermore, 35% of doctors feel placed in this position more frequently in the past 5 years. Of course, interpretation of the small survey varies, but failing to inform patients about useful treatments denies them the opportunity to challenge insurance restrictions.

On the other hand, we are pragmatic and realize that practicing health care providers of all independent degree designations (allopathic, osteopathic, and podiatric physicians; dentists; optometrists; chiropractors; psychologists; and nurse practitioners) must learn to better compete in the next decade. Ultimately, practitioners who are clinically *and* economically responsible are the wave of the future. It is the physician/ executive with professional managerial training who can best direct future systems of autonomous care, with improved outcomes for patient, payer, and doctors alike.

The information in this text will help achieve this goal and is most applicable to the solo, small, or medium group practice and for those physicians who aspire to be decision makers and administrators. For the employed physician or resident, it will also serve as a blueprint for what can still be achieved. And for practice administrators, it will serve as a guide to the next generation of medical networks or more complex large group-management endeavors.

This new edition, like the first edition, is written in plain prose form, using nontechnical jargon, without the need to document every statement with a citation from the literature. This allows a large amount of information to be condensed into a single and practical volume. It also allows the reader to comprehend important concepts in a single reading session, and a deliberate effort is made to include germane examples. The interested reader is then able to research selected topics. Overlap of material has also been reduced, but important concepts are reviewed for increased understanding.

The textbook itself is divided into three major sections, written by 20 contributing authors, and with the concepts developed in Section II (quantitative) and Section III (contemporary) building on those of Section I (qualitative). Each section is then divided into multiple parts, for a total of 27 logically progressive, yet stand-alone, chapters.

Chapter 1 briefly reviews the history of health care economics in the United States, from the days of private pay to indemnity insurance and the "golden era of medicine" to contemporary managed care, offering several ideas for re-creation and retooling. Chapters 2 and 3 are new to this edition, and they discuss how to write a medical office business plan to obtain office capital and create a strategic plan to run back-office operations. Chapter 4 is also new; it discusses medical-office relationships, partners, and personalities, while chapters 5 and 6 explain compliance methods, risks, and programs, and the insurance CPT coding issues that are increasingly arcane in a skeptical payer climate. Section 1 concludes with three entirely new chapters: 7, 8, and 9, which deal, respectively, with six-sigma initiatives, quality and medical processes improvement, and the use of futuristic information technology to track clinical outcomes, treatment results, and medical care.

Section 2 begins the quantitative aspects of the book, as chapter 10 presents a fresh look at capitation econometrics, and chapter 11 documents the perils of indiscriminate cash-flow control in rising, declining, and neutral growth environments. Chapter 12 presents basic economic concepts of fixed and variable office-cost behavior and expense modeling, while chapters 13 and 14 explore the disciplines of mixed cost analysis, linear regression analysis, and activity-based cost management (ABCM), a watershed concept to most physicians that has become the costing method of choice in the present hypercompetitive environment. Chapter 15 explores financial-ratio analysis and benchmarking and surveys the typical office for lost sources of additional profit or ways to avoid burdensome expenses. Chapter 16 demonstrates how to calculate and augment your return on office investment, resulting residual income, and the advantages/disadvantages of the novel meter of medical enterprise value added (MEVA). Chapter 17 explains the elusive concept of business value and the philosophy required to create real practice equity in an era of health care mergers and acquisitions, while chapter 18 discusses practice-valuation techniques, concluding the section with an emphasis on Uniform Standards of Professional Appraisal Practice (USPAP) protocols and discounted cash-flow analysis, as office bricks and mortar are becoming increasingly worthless. It is an important chapter for the new practitioner seeking to purchase an existing practice or the retiring practitioner in the quest for proper payoff after years of hard work.

Section III begins with chapter 19 and a comprehensive look at the Health Insurance Portability and Accountability Act (HIPAA) and the information systems and medical office business equipment required for its full understanding and implementation in an increasingly unwired, unsecured, and mobile WiFi world. Chapter 20 presents updates to the outsource versus in-house dilemma of human-resource management, in an attempt to reduce risk, while the contentious issue of restrictive covenants and practice noncompete agreements is reviewed in chapter 21. Chapter 22, which is on physician recruitment, is new, as is the case for concierge medical practice outlined in Chapter 23. Customer (patient) relationship management (CRM) is extensively detailed in Chapter 24, and it presents a controversial concept to traditionally educated physicians. Chapter 25 opines on the ethical and moral issues of managed medical care. Chapter 26 dissects the civil battleground of a medical malpractice trial with its myriad legal tactics, maneuvers, and machinations. Finally, chapter 27 rightly concludes the third section—and the book—with a discussion on choosing the business management advisor that represents the best fit for both office environment and individual physician.

In conclusion, as you read, study, and reflect on this challenging textbook, remember the guiding philosophy of Eric Hoffer: "In a time of drastic change; it is the learners who will inherit the future. The learned find themselves equipped to live in a world that no longer exists."

INSTRUCTIONS FOR CONDENSED READING AND REVIEW

To the new physician, midcareer practitioner, seasoned health care provider, or those practice managers and administrators who find that mastering business topics is a difficult endeavor, this book is a useful source of information, even if you recoil at the thought of cost-volume profit analysis or contribution margins in conjunction with a medical practice.

If you are of this ilk, I urge you to begin your reading with chapters 1, 2, 3, and 6, which will encourage you to learn the basics of management theory and insurance as it relates to the practice of medicine today. After reading this much of the book, you are sure to find enough business material communicated in Section I that you will want to give the mathematical portions of the book another try. All theories are explained in plain language, with easily understood spreadsheet calculations and tables to reinforce vital concepts in Section II. Chapters 12, 13, 14, and 15 are the most difficult of the book, but they are also the most worthwhile, especially to larger group practices. Moreover, chapters 19, 20, 23, and 24 (in Section III) offer the modern information technology (IT) and human-resource guidelines, concierge practice philosophy, and CRM issues of an economically driven society. Beware, chapter 26 is mentally caustic, so take your time and read slowly to consider and digest the chilling material thoroughly.

Finally, study and enjoy the remaining chapters of the book at your leisure. There is something in them for all medical professionals, regardless of specialty or degree designation. The effort will be well rewarded with enhanced revenue, decreased personal stress, and improved patient care, which are the ultimate goals of any contemporary health care reform or futuristic medical business model.

Your thoughts, suggestions, and opinions after reading *The Business of Medical Practice: Advanced Profit Maximization Techniques for Savvy Doctors* are most appreciated and welcomed.

Hope Rachel Hetico, RN, MHA, CMP© cand.
Author's Editor

Qualitative Aspects of Medical Practice

CHAPTER 1

Healthcare Economics in Medical Practice

David Edward Marcinko, Hope Rachel Hetico, and Rachel Pentin-Maki

> The fragmented-by-design healthcare delivery system, rising consumer expectations, and rampaging information technology advances all serve to compound the degree of difficulty in effective use of information technology. The industry's track record regarding information systems in terms of increased efficiency, ease-of-use, and improved margins has been short of expectations. Information systems aimed at improving workflows, connecting to trading partners, and taking advantage of new technologies are still in development. The opportunity remains attractive to information technology providers, as evidenced by a near-continual flow of business venture announcements from technology companies and various industry participants.
>
> —Richard D. Helppie, Chief Executive Officer and Founder, Superior Consultant Company, Inc. (SUPC-NASD)

A basic, but hardly promoted, premise of all healthcare economics is imprecision. Nevertheless, we may define traditional healthcare economics as how the medical-industrial complex allocates its limited resources (cerebral input, equipment, technology, infrastructure, and monetary assets) to the insatiable appetites of the U.S. consumer through the natural laws of supply and demand. This occurs because physicians are willing to sell their services, and patients are willing to buy these services. At some point of equilibrium, supply equals demand; this point is known as *market equilibrium.*

For example, let's take a look at the medical practice of Dr. Jane Smith and her competitor Dr. Harry Jones. When the price of a noncovered Medicare service is lowered by Dr. Smith, her patient load increases and Dr. Jones's volume slows. Conversely, if she raises her fees, Dr. Jones's practice flourishes. This phenomenon, illustrated by market forces, or the "invisible hand" of Adam Smith, can be reviewed from the traditional, contemporary, and futuristic healthcare economic perspectives outlined in the following text.

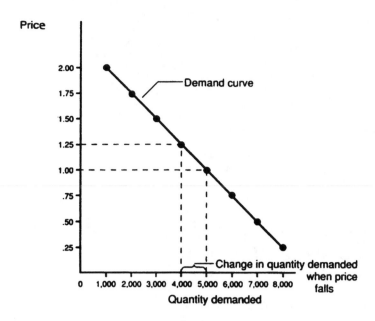

FIGURE 1.1   Typical downward sloping demand curve for health services.

TRADITIONAL HEALTHCARE ECONOMICS

Demand-Side Considerations in Medical Care

Medical care may be defined as the examination and treatment of patients. Implicit in this definition is the fact that the lower the direct out-of-pocket price offered to the patient (all other factors held constant), the greater the number of units of medical commodity the patient will demand. In this relationship, *"demand"* is defined as the set of service quantities (outputs) demanded at various prices, while the *"quantity demanded"* is the amount of care requested at a specific price. Changes in demand occur as a result of personal income and tastes, physician shortages and surpluses, personality and perceptions, and a host of other factors. A graphical representation of this relationship is the classic downward sloping demand curve, and the rationale behind the curve lies in the possibility of substitution, since very few, if any, commodities are absolutely identical and necessary.

Supply-Side Considerations in Medical Care

Historically, physician suppliers were motivated to maximize their profits by augmenting services and minimizing costs. Implicit in this definition is the fact that physician suppliers will endeavor to provide as many services as possible. In this relationship, *"supply"* is defined as the set of services quantities (outputs) provided at various prices, while the *"quantity supplied"* is the amount of care rendered at a specific price. Changes in supply occur as a result of similar, but opposite, factors

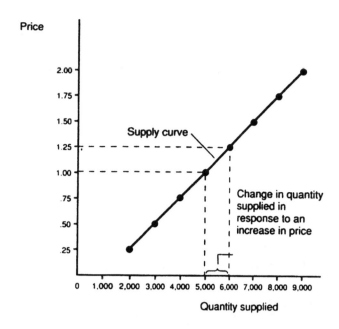

FIGURE 1.2 Typical upward sloping supply curve for health services.

as found in the demand relationship. A graphical representation of this relationship is the classic upward sloping supply curve, while equilibrium is reached when the supply and demand curves intersect at the historic usual, customary, and reasonable price point.

Marginal Revenues and Marginal Cost

If a doctor has the opportunity to see even a single additional patient at a profit, he will rationally do so. The marginal revenue (MR) from the extra office visit exceeds the marginal cost (MC) of the visit. Once the cost of the visit equals the revenue it produces, the incentive to see more patients is lost. In other words, no additional profit is left at the point where $MR = MC$. This is a standard business concept that always hold true, absent situations such as monopolies or oligopolies. Once satisfied, healthcare gratification, or *utility,* diminishes and more care has a lower return on health and productivity.

Marginal Utility and Medical Price Elasticity

If utility is a word used to describe the value of medical service to a patient, then *marginal* utility (MU) is the value of treating one additional patient. At some point, the treatment plan is completed, the patient is satisfied, and additional services are of no value. Another example of this is the inadvisability of having two offices in the same neighborhood rather than in different geographic locations. The marginal utility of the second neighborhood office is often negligible.

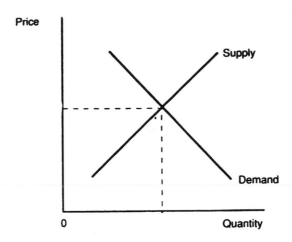

FIGURE 1.3   Market equilibrium for health services.

   In our initial example involving Dr. Smith, some patients may not decide to leave her practice despite the fee increase. Patients may consider such intangibles as demeanor, location, or quality of service and elect to continue their relationship with her. When this occurs, we say patient demand is *inelastic* to price change or price increases. On the contrary, if patients quickly go to Dr. Jones, demand is said to be *elastic* to price pressure, and some studies show that a mere 18–21 dollar monthly increase in out-of-pocket costs is enough to send patients elsewhere. Medical service elasticity is affected by insurance deductibles, copayments, physician's reputation and communication skills, waiting-room time, and the like. When an industry becomes more competitive, as in health-care today, fees tend to become more elastic and patient volume becomes very sensitive to even small changes in price. In a managed-care environment, every noncovered service will have its own level of pricing elasticity, and every doctor should estimate that level for all fees to achieve optimum patient volume.
   Traditionally, medical services and food were inelastic to price changes, while automobile sales are very elastic to price sensitivity. This relationship is rapidly changing, and there is even a mathematic equation stating this phenomenon in ratio form:

$$\text{Elasticity of Medical Supply} = \frac{\%\ \text{Change in Total Revenue}}{\%\ \text{Change in Price}}$$

For instance, if a 20 percent increase in an office visit charge resulted in a 30 percent increase in quantity of services supplied, the price elasticity would be $30/20 = 1.50$. Therefore, a high elasticity coefficient equates to higher price elasticity. Generally, a coefficient greater than 1 is considered elastic, while a coefficient less than 1 is inelastic. Interestingly, exact unity prevails when elasticity of supply is exactly equal to 1.
   In addition to price elasticity of demand, the competitive marketplace drives supply and prices. For example, there is usually more medical competition in large

metropolitan areas than in rural areas. Prices tend to rise and fall, respectively, while the market is more sensitive to price fluctuation due to this structure. In the traditional medical community, this led to the development of four basic medical marketplace types.

The Four Traditional Models of Medical Competition

In a discussion of competitive medical models, assumptions must include normal demand quantities, many fully informed patients, and the fact that physicians cannot directly influence demand for care. These assumptions, although fluid, also preclude the possibility that patient buyers are large enough to have any influence over price. This results in the following structures:

- In a *pure monopoly*, there is only one provider with a unique service. The doctor is a "price maker" and charges whatever he wishes.
- In an *oligopoly*, there are a few physicians who provide similar services. For example, when it becomes clear to Dr. Smith and Dr. Jones that neither can win their price war, oligopolists return prices to prior, but still inflated, levels.
- In *monopolistic competition*, there are many providers with differentiated services. For example, should Dr. Jones decide to have evening hours, she may charge a premium for her fees if Dr. Jones doe not follow suit.
- Finally, when *pure competition* occurs, there are many physicians providing similar and substitutable services. Marketing and advertising does not affect fees, and prices are determined by supply and demand. The doctors become "price takers" by accepting fees arrived at by practicing competitively.

Externalities that Defy Traditional Medical Supply and Demand Economics

The above marketplace structures, while efficient, are not necessarily timely. This is particularly true in medicine and is attributed to various externalities that seemingly deter competition. Formally, *externalities* are defined as the cost or benefits of market transactions that are not directly reflected on the price buyers (patients) or sellers (doctors) use to make their decisions. They represent defects, or inefficiencies, in the pricing system and can be either positive or negative. Pertinent externalities for the physician and the healthcare practitioner include but are not limited to the following:

1. *Barriers to Entry:* Physicians and other learned healthcare professionals receive an extended formal education. This not only ensures competence and protection of the public, but it also reduces competition.
2. *Competitive Advantage:* Once school is over, a medical degree is an effective strategic advantage over a nondegreed practitioner.
3. *Monopsony and Oligopsony* occur when discounts are extracted from healthcare providers because of supply-and-demand size inequalities. This may lead to running afoul of antitrust laws.
4. *Barriers to Exit:* The increased cost of doing business, effectively precludes many physicians from terminating practice until all fiscal investments are

recouped. Observe that few doctors can practice part time and still afford their overhead.

5. *Moral turpitude:* Since physicians take the Hippocratic Oath, they are expected to place patient welfare above their own. This is not necessarily true with business entities that must adhere to legalities only.

6. *Moral Hazards:* Everyone knows that cigarettes, dietary indiscretions, drinking, drug use, and promiscuous behavior are unhealthy. Yet, many pursue this lifestyle, which drives up healthcare costs for society as a whole.

Other externalities that drive up the cost of healthcare are well known but not easily changed. First, most Americans have group insurance through their employment and don't have to pay for medical expenses, making them fairly indifferent to the cost or need of individual health care purchases. Second, acquiring health insurance is not like buying a commodity, and it is difficult for a layman to know which purchases make sense and at what price. Third, most health-insurance purchasing decisions are made by the doctor (e.g., referral to a specialist or to have surgery), not the patient/consumer, and, hence, there is a vested interest in increasing service demand. Last, what well informed person would try to bargain when his or her health is at stake? Who is going to negotiate fees with a neurosurgeon?

During the so-called golden age of medicine (1965–1985), Medicare, Medicaid, and all the previously named factors worked to isolate American medicine from financial reality. In the last decade, however, the private sector has demanded cost containment in the form of negotiated prices for medical services.

Medical Profit Maximization

Now that something about marketplace inefficiencies has been reviewed, it is time to consider how these externalities are applied to the profit maximizing medical practice marketplace. Realize that the imperfect fee-for-service marketplace is now more perfectly competitive in the managed care environment. For example, consider the following economic scenarios.

1. A glut of good physicians causes them to become price takers, selling a homogenous (commoditized) service. An appendectomy is an appendectomy! Or is it? Financially, many doctors are "taking what they're given" *(by Managed Care Organizations), because they're working for a living"*. Younger doctors (those under 40) are especially inclined to work for less since they have had little exposure to fee-for-service compensation. Perhaps providers need to differentiate themselves from the competition? Ponder the MD vs. DO controversy, since one of the fastest growing areas of specialization is osteopathic family medicine. Or consider the potential economic impact of *any willing provider* laws allowing any doctor, to participate in any plan under its clinical guidelines and compensation rules, at will.

2. Physicians have an increasingly smaller share of the medical marketplace because of extended-care providers. Does this help or hinder them? Price information is freely available to all MCOs because of computerization. Recall

all the fee schedule surveys that were popular several years ago? How does this knowledge impact medical care today?

3. Doctors have been defeated in their ability to influence the marketplace by selling a quality, but nevertheless standardized, service. Consider the economic effects of practice guidelines in this light.

4. As medical care becomes efficient, each doctor becomes a perfect substitute for the other. This may either be an accolade or a curse, since patient demand becomes perfectly elastic at the HMO's capitated set price. This being the case, there is no incentive to lower fees in an attempt to attract more patients, since doctors would not be able to treat any more patients than they would otherwise. The price decrease just lowers income but has no effect number of patients treated. It simply decreases profits.

5. Since marginal revenue is the fee obtained from seeing one extra patient, marginal revenue becomes equal to HMO price, and marginal profit is zero when marginal revenue only equals marginal cost. Will the MD still want to wait another hour just to see that last late HMO or Medicaid patient?

6. A profit maximizing office will operate at a short-term loss as long as its minimum average cost is less than its minimum possible average variable cost. But just how long *is* short term?

7. Efficiency prevails when medical services are made available just up to the point that marginal benefits equal marginal costs. When efficiency is achieved, it is not possible to make more money without decreasing another doctor's income in a risk-pool situation. Voila! Managed competition, anyone? It is estimated that more than a quarter of all physicians may leave practice by the year 2008!

Regardless of the technical nature of the above arguments, practical attention must be directed toward the possibility of governmental (i.e., national healthcare) intervention or marketplace (i.e., HMO) intercession, relative to two other concepts that directly affect medical practices, namely, *price ceilings* and *price floors.*

Price ceilings are the legally maximum charges and always result in shortages when set below market equilibrium prices. How long is the wait at a local charitable hospital vs. a local for-profit medical center? Price ceilings often result in an underground black-market economy that exceeds legal limits.

Non–price rationing (i.e., free medical care), on the other hand, distributes available services to patients on a basis other than ability to pay. The most common non–price rationing device is, "first-come, first-served."

Price floors establish minimum prices, which often result in surpluses when they exceed equilibrium price levels. The minimum wage is a good example of a price floor.

Price ceilings and floors benefit certain groups but impair the distribution of goods and services by the price system in free competitive markets. Government intervention interferes in the functioning of competitive markets and is likely to result in resource allocation problems. Remember Keynesian macroeconomic philosophy? In evaluating managed-care price controls, the gains to beneficiaries of price ceilings and floors must be weighed against the resulting allocation problems. Alternative methods that will make the gainers just as well off without impairing the rationing

2003 Market Basket of Goods			
Food and beverages	16%	Recreation	6%
Housing	41%	Education	3%
Clothing	4%	Communication	3%
Transportation	17%	Other goods and services	4%
Medical care	6%		

FIGURE 1.4   Market basket of goods and services representing the domestic CPI.

function of medical prices can be considered as ways to increase efficiency in the medical economy.

Traditional Methods of Healthcare Delivery

Prior to 1970, the healthcare reimbursement system was not a monolithic complex, and most Americans received their healthcare through one of five third-party organizations: (1) Blue Cross/Blue Shield (prepaids), (2) Commercial insurance (private) companies, (3) Medicare (federal program for the elderly), (4) Medicaid (state program for the poor) and (5) Military, through the Civilian Health and Medical Program Uniformed Service (CHAMPUS).

The four participants in this fragmented system were the patient (consumer), the physician (provider), the employer (buyer or payer), and one of these third-party intermediaries. Moreover, the doctor-patient relationship was often muddled by the third parties who became brokers between MD and patient; both of which merely sought to understand (a) who was responsible for payment, (b) how the MD would assist the patient obtain reimbursement, and (c) how to establish the ultimately responsible party.

In the meantime, commercial insurance medical costs were accelerating at a rate greater than three times the Consumer Price Index, a measure of goods and services in a market basket intended to be representative of a typical patient's purchases.

There was no single reason for medical cost escalation, but many economists believed the following circumstances conjoined at one point in time to increase health care costs dramatically:

1. **Law of Supply and Demand** (increasingly, too many doctors chasing too few patients). For example, Milliman & Robertson, the actuarial firm, estimates that only about 70% of physicians actively practicing medicine in the United States are necessary. The same situation is true for other healthcare employees. Mergers, acquisitions, outsourcing, closings, and consolidations have only exacerbated the situation.
2. **The US federal budget deficit** is about 3.5 trillion dollars, since income is 1.5 trillion Dollars and outflow is 5 trillion dollars. On the other hand, the budget surplus that existed several years ago was dissipated by 2004, thanks to the flagging economy and war with Iraq. Additionally, the federal budget further

demonstrates the severity of the healthcare-cost problem as a percentage of the national budget: (social security = 21%; national debt interest = 20%; Medicare and Medicaid = 16%; defense spending = 15%; domestic spending = 15%; miscellaneous spending = 11%, and international spending = 2%.

3. **Increased administrative costs and advancements in technology.** The primary use of new technology has been in the areas of diagnosis and treatment. However, MMOs also use technology to increase operational efficiency and to reduce costs. The price paid is in the loss of jobs or reduction in the skill level needed to perform certain tasks that were formerly done by trained technicians, nurses, or physicians.

4. **Malpractice phobia, misinformed patients, hungry trial lawyers and class action lawsuits.** The median malpractice award for all medical negligence claims has increased by 14% since 2000, and in childbirth cases, the increase is $1.3 million, more than double the median for any other type of medical malpractice verdict. Other median awards:

   - More than $650,000 for medication errors.
   - More than $550,000 for misdiagnosis cases.
   - More than $265,000 for surgical negligence.
   - More than $275,000 for non-surgical treatment cases.
   - More than $255,000 for cases involving doctor/patient relations.
   - More than $590,000 median award for all medical-malpractice cases.

5. **Cultural and socioeconomic timing** ("medical care is a right; not a privilege"). Some patients or employers are not willing to pay the price for good medical care.

According to Steven Wetzell, of employer-initiated Buyers Healthcare Action Group (BHCAG) in St. Paul, MN, even seemingly small healthcare premium amounts matter. For example, the difference between his group's high and lost cost health care plan is about $2025 per member/per month, yet his low cost provider groups continue to gain enrollment as high cost providers lose enrollment. It was the BHCAG experience that price was the driver of enrollment in health plans more than was patient satisfaction.

Domestic Productivity Crippled by Exploding Healthcare Costs

Traditional organizations, except for the military, provided a type of insurance known as *indemnity insurance*, which has the following features: *(a)* An insured individual has the ability to choose the physician and the hospital he or she wants to visit. *(b)* Medical providers are paid a separate fee, for every service provided, as long as it is covered by the patient's benefit plan. Under the system of indemnity (fee-for-service) reimbursement, the implication was that it was the MD's fault if he or she was not paid, and it was the doctor's problem if the medical needs of the patient were not met.

Although confusing, the system gave patients great freedom and MD's great incentive to supply care, but insurer's have little control over the care rendered and its associated costs. Healthcare costs skyrocketed to more than one trillion dollars, or 15–16% of GNP, by 2004–, crippling US productivity.

For example, consider that Medicare in 1999 cost $ 250 billion dollars and is projected to be fiscally insolvent by the Year 2008, when health care spending reaches 2 trillion dollars or 16–17% of US GDP. Currently, it has enough to "pay" medical benefits for several years, but in reality it cannot pay anything. This creates a rising burden on the young, who subsidized treatment for the old and middle-aged. Workers under 65 pay most taxes, and, even among workers, there are generational subsidies. In 2000, workers 45–64 years old with employer-paid insurance had health costs twice those of workers 18–44, since the young have their real wages reduced because of elder insurance costs.

Moreover, consider that since 1963, in the Medicare system alone, the following happened:

- Workers contributing to the system decreased from 6:1 to 2:1 since.
- Enrollees increased from 20 million to 42 million, and the number is climbing.
- The elderly population increased from 10% to 14% of the US population.
- The average life Span increased from 70 to 78 years.
- The Medicare Trust Fund increased from 3 Billion to 132 Billion dollars. (This is not really a trust fund but is actually an accounting fiction, since, technically, the fund holds interest-earning US government bonds, representing a $ 200 million accounting surplus of payroll taxes collected in 2003 minus benefits paid. But these are very special government bonds, as the trustees cannot sell them on Wall Street and can only hand them back to the US Treasury. This does not increase the size of Uncle Sam's wallet, since every trust fund asset is a treasury liability. For the government as a whole, the assets and liabilities net out to zero, and, if the trust fund was abolished, there would be no effect on private bondholders or economic activity. The government would not be relieved of any existing obligations or commitments. The bonds are essentially IOUs the government has written to itself).
- For patients, the Medicare Part B monthly premium, which accounted for 25% of estimated program costs, rose 8.7%, from $54 to $58.70. The Medicare part B deductible remained $100, while the part A deductible rose 3.4%, from $812 to $840, in 2003.

Furthermore, the rising cost of healthcare can also be contributed to wide variability in treatment patterns that could be ascribed only to style and not to patient differences.

For example, John (Jack) Wennberg, MD, in the early 1970s at Dartmouth Medical School, shocked the health care community when he discovered that differences in hysterectomy, tonsillectomy, and prostatectomy rates in one county were 30%–50% higher than were rates in adjacent counties. By the early 1980s, Wennberg's studies concluded that new physician incentive were needed if doctors were to provide appropriate care at acceptable costs. Nevertheless, iatrogenic factors contributing to health care cost escalation continued into 2004–. For example, it is now estimated that

- More than half of all surgeries may be unnecessary.
- One third of all medical office visits may not be needed.
- One third of all hospital admissions may be iatrogenic.

- Medication errors abound, according to the Institute of Medicine (IOM), resulting in more than 98,000 deaths during the last reporting period.

Other causes of spiraling costs included: voracious consumer appetite, lifestyle drugs and medical interventions, inflation, cost shifting, and the relative insulation of consumers to the true cost of medical care due to the business deductibility of health insurance premiums (starting in 2003, self employed workers were are able to deduct 100% of health-insurance premiums).

Not coincidentally, corporate America, insurance companies, and even the federal government looked for methods to contain costs and to provide proactive, rather than retroactive, medical care.

Medicare Cost Containment Policies

In the past, Medicare efforts to control the cost spiral included (1) increasing Medigap premium taxes making copayment and deductibles more expensive and discourage enrollees from obtaining first-dollar insurance coverage on medical expenses, (2) increasing supplemental medical insurance (SMI) premiums, copayments, and deductibles (cost sharing), (3) lowering physician assignment fees, (4) screening out unhealthy patients ("cherry picking" and "adverse selection"), (5) reducing beneficiary benefits (rationed care), (6) incorporating utilization review (prospective, concurrent, and retrospective) programs, (7) precertifying hospital and ambulatory surgery center admissions with reduced Diagnosis-Related Groups (DRGs)and Ambulatory Payment Classification (APC) payments, (8) increasing the use of second opinions for surgical procedures, (9) implementing the case management of expensive disease processes, (10) organizing corporate self insurance, (11) using direct employer contracting, (12) pushing back the age of eligibility to 67, (13) increasing the use of prepaid managed care organizations, (14) encouraging the use of high deductible medical savings accountants (MSAs), and (15) since 1999, the promotion of Medicare HMOs, known as Medicare+Choice plans, which has proven to be a dismal failure.

Needless to say, the above cost reduction attempts were largely ineffective, and now the Medicare/HMO precursors and their 7 million enrollees are still projected to lose money and benefits. Moreover, as the US Congress tinkers with future budgets to augment the above measures, there is always the potential for the incorporation of onerous medical practitioner user fee(s), as proposed below:

- $1 fee on any medical claim not submitted electronically.
- Fees for unprocessible "dirty" medical claims submissions.
- Provider registration fees.
- HIPAA electronic date interchange fees, since implementation in October 2003.

In addition, until about 15 years ago, traditional fiscal output-maximizing models were used by most hospitals to maximize reimbursement, in a manner somewhat like the following formula.

Hospital Cost = Costs Per Service ($\times$) Services Per Patient / Per Day ($\times$) Days Per Admission ($\times$) Number Admissions.

That is to say, third parties reimbursed hospitals for expenses already incurred calculated by some retrospective formula based on a lower of cost or charges (i.e., cost plus) basis. Regardless of how costs were defined, this encouraged hospitals to expand, adding facilities, technology, and expenditures.

Diagnosis-Related Groups

In 1983–1984, the federal government introduced a prospective payment system for hospital, known as *Diagnosis-Related Groups* (DRGs) for Medicare patients. According to this system, all charges were reimbursed on a per diem diagnosis-case basis. The model suggested that a given hospital would minimize costs because they were at risk for any expenses incurred above the given reimbursement rate, and that the hospital would strive to reduce costs to an efficient level. This was unlike the behavior of any hospital that was reimbursable under the older retrospective system, and, recognizing that the model predicted a tendency for hospitals to maximize the number of patients admitted, Medicare regulations made provisions for professional review to determine the necessity of care.

Under current reimbursement rules, the Health Care Finance Administration (HCFA) mandates that patients must now stay the national average length of stay for the specific DRG, for hospitals to earn a full DRG payment. Hospitals that normally discharge faster than average have two choices: (1) retain the patient until the national average is reached (this is most likely), or (2) discharge the patient earlier (this is least likely) to incur the full cost of treatment and get a serious reduction in revenue.

Unfortunately, not being an all-payer system, hospitals shifted services and costs to non-Medicare patients, and so the DRG system had systemwide ramifications beyond its intended population. Additional modification made the DRG system increasingly unwieldy, and, ultimately, this cost-containment strategy was not enough. Therefore, even prior to the 1973 HMO Act, it was apparent that the healthcare delivery system needed more dramatic changes. A new strategy, known as *managed care,* which is an approach that links the delivery and financing of healthcare in order to coordinate care, was adopted.

This new approach caused insurers and providers to renounce the traditional incentives of indemnity insurance to control costs and eliminate inefficiencies. The ideology produced what is known as the *medical reimbursement paradigm shift,* because it was a dramatically different way of thinking about medical-care payments. Whether this lofty goal has indeed been achieved, however, is still debatable. Nevertheless, the following types of formal and informal models exist in the managed-care system, and they must be understood in order to economically survive as a business unit into the next millennium.

MANAGED CARE ECONOMICS

The physician activist Dr. Paul Ellwood coined the term *health maintenance organization* (HMO), which he aggressively advocated. An HMO is a group responsible for both the financing and the delivery of health services to an enrolled population.

Managed care is a prospective payment method (providers, hospitals, out-patient centers, vendors and ancillary care givers) whereby medical care is delivered regardless of the quantity or frequency of service for a fixed payment, in the aggregate. It is not the individual care of the traditional indemnity insurance. It is essentially utilitarian in nature and collective in intent.

Prepaid medicine is not new but, rather, was promoted extensively by the precursors of today's managed care revolutionaries, the so-called Four Horseman of the Apocalypse (Walter McClure, Clark Havighurst, Alain Enthoven, and Paul Ellwood). Since passage of the HMO Act in 1973, the growth of HMOs and managed care organizations (MCOs) have increased enrollment to more than 100 million. This represents an increase of 20 fold within the past few years, with a 10% commercial growth rate in prior years. Medicare enrollment is also expected to accelerate in the future.

The Pacific region accounts for 17% of all HMO medical group practices, followed by the Mid-Atlantic (12%) and the South-Atlantic (17.8%) regions, New England (6%), Mountain region (6.6%), South Central (14.3%), and the West North-Central region (9%).

Individual states with the most HMO penetration are: Oregon (48%), Massachusetts (45%), California (44%), and Utah (41%). States with the least penetration are Alaska (1%), Vermont (1%), Wyoming (1%), North Dakota (2%), Mississippi (2%), Montana (3%), South Dakota (3.5%), and Idaho (4%).

According to Alain Enthoven of Stanford University, the term *managed care* covers a wide range of options that differ dramatically in incentives offered to physicians and the methods used to control utilization and expenses.

Structurally, HMOs are often divided into two types, and six subtypes. The two basic HMO types include the *command control* and *empowerment* models. In the former, it is assumed that the doctor's need to be strictly controlled, dominated, and micromanaged because they will not take responsibility for managing the quality and cost of medical care. The latter HMO type assumes the exact opposite in regard to its physicians, giving them more latitude for independent thought and decision-making skills. The six traditional HMO subtypes follow:

- A *Staff Model* HMO is the most restrictive plan for both doctors and patients, and it requires that physicians be considered as employees who treat only the HMO's own members at centralized locations in coordination with a closed panel of providers. This model is in market decline because of its lack of flexibility.
- In a *Group Model*, the doctors are not employees but may treat non-HMO members and work out of a private office.
- In a *Network Model*, the HMO contracts with the MDs who may or may not have an exclusive relationship with it, and may be in a closed or open panel.
- An *Independent Practice Association (IPA Model)* is built around a group of independent physicians who retain the right to see other patients and exist in an open panel. The doctors retain their own separate self administered offices.
- In a Direct *Contract HMO*, the provider's practice is similar to the IPA model, but the HMO administrators have a direct contract with each participating MD, who may or may not retain the right to see non-HMO patients and practice in a variety of settings.

- Finally, the least restrictive model is the *Mixed Model* HMO, which represents a combination of the other five HMO types.

Employee Retirement Income Security Act

When dealing with the major medical programs, one must be cognizant of the Employee Retirement Income Security Act of 1972 (ERISA-IRC 404[c]), which determines whether the third party is an insurance company or an ERISA organization, since state laws through the Freedom of Choice Act (FCA) preclude discrimination on the part of insurance companies. Since ERISA programs are covered under federal law, they are not subject to the FCA. Generally, patients can sue health plans and employers in federal court, though not in state court, for the cost of a denied benefit, legal fees, and court costs, but not for compensatory or punitive damages. They can also sue doctors for malpractice in state court. Federal employees may sue the Office of Personnel Management (OPM) in federal court only for the amount of denied coverage, plus attorney and court costs. If it loses, the OPM can obtain a court order to require the insurer to pay. Thus, ERISA has shielded nongovernmental health plans from punitive and compensatory damages in state courts. This is known as the ERISA exemption, and it has allowed MCOs to flourish.

Preferred Provider Organizations

A preferred provider organization (PPO) is a bridge between traditional indemnity insurance and an HMO. There are several different types of PPO; most of them attempt to give the provider choices seen in indemnity insurance with the nonrisk cost reductions seen in HMOs.

Two similar entities, known as an exclusive provider organization (EPO), or point of service or swing out (POS or SOP) plans, consist of an exclusive provider panel that have agreed to accept a deep discount in medical fees in return for the volume of patients the plans can provide to them. A combination of the models described earlier has been very successful for many employers, and this model is not as restricted by the HMO Act. A payment timeline for a typical PPO may look something like the following:

Healthcare Provider bills PPO → PPO bills company → Company pays PPO →
PPO pays Provider

Changes in Medical Payment Delivery Models

As payments have shifted from the older fee for service model to the newer managed-care capitation model, the following differences were observed.

Traditional (Fee for Service) Methodology

Characteristics include the following:

- Full fee for service rendered as medical payment.
- Illnesses and diseases were treated, retroactively.

- Individual patients were treated.
- Active and acute diagnoses were made.
- Medical care was rendered in the office or hospital setting.
- Referrals to specialist were made in difficult cases.

Contemporary (Managed Care-Capitation) Methodology

Per Member/Per Month Capitation: The per member/per month (PM/PM) medical capitation model requires the payment of a fixed sum of money to a medical provider to cover a defined set of health care services for an individual enrollee over a defined period of time. Under PM/PM capitation, the doctor assumes the risk for the incidence (utilization rate) of medical conditions requiring procedures specified in the MCO contract.

Characteristics:

- Discounted payment from HMOs and MCOs.
- Illnesses are prevented proactively.
- Population cohorts are treated collectively, not individually.
- Chronic diseases are intervened before acute disease exacerbates.
- Care rendered in networks, the home, or other subacute care facility.
- Outcomes are evaluated based on results, not specialty care.

Under PM/PM capitation, the MD is at risk for: *(a)* utilization and acuity, *(b)* actuarial accuracy, *(c)* cost of delivering medical care, and *(d)* adverse patient selection.

MCO Carrier Benefits

Some of the benefits for corporate America (payers), who supply the majority of health insurance to its employees (insureds), are listed below:

- Known medical expenses (fixed, not variable, costs) to companies.
- MD/provider's bear the risk and benefits of patient compliance, not corporations.
- Less administrative staff needs since medical claims are no longer reviewed.
- Costs are reduced through economies of scale.
- Patients are controlled and MDs carefully managed.

Medical Provider Benefits

The following is a brief list of the benefits physicians supposedly may derive by participating in managed care plans.

- Stable patient load and predictable cash flows.
- Potential referrals and community visibility.

- Reduced office expenses, liability and utilization review.
- Reputation equivalency (i.e., all doctors in the plan are considered good).

Why Healthcare Practitioners Are Disenfranchised

Despite the above purported benefits, anecdotal evidence suggests that MDs are less happy about managed care, compensation, and their profession than ever before.
There are other reasons, as well:

- Fewer fee-for-service patients and more discounted patients.
- More paperwork and scrutiny of medical decisions.
- Lost independence and medical morale.
- Healthcare providers are making less money, as Medicare reimbursement was cut 5.4% in 2002 and 4.4% in 2003. Furthermore, such cuts also stand to hurt physicians with private payers, since commercial insurers often tie their reimbursement schedules to Medicare's resources.
- The profession of medicine is no longer satisfying.

And in the past few years, the following occurred:

- The Health Care Financing Administration (HCFA) became known as the Centers for Medicare and Medicaid Services (CMS: www.cms.hhs.gov). Administered by Thomas Scully, it was reorganized into three parts. The Center for Medical Management runs the traditional fee-for-service program. The Center for Beneficiary Choices expands the number of Medicare beneficiaries belonging to private plans. The Center for Medicaid and State Operations shares responsibility with state governments.
- Certain administrative requirements for the Health Insurance Portability and Accountability Act (HIPAA) went into effect in April 2003 and in October 2003. And, for many doctors, their biggest liability may be a single unfortunate event that could result in a lawsuit, an HHS investigation, and/or bad publicity.
- The executive committee of the Pharmaceutical Research and Manufacturers of America (PhRMA) adopted a new marketing code to govern PhRMA's relationships with physicians. Although now voluntary, DHH is urging compliance as critics charge that direct to consumer (DTC) advertising results in appropriate prescription patterns, frustrated patients, and increased costs.

Manipulating the Capitation Payment Numbers

Since MCO's pay a fixed amount of money regardless of the quantity of care provided (i.e., capitation), we can begin to explore how reimbursement issues have been dramatically changed under this new payment paradigm.

Example

For simplification, suppose Dr. Kosmicky received a capitated MCO contract to evaluate, and the following numbers were supplied to him by the MCO:

- Capitation Range = 5 per 125 cents ($1.25) PM/PM
- 10,000 Lives @ 30 cts. / Pt / Month / Year
- 5% Patient Encounter Rate (range = 2.5–7.5%)

The following is the financial yield possible from this contract:

- $10,000 (5%) = 500 Visits / Yr. or 41 Visits / Mo. or 10 / Week
- $10,000 × .30 = $-3-K Month or 36-K/Year
- **$72 dollar average per New Patient**

NP = 3 Visits/Year average = **$24 per old patient visit.**

Now, a capitation analysis might evolve to look something like the following, if he is able to treat the numbers of patients given in the following example, by accepting additional similar contracts.

- $24/Patient × 3 Patients/Hour = $72 Hour.
- 72 Patients × 8 Hours = $576/Day
- $576 × 5 Days / Week = $2,880/Week
- $2,880 / 4 Weeks / Month = $11,520/Month
- **$11,520 × 12 Months = $138,240 / Year**

In other words, the provider becomes a quasiemployee of the HMOs and is reduced to an hourly worker; even though he may receive increased compensation at the indicated volume demonstrated below:

- 6 Patient / Hours / 48 Day = $276 (480 per Year)
- 9 Patient / Hours / 72 Day = $414 (720 per Year)

Also realize that, many times, the doctor does not even derive the full $72 economic benefit from new patient visits, since most patients have already been in the existing practice. The result is simply an across the board wholesale fee reduction for the practice.

Dr. Kosmicky also recognizes that this rate is based on averages and he will receive no additional payment if all members of a single contract visit him more than three times a year; nor is his payment reduced if they don't visit him at all. The rate is reasonably close to his normal office fee of $30, so he accepts the financial risk of the contract.

To further illustrate the contentious point of physician compensation reduction, consider the futile AMA sponsored lawsuit, by the Medical Association of Georgia in 1998 on behalf of its physicians when Blue Cross and Blue Shield of Georgia reduced reimbursement rates on its indemnity insurance plan, which affected 13,480 doctors. In effect, older methods of compensation are being made obsolete by capitation. These include:

- Productivity based systems (majority of practices).
- Fixed-salary system.
- Equal distribution of revenue among partners.
- Individual contracts for each MD.

Point of Service Plans

Capitation offers the same advantages to Point of Service (POS) plans as it does to HMOs, but it is riskier for the provider. The main reason for the discrepancy is medical risk acceptance without considering POS peculiarities. For example, these plans, unlike HMOs, allow out-of-network services; POS managers and providers must then pay the unmanaged outside contractors in addition to the discounted in-service physicians. Reinsurance is useful, but these plans tend to be chronically short of capital and, as a result, should expect higher operating costs than traditional HMOs.

Physician Hospital Organizations

A physician-hospital organization (PHO) is a blend of private doctors and hospitals, maintaining its concentration and control of surgical rather than of medical care. Ownership may be divided by a governing board, according to a prorata basis with the larger partner having most organizational strength and bargaining power in the corporate structure. Typically, this favors the hospital. From a strategic standpoint, most MDs are still not currently aligned with many PHOs, since surgical care is increasingly being delivered in private offices or ambulatory care centers (ACs). Additionally, PHOs may become potential MD competitors, and they often lack managed care contracting experience, have inflexible provider networks, and require MD exclusivity in their organizations.

Nevertheless, the function of a PHO is to

- Negotiate managed care contracts.
- Negotiate on all health insurance contracts.
- Establish insurance product(s).
- Employ doctors and support staff.
- Consolidate and acquire physician practices.
- Acquire alternative medical practices.

Medical Networks and IPAs

In an attempt to increase market share and augment profits, some doctors contemplate forming independent physician associations (IPAs). Some of the benefits of these organizations include (1) marketing and advertising benefits, with reduced equipment costs through economies of large scale for equipment, (2) the network pays the MD/DO directly, (3) there is no need for individual negotiations, (4) a patient and cash flow stream is available, and (5) collective group autonomy exists.

On the other hand, potential risks include (1) the MD/DO is not capitated, but the physician pool likely will be; this merely means that the per unit price of each medical intervention will likely decrease as individual doctors in the pool competed for its limited resources (managed competition), (2) variable income due to the managed competition described above. 3. 10%–20% administrative fee, payable in cash, to the IPA managers, (4) reduced and discounted fee schedules, and (5) lost personal autonomy.

Obviously, signs of insolvent networks include (1) delayed data entry, (2) telephone or facsimile delays, (3) slow payment schedules, (4) poor expense tracking, (5) insufficient MIS and software, (6) sparse interest statements or financial information.

Management Service Organizations

Most management service organizations (MSOs) for doctors are organized as IPAs. Under such plans, the MDs make the rules, regulations, and medical care guidelines, while MSO executives (MBAs, CPAs, CCAs, MHAs, CFAs, PhDs, MHAs, JDs, CFPs©, CMPs© and CMAs) administer those policies. Centralized data is collected, and the organization is responsible for utilization review, quality control, and eligibility verification and payment. The MSO is more of a broker, who works for the physicians in the plan, marketing, selling, and running it on a daily basis. This leaves the MDs unfettered to provide patient care; for a price that is typically 10%–18% of net patient revenues per month.

A practitioner may be a candidate for an MSO organization, if he or she possesses most of the following characteristics: has excellent medical education and management and leadership skills; practices in a large multidoctor group with rising net income; possesses current management information; uses technology systems with gross margins exceeding 50%–55%; provides ancillary services such as a wound care center or ambulatory surgery center; is under 45 years of age and desirous of practicing medicine in the future.

Finally, the provider should have some business savvy and practice in an area with relatively weak MCO market penetration. A provider should also consider joining an MSO if his or her future professional outlook is optimistic and positive.

FUTURISTIC HEALTHCARE ECONOMICS

Uwe Reinhardt, PhD, James Madison Professor of Political Economics of Princeton University in New Jersey, and an opponent of MCO liability, opined that in the near future, there will be a three tiered system of medical care in the United States. The bottom tier will consist of the uninsured and uninsurable (46 million, January, 2004), the middle tier will be served by managed care organizations, and the top tier will continue to demand traditional (indemnity) fee-for-service medicine.

Regardless of future model(s) of care, the goals of any optimal healthcare economic policy should include the following characteristics: (1) low demand barriers of price, travel, wait time, referral ease, and paperwork, (2) adequacy of supply regarding medical personnel, clinics, drugs, and equipment, (3) technical efficiencies such as service mix, (4) public expenditure control with tax reductions, and (5) quality of care for the common social good. The following machinations might prove useful in the future.

Medicaid Cost Containment Policies

Some state governments have applied for, and received, special waivers from the federal government (Department of Health and Human Resources), forcing more

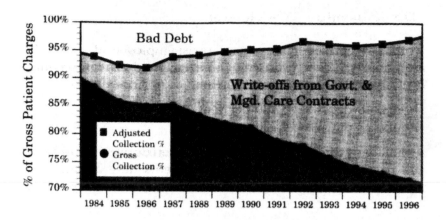

FIGURE 1.5   Bad debt; write-offs from government and managed care contracts; gross fee-for-service collections.

than 22 million Medicaid enrollees to various managed care-risk plans. The resulting fixed payment methodology is usually varied, with states using a "take-it-or-leave-it" or "bid" payment methodology to further reduce costs. Under the former method, states offer the same payment structure to all HMO plans. Under the latter method, HMO plans submit a proposed payment schedule within the state's predefined range, preventing lowball underbidding (promoting under utilization) or overbidding (promoting excessive profits). Pricing floors and ceiling are effectively created in this manner as bad debt expenses slowly increase.

Ambulatory Payment Classifications for ASCs

Most doctors are aware of the Medicare payment regulations implemented in 2001–2002. Ambulatory Payment Classifications (APCs), originally termed ambulatory payment groups (APGs), replaced cost-based and cost-plus reimbursement contracts for all outpatient services, especially for ambulatory surgery centers (ASCs). Much like diagnostic related groups (DRGs), which were enacted for hospitals in 1983 and divided disease management into 497 groups (based on ICD-9-CM diagnoses, procedures, age, sex, and discharge disposition), APCs changed the hospital and IPA landscape forever

For more than a decade, the Federal Government and the Health Care Financing Administration (HCFA), now the Centers for Medicare and Medicaid Services (CMS), had planned this shift to prospective payments through its Outpatient Prospective Payment System (OPPS), which came about as a result of the Omnibus Budget Reconciliation Act (OBRA) of 1986. Unlike DRGs however, with their multiyear phase-in period, APCs had no similar grace period, and hospitals, IPAs, and other out-patient centers needed to be compliant immediately.

Ambulatory Payment Classifications

The APCs system is designed to explain the amount and type of resources utilized in outpatient ambulatory visits. Each APC consists of patients with similar characteris-

TABLE 1.1

PROCEDURE		ASC	HOSPITAL
1.	Cataract removal	$942	$1,334
2.	After-cataract laser surgery	429	246
3.	UGI endoscopy with biopsy	429	359
4.	Diagnostic colonoscopy	429	401
5.	Epidural injection	320	183

tics and resource usage and includes only the facility portion of the visit, with no impact on providers, who will continue to be paid from the traditional CPT-4 fee schedule and modifier system. This will effectively eliminate separate payments for operating, recovery, treatment, and observation-room charges. Anesthesia, medical and surgical supplies, drugs (except those used in chemotherapy), blood, casts, splints, and donated tissue will also be packaged into the APC. Unbundled, fragmented, or otherwise separated codes will be eliminated from claims prior to payment.

APCs group most outpatient services into 346 classes according to ICD-9-CM diagnosis and CPT-4 procedures. This includes 134 surgical APCs, 46 significant APCs, 122 medical APCs, and 44 ancillary APCs. Surgical, significant, and ancillary APCs are assigned using only the CPT-4 procedure codes, while medical APCs are based on a combination of ICD-9-CM and E&M CPT-4 codes.

The full impact of this regulation on facilities and IPAs is unknown, but it is expected to decrease reimbursement for more than 75% of all ambulatory facilities. This may occur because the initial variable used in reimbursement determinations is the principle procedure. Payments are then calculated for each APC by multiplying the facility rate times the APC weight times a discount factor (if multiple APCs are performed during the same visit). Total payment is the sum of the payments for all APCs. However, no adjustment provisions are made for outliers or teaching facilities, rural hospitals, or disproportionate share or specialty hospitals or facilities.

Estimated Potential APC Economic Impact

In 2003, the Medicare Payment Advisory Commission (MedPAC) asked Congress to reduce ASC payments in 2004, because escalating payments were based on growth and not cost issues. The Centers for Medicare/Medicaid Services itself has not conducted a cost survey, since 1994. But the following table lists the five highest volume procedures and an ASC versus hospital Medicare payment comparison, according to federal data in 2001.

Facilities affected by Medicare's OPPS include those designated by the Secretary of Health and Human Services, such as hospital outpatient surgical centers, hospital outpatient departments not part of the consolidated billing for skilled nursing facility (SNF) residents, certain preventative services and supplies, covered Medicare Part B inpatient services if Part A coverage is exhausted, and partial hospitalization services in community mental health centers (CMHCs).

Exempted facilities include clinical laboratories, ambulance services, end stage renal disease (ESR) centers, occupational and speech therapy services, mammography centers, and durable medical equipment (DME) suppliers.

The remaining facilities may experience a slight payment increase if they convert their management information systems (MIS) to APC compliant hardware and software. Compliance measures include electronic interconnectivity, data storage, retrieval, and the security features mandated by HIPAA.

Although the Balanced Budget Act (BBA) of 1997 required HCFA to implement an OPPS by January 1, 1999, Y2K concerns delayed implementation until "as soon as possible after January 1, 2000." This delay meaningfully led to a functional 2002 date. But they are fully functional today.

Utilization of Medicare Private Accounts

According to Texas A&M healthcare economists Thomas R. Saving and Andrew J. Rettenmaier, toddy's young people could replace Medicare with private insurance if they saved about $600/year (2% average earnings) into private accounts. For each dollar deposited into the account, the Medicare payroll tax could be reduced by a dollar. The government would deposit the difference for those not able to afford the contribution. The accounts would be conservatively invested to grow with the economy as a whole. Upon retirement, participants could then choose from options such as traditional or managed Medicare, HMOs, PPOs, or whatever model existed at the time of enrollment. This private account option would secure health benefit if begun now. If not, according to Boston University economist Laurence Kotlikoff, Medicare payroll taxes could be increased up to 55% (probably uncollectable) and/ or severe rationing would occur for the future elderly.

Medical and Health Savings Accountants

Despite managed care, health insurance premiums soared up to 35% in some cases, in 2004. This placed a significant burden on individual patients, as well as small medical practices.

Enter the medical savings account (MSA) (still an experimental separate federal account), which can be set up in conjunction with your practice's health insurance account, thus enabling the doctor-employer or employee to contribute money tax deferred into a savings account to be used at a later time for a variety of health care costs. The money in an MSA can be used to pay an employee's deductible and copays, as well, a number of other health insurance costs not normally covered under traditional small practice health insurance plans.

According to R. DeFrancesco, JD (*www.wealthpreservation123.com*), there are three main reasons for a practitioner to use an MSA.

- First, there is the possibility of lowering your health insurance premiums.
- Second, you can offer added benefits without any extra out-of-pocket costs.
- Third, if the money contributed to the MSA is not used during a calendar year, it not only rolls for use during a later year, but at age 59, the money can be

used as a supplemental retirement benefit (similar but more flexible then an IRA).

Today, most offices have health insurance deductibles between $250–$500 per person. That means the maximum exposure to the employee is that $250–$500 (plus any copays). Based on the health of your employees and the deductible, a health-insurance company quotes your practice a premium for families and individuals.

MSAs are based on the concept of high deductibles. Employee-only deductibles must be between $1,600–$2,400 a year and family deductibles are between $3,400–$5,100, indexed annually. The key is that with the higher deductibles the employee and family insurance premiums will be significantly lower.

The first impression of a change to a high deductible plan is seen as negative by the employee and doctor-employer. This is because no one wants to be responsible for that extra high deductible. The key to success with a high-deductible plan is through the incorporation of the MSA. A doctor-employer or employee can fund the MSA to cover the extra cost of the deductible.

Why would anyone entertain such a model? The simple answer is long-term savings and extra benefits. Right now, once health insurance premiums are paid, the money will never come back to the employer-doctor or employee. With an MSA, if the money is not used inside the MSA, the employee gets to keep the money as their own for future medical expenses. Once enough money is deferred into the MSA to cover the deductible, an employer can choose to stop contributing to the MSA thereby significantly decreasing the annual health insurance/MSA expenses.

Example of a Medical Savings Account

Assume with a small medical-office health plan that the family premium is $600 a month with a $500 deductible. Also assume that a family premium with a $5,000 deductible is $250 a month. Assume the family premium is for a doctor/owner of a medical practice.

Total premium for Doctor Smith for 1 year	$7,200 for 1 year with a $500 deductible plan $3,000 with a $5,000 deductible plan
Total annual savings in premium for Dr. Smith	$4,200

Note. Annual health insurance premiums were 60% deductible in 2001 and were 70% deductible in 2002 for a doctor/owner of a PC, LLC, or Sub S corporation. Employee premiums are 100% deductible to the corporation.

Dr. Smith's total contribution to a MSA for 1 year	$3,600
Total out of pocket cost for Dr. Smith, including the MSA contribution	$6,600 ($3,000 + $3,600)
Dr. Smith's tax deduction for normal $7,200 premium/$500 deductible plan	$7,200 × 60% = $4,320
Dr. Smith's tax deduction for $3,000 premium/$5,000 deductible plan	$3,000 × 60% = $1,800

Dr. Smith's Tax deduction for MSA Contribution	$3,600 × 100% = $3,600
Additional tax savings by using the MSA in conjunction with a high deductible plan	$1,080
Annual out of pocket savings using an MSA plus a high deductible plan over the $500 deductible plan	$7,200 − $6,600 = $600
Total overall savings for the doctors at the end of the year	$1,680

Many doctors are unaware that they can only deduct 70% of their family health insurance paid for by the office. The CFP™/CPA for every doctor's office knows this, but it is often not communicated to the physician.

Medical Savings Account Benefits

In the above example, three good things happen. First, the total out of pocket expenses for the health insurance and the MSA costs are $600 lower than the traditional $500 deductible non-MSA plan. Second, the money contributed to the MSA is 100% deductible thereby saving the doctor an additional $1,080 in taxes. Third, and just as important, is the fact that if the owner's family is relatively healthy and does not use all the money in the MSA, that money can roll to the next year thereby cutting the next year's out-of-pocket costs of the owner. The owner could also continue to fund the MSA at $3,600 a year to stockpile money in the MSA for other medical expenses (orthodontics) or for supplemental retirement benefits.

Yet, MSAs are underutilized for three reasons:

- First, many insurance agents despise the concept of MSAs. When an insurance agent lowers the premium for a doctor-client, the agent takes a significant pay cut. The agent makes nothing on money contributed to the MSA.
- Second, most employer-doctors don't have the guts to implement a plan that raises their employee's deductibles to $1,600 a year. If fully explained to the employees, the employees should jump at the chance to have an MSA implemented by their employer-doctor. Why? The employer is going to cover the difference between the old deductible and new deductible; and if, at the end of the year, the employee didn't need to use the money in the MSA for deductibles, then that money becomes the employee's.
- Third, offices with several sick employees (employees who always hit their deductible and then some every year) will have a hard time making the MSA concept cost effective due to prohibitively high insurance premiums.

Nevertheless, when appropriately used, MSAs can fill the special needs of many medical offices and patients.

HEALTH SAVINGS ACCOUNTS

A bill to create another vehicle, known as a health savings account (HSA), for patients to pay for medical care, was passed in late 2003 (HR 2351). The legislation amended the Internal Revenue Code of 1986 to allow patients to deduct contributions to a health savings account. The plan is portable and allows a tax-free rollover of up to $500 of unspent flexible spending-account balances, which currently are forfeited at the end of each year. Other elements of the health savings account legislature include the following:

* Availability to all individuals with a qualified deductible plan.
* Establishment with a health-insurance plan establishing a minimum deductible of $1,000.
* Allowance of annual contributions to equal 100% of the deductible.
* Allowance of both employer and employee contributions.
* Marketing by PPOs and cafeteria plans.
* No cap on taxpayer participation.

But like MSAs, critics contend the plan could harm more than help because HSAs are likely to be more attractive to younger and healthier populations than to older or sicker ones.

Spread of Specific Episode Capitation

Under the *Specific Episode of Care* (SEC) capitation model, MD-providers deliver care for covered enrollees with a specific medical condition or who require a particular treatment intervention on a fixed basis per episode. Many believe this concept will grow in the future.

Adoption of Full Risk Capitation

For many physician's, the future might include "full risk" medical care contacts. This is because of market pressure and the expansion of partial risk PPO contracts

In the full-risk payment system, the participant agrees to provide "all" of the care for a given patient population or contract. In other words, the MD would have to include services such as diabetic management, traumatology, radiology, emergency care, pediatric immunizations, geriatrics, home IV antibiotics, DME, and all specialty care in the consideration of this "full risk" contract. Of course, increased benefits accompany the increased risk.

The risks: all medical and surgical care necessary for the contracted population. Since there is the potential for more reward but with much more risk, the physician/ business executive must carefully consider these contract types and maintain the following relative contingencies:

* Stop-loss reinsurance.
* 15–50 mile coverage radius.
* Subcapitated medical specialists with deep discounts.
* 25–100 providers in the network.
* 100–250,000 patient population, or more (more patients mean less risk).

- Subcapitated hospitals, surgical centers, pharmacy, and DME vendors with discounts.
- Encompass a small (< 20%–25%) portion of the practice.

Certainty, this system does not bode well for the solo practitioner or even for small medical-group practices.

Development of Social HMOs

This type of HMO offers extended coverage for some of the unconventional expenses associated with senior healthcare, such as transportation and in-home daycare not covered by traditional MCOs. One such plan is Elderplan, in Brooklyn, NY. According to the American Association of Health Plans (AAHP), social HMOs provide coordinated services by uniting federal and state funds and services to benefit the elderly.

Proliferation of Fraudulent Silent ("Mirror") Healthcare Models

A silent, *faux,* or "mirror" PPO, HMO, or other provider model is not really a formalized managed care organization at all! Rather, it is simply an intermediary attempt to negotiate practitioner fees downward by promising a higher volume of patients in exchange for the discounted fee structure. Of course, the intermediary then resells the packaged contract product to any willing insurance company, HMO, PPO, or other payer, thereby pocketing the difference as a nice profit. Sometimes, these virtual organizations are just indemnity companies in disguise. Physicians should not fall for this ploy, since pricing pressure will be forced even lower in the next round of "real" PPO negotiations!

Occasionally, an insurer or bold insurance agent will enter a market and tell its practitioners that they have signed up all the local, or many major, employers. Then, they'll go to the employers and give them the same story about signing up all the major providers. The real case is that they haven't signed up either, and a Ponzilike situation is created! Providers should be on guard for silent HMOs, MCOs, and any other silent insurance variation, since these virtual organizations do not exist except as exploitable arbitrage situations for the middleman.

Use of the "Hospitalist" or Hospital-Based Medical Group

The usual role of inpatient care in this country saw hospitalized patients cared for by their primary-care or admitting physician. Although this model has the advantage of continuity, and perhaps personalization, it often suffered because of the limited knowledge base of the physician, as well as familiarity with the available internal and external resources of the hospital. Furthermore, the limited time spent with each individual patient prevented the physician from becoming the quality leader in this setting. These shortcomings have led hundreds of hospitals around the country to turn to the hospitalists as dedicated inpatient specialists. The National Association of Inpatient Physicians (NAIP) estimates that the model could result in up to 40,000 hospitalists by the year 2005.

The term *hospitalist* was coined by Dr. Robert M. Wachter of the University of California at San Francisco. It denotes a specialist in inpatient medicine. At its center is the concept of low cost and comprehensive broad-based care in the hospital, hospice, or even extended-care setting If well designed, hospitalist programs can offer benefits beyond the often cited inpatient efficiencies they bring. For example, the average length of stay for patients on the medical service of UCSF's Moffitt Long Hospital fell by 15%, compared to concurrent and historical controls adjusted for case mix. There was no reported decrease in patient satisfaction or clinical outcomes.

Similarly, another integration model is "on-site" employee affiliations that represent an adjustment of the hospitalist concept. This redeployment of existing MDs into the workplace (factory, police station, office building) or retail setting (Walmart, Intel Corp, Micro-Soft, IBM, etc.) is another exciting challenge in heath care today. The keys to success are thoughtful implementation and a commitment to measure the results of change and use the data to produce further changes.

Physician Practice Management Corporations

Physician Practice Management Corporations (PPMC), left for dead by the year 1999, may make a comeback by 2005. They are evolving from first-generation multispecialty national concerns to second-generation regional single specialty groups to third-generation regional concerns, and finally to fourth-generation Internet-enabled service companies, providing both business-to-business solutions to affiliated medical practices and business-to-consumer health solutions to plan members.

PPMC From:	To: Current Entity
Coastal Physicians	PhyAmerica Physician Group
MedPartners	Caremark and Team Health
PhyCor	Aveta Health
Physicians Resource Group	MediNetwork
Raven Healthcare Management	STAT Solutions
Specialty Care Network	Healthgrades.com

But survivors like Pediatrix Medical Group saw its stock drop 23.5% at one point in 2003, and the group is floundering following disclosure that federal officials were investigating its Medicaid billing practices. On the other hand, many private medical practices are now being bought back by the same physicians that sold out to the PPMCs originally. But if an entity is being bought back and accounts receivable is being purchased, be careful not to pick this item up as income twice. The costs can be immense to the practice

For example, a family practice recently purchased itself back from a PPMC. Part of the mandatory purchase price, approximately $200,000 (the approximate net realizable value of the accounts receivable), was paid to the PPMC to buy back accounts receivable generated by the physicians buying back their practice. The office administrator unknowingly began recording the cash receipts specifically attributable to the purchased accounts receivable as patient fee income. If left uncorrected, this error could have incorrectly added $200,000 in income to this practice and cost it (a C Corporation) approximately $70,000 in additional income tax ($200,000 in fees × 35% tax rate).

The error in the above example is that the PPMC must record the portion of the purchase price it received for the accounts receivable as patient fee income. The buyer practice has merely traded one asset, cash, for another asset, the accounts receivable. When the practice collects these particular receivables, the credit is applied against the purchased accounts receivable (an asset), rather than to patient fees.

Medical Malpractice Insurance Crisis

By early 2004, the American Medical Association announced six more states had reached a medical malpractice crisis, with patients losing access to care due to physician attrition. The AMA's list of crisis states now totals 18. The new states are Arkansas, Connecticut, Illinois, Kentucky, Missouri, and North Carolina. The 12 states previously identified are Florida, Georgia, Mississippi, Nevada, New Jersey, New York, Ohio, Oregon, Pennsylvania, Texas, Washington, and West Virginia. Meanwhile, the Medical Group Management Association (MGMA) reported that medical malpractice premiums for its members increased by more than 53% between 2002 and 2003. About 26% of the physicians planned to retire, relocate, or restrict their services over the next three years. Massachusetts was especially hard hit as the practice environment worsened for the ninth consecutive year, driven primarily by rising premiums for medical malpractice coverage.

Boutique Medical Practices

The boutique or concierge medical practice business model requires an annual fee for personalized treatment that includes amenities far beyond those offered in the typical practice or suggested by physician medical unions. Patients pay annual out-of-pocket fees for top-tier service but also use traditional health insurance to cover allowable expenses, such as inpatient hospital stays, outpatient diagnostics and care, and basic tests and physician exams. Typical annual fees can range from $1,000 to $5,000 per patient, to family fees that top $20,000 a year or more. The concept, initially developed for busy corporate executives, has now made its way to those desiring such service.

Patient Bounty Hunters

Under the Health Insurance Portability Accountability Act, the Department of Health and Human Service (HHS) has operated the Incentive Program for Fraud and Abuse Information since January 1999. Under this program, HHS will pay $ 100–1,000 to Medicare recipients who report abuse in the program. To assist patients in spotting fraud, HHS has published examples of potential fraud, which include the following:

- Medical services not provided.
- Duplicate services or procedures.
- More expenses, services, or procedures than were provided (upcoding/billing).
- Misused Medicare cards and numbers.

- Medical telemarketing scams.
- Nonmedical necessity.

And, there is no question that real fraud exists. The Office of Inspector General of HHS saved American taxpayers a record $21 billion in Fiscal-Year 2002, according to Inspector General Janet Rehnquist. Savings were achieved through an intensive and continuing crackdown on waste, fraud, and abuse in Medicare and over 300 other HHS programs for which the Office of Inspector General (OIG) has oversight responsibility. The agency performed or oversaw 2,372 audits, conducted 70 evaluations of department programs, and opened 1,654 new civil and criminal cases, bringing to more than 2,700 the number of active OIG investigations. Additionally, the OIG excluded 3,448 individuals and entities from participation in Medicare, Medicaid, and other federally sponsored health care programs, and its enforcement efforts resulted in 517 criminal convictions and 236 successful civil actions. Source: http://oig.hhs.gov/publications/docs/semiannual/2002/fallsemiannu al02pr.pdf.

To discourage flagrant allegations, regulations require that reported information directly contribute to monetary recovery for activities not already under investigation. Nevertheless, expect a further erosion of patient confidence as they begin to view healthcare providers in the same light as bounty hunters.

Governmental Antifraud Success

The federal government has grown increasingly effective at Medicare fraud recovery, but state Medicaid programs lag behind, according to New Directions for Policy, a Washington, DC, research firm. In the case of Medicare fraud recoveries, the federal government's return on investment improved to nearly 9-to-1 in 2001 from 8-to-1 in 2000. Medicare fraud recoveries from healthcare providers grew 71% to $1.20 billion in 2001, while enforcement costs increased 6.30% to about $72.8 million. State Medicaid fraud collections, totaled $43.00 million in 2001. And the federal government, which recovered $2.85 billion from Medicare fraud from 1997 to 2001, collected $115 million in Medicaid fraud recoveries during the same period, according to Medicaid Policy, a Washington consulting firm.

Managed Care Backlash

According to a study by The MEDSTAT Group and JD Power and Associates, which surveyed nearly 30,000 physicians participating in 150 healthcare plans located in 22 different markets; nearly 7 out of ten physicians considered themselves anti–managed care, with capitation accounts declining in nearly every HMO category.

Dissatisfaction with financial reimbursement was the leading factor, but four other major factors drive a physician's rating of health plans:

- Satisfaction with financial reimbursement.
- Administration.
- Policies impacting on care quality.

- Support of clinical practice.
- Limits on care.

The number of operating HMOs is declining, as well.

Nevertheless, HMOs have not been unresponsive to this managed care backlash. Since 1998, managed care companies and their allies fought against restrictive new proposed regulations and spent more than $ 112,000 per lawmaker to lobby Congress. This 60 million dollar outlay was four times the $14 million plus spent by medical organizations, trial lawyers ($1 million), unions ($1.4 million) and consumer groups ($8 million) to press for passage of the failed Patients Bill of Rights. The $60 million dollar lobbying tab is 50% higher than the $40 million dollars that tobacco interests spent to kill legislature to raise cigarette taxes to curb teenage smoking!

But there have been some physician victories. For example, the Independence Blue Cross (IBC) and the Pennsylvania Orthopaedic Society agreed to settle a class action lawsuit about its payment policies, in July 2003. Members of the class were to receive benefits worth an estimated $40 million, but, more important, IBC will disclose its standard fee schedules, changes applicable to provider's specialty, and policies that may have an effect on reimbursement. IBC will also replace its independent procedure designation with Current Procedure Terminology's (CPT) separate procedure designation and will process claims in accordance with established standards. Finally, the insurance company will establish a formal resolution process for provider payment appeals. IBC subsidiaries include QCC Insurance Company, Keystone Health Plan East, Amerihealth HMO, Amerihealth, Amerihealth HMO New Jersey, and Amerihealth New Jersey.

"Don't Give Up Your Practice Yet!"

It is no wonder, then, that according to Dr. Regina E. Herzlinger, the Nancy R. McPherson professor of business administration chair at Harvard Business School and author of *Creating New Healthcare Ventures* and *Market Terms in Healthcare,* many medical professionals become depressed and want to give up their careers entirely.

For example, Gigi Hirsch, MD, a former ER physician and instructor at Harvard Medical School, grew so disenchanted with clinical medicine, that she ditched her career and started her own business, MD IntelliNet, in Brookline, MA. The company places doctors in nontraditional jobs by pairing them with venture capitalists and other businesses seeking physicians.

In the same light, Michael Burry, MD, a promising young neurologist from Stanford and Vanderbilt, rejected his medical career to become a private portfolio manager for Scion Capital Management, as did Harvard trained radiologist, Faraz Naqvi, MD, the fund manager for Dresdner RCM Biotechnology Fund, along with Dr. Dimitri Sogoloff, MBA, of Alexandra Investment Management, LLC, and Dr. Kenneth Shuben-Stein, CFA©, of Spencer Capital Management, a hedge fund in New York City.

But Herzlinger implores in her book *Market Driven Healthcare,* "Don't give up [your] practice yet!"

The *Real* Insurance Solution

According to Michael K. Evans, chief economist for American Economics Group, Washington, DC, a real market-driven insurance model may be a solution to the current crisis. It would work like an MSA, HSA, or any other insurance plan by using self-payment for routine visits and medications and using the insurance only for catastrophic illness. Ironically, this was the plan in the original Medicare legislation. This is he reason prescription drug costs are not currently covered. However, many older patients claim that the cost of doctors, hospitals, and medications has risen so much that they are often forced to choose between food and medical care, since the CPI grossly understates the cost of living for the elderly. A one-time adjustment is needed to put those payments back where they actually cover the average market basket of goods and services they buy. But with that adjustment must come an ironclad agreement that government aid for medical care should be used only for major costs associated with catastrophic illness, not for routine care.

Furthermore, Evans believes that when drug companies, hospitals, and physicians find that consumers are spending their own money, they will then work out more reasonable price schedules—or they won't get paid. Just as not everyone can live in the most expensive neighborhood, not everyone can afford to see the most expensive doctor. As lower prices work their way through the system, employers who offer health-care benefits will find their financial situation also will benefit, because costs incurred by employees will rise less rapidly. In the long run, even though the initial effect will be to boost government spending, the net result will be lower medical-care costs, more covered recipients, less bureaucracy, more content physicians, smaller government outlays, and a greater chance that some manufacturing firms will remain in the United States instead of outsourcing to countries where labor costs are much lower.

Physician Education and Re-engineering

Absent the above reforms, it is important for healthcare providers to stay informed and current as to the volatile direction that health care is taking in this country. It is vital for every physician to learn as much about medically related business and financial topics as possible.

Several medical schools have even initiated business certification and degree programs, and, going forward, other medical colleges along with the private sector will do the same. This will allow the profession to make the transition from a supply-based medical system, to a demand-driven one. It will also ensure that practices are operated as a strategic business unit (SBU) and not like the "home office" medical practices of the past. In fact, the trend in managed care now appears to be moving toward giving control back to physicians who stay the course and continue to practice medicine.

However, many physicians, nurses, and healthcare workers don't see it this way and become depressed. Pragmatically, the future healthcare industrial complex will offer great opportunities to change medicine for the better. The way to accomplish this goal is to run your practice like a business and integrate management concepts with a team of trusted advisors—or, formally re-educate yourself.

Online master's degree programs for medical professionals, like those offered at Regis University (303-964-5447), the University of Tennessee (423-974-1768), Washington University (Olin) in St. Louis (888-273-6820), and the University of Wisconsin (608-263-4889), can be utilized. More traditional MBA programs are listed here:

Auburn University, Auburn, Alabama
www.pemba.business.auburn.edu

University of South Florida, Tampa
www.coba.usf.edu/programs/docs

University of Tennessee, Knoxville
www.pemba.utk.edu

University of Colorado, Denver
www.colorado.edu/execed

University of California, Irvine
www.gsm.uci.edu/programs/index.asp

University of Massachusetts, Amherst
www.intra.som.umass.edu/mba/acpe/

University of St. Thomas, Minneapolis
www.stthomas.edu/chma

Carnegie Mellon University, Pittsburgh
www.heinz.cmu.edu/mmm

Tulane University, New Orleans
www.hsm.tulane.edu

University of Southern California, Los Angeles
www.marshall.use.edu/web/execdev.cfm?doc_id=1325

Oregon Health & Services University, Portland
www.ohsu.edu

University of Utah, Salt Lake City
www.uuhsc.utah.edu/medinfo

Still, since an MBA is a huge time and money investment ($30,000–$90,000), it is not for everyone. And do not expect increased earnings or an automatic managerial position without experience. However, total compensation for a full time experienced chief medical officer (CMO) increased 8% last year, and more than half the CMOs were working toward an advanced management degree.

Therefore, a less costly but efficient alternate is the online Certified Medical Planner© designation program from the Institute of Medical Business Advisors, Inc. This is a 500-hour, 12 month long program designed to support medical and financial professionals working in the conjoined medical practice, healthcare management and/or financial planning space. CMP© professional certification provides an opportunity to further develop a deep subject matter understanding of the health care business industry, medical community, and related management delivery system, along with consulting and leadership skills (www.MedicalBusinessAdvisors.com).

CONCLUDING REMARKS

In the short term, the most practical way for physicians to regain their place as conductors of the nation's health care symphonies is to master the concepts of third-party reimbursement, insurance coding and compliance, accounting, business, management, capitation econometrics, marketing, medical advertising, and information technology. The remaining chapters of this book are designed to assist in the endeavor.

ACKNOWLEDGMENTS

Thanks to Jerry Belle, President, Aventis Pharmaceuticals North America, for granting permission for all illustrations from the *Managed Care Digest Series*.

CHAPTER 2

Medical Office Business Plan

David Edward Marcinko, Hope Rachel Hetico, and Rachel Pentin-Maki

> The business plan is a necessity. If the person (physician) who wants to start a small business can't put a business plan together, he or she is in trouble.
>
> —Robert Krummer, Jr., Chairman, First Business Bank, Los Angeles

The business plan is a key tool for raising start-up capital for a new medical practice. It is also used for acquiring loans to finance growth of an existing practice. Although long recognized as a quintessential business tool, its formal structure and mental rigor are only now being recognized in the medical community as competition increases in the health care industrial complex.

There are many reasons to write a medical-practice business plan. The process of gathering, compiling, and analyzing information is an invaluable experience to the beginning practitioner or the experienced veteran. Some specific reasons for writing a plan follow:

- Determine the feasibility of a new practice start-up.
- Raise money from investment bankers for a new practice.
- Obtain financing to expand an existing office or turn-around a declining satellite.
- Develop an operational strategic plan and conduct due diligence.
- Create a budget, time frame, or business direction for a practice.
- Unmask potential problems, risks, or benefits of a medical practice.
- Focus on market opportunities by determining revenue centers or cost drivers.
- Persuade Third Party Payers, networks, and insurance carriers that your practice has a future and represents a viable synergistic partner for their organization.

A STANDARD FORMAT

Physician Executive Summary

The physician executive summary (PES) is always included at the beginning of a formal business plan. It represents a brief synopsis of the entire plan. Its appearance, grammar, and style should be sharp and crisp, as it represents an enticement for the reader to maintain interest and contribute intelligent or economic input into the new venture.

The PES should contain information about the practice, advertising and marketing opportunities, physician management, proposed financing with pro forma financial statements, business operations, and exit strategy. This last point, while unpleasant, is often overlooked by naive practitioners. Business experts, however, look favorably upon an escape plan and view it as the mark of mature professional that realizes the possibility of success as well as failure.

Ultimately, the plan must explain to potential investors how you will make the practice profitable and produce the required return on investment (ROI) for them. It must describe medical services, patient acceptance and benefits, provider qualifications and accomplishments, the amount of capital required, market size, potential practice growth rate, and market niche. Additional information may include office location, proximity to labor, transportation, license requirements, business entity status, proprietary technology and potential working agreements with various insurance, managed care, and HMO plans. If all of the above seem bewildering to the uninitiated, you are correct. Remember, however, that if you do not have, or can't borrow, the funds to begin a private practice, you will just have to become an employed practitioner until you can. It is therefore imperative to start off on the right foot with a sound business plan as you begin your medical career.

Marketing and Sales Analysis

Marketing generally describes your strategic competitive advantage and/or professional synergy that is unique to the practice and not necessarily a significant cost driver. Generally, this may be evaluated through a SWOT analysis of the practice: (S)trengths, (W)eaknesses, (O)pportunities, and (T)hreats.

Sales, on the other hand, represent the act of transferring service ownership to a willing buyer, for compensation. In the past, the four components of marketing were considered to be (1) product (medical service), (2) price (inelastic), (3) place (office), and (4) promotion (demand and supply induced). These four Ps are much less important in today's managed-care environment (especially price), because this simplified secular concept has been replaced with more scientific and quantitative concepts of medical marketing, along with managed-care fixed compensation schedules.

The science of such modern marketing and sales analysis is based on intense competition largely derived from the interplay of five forces. In the early 1980s, Professor Michael F. Porter of Harvard Business School codified these forces, which are often used in medical business and marketing plans today. Although they vary among and within industries, their mix may explain why some practices fail while others succeed. These important marketing forces will be addressed and demonstrated in this section of the business plan.

Power of Buyers

Corporate buyers of employee healthcare are demanding increased quality and decreased premium costs. This has affected competition within the entire healthcare industry. The extent to which these conduits succeed in their bargaining efforts depend on several factors:

- **Concentration:** Insurance companies, managed care organizations, and HMOs represent those buyers that can account for a large portion of a practice's revenue, thereby bringing about certain concessions. These concessions are, typically, price reductions, but they may also include service reductions, such as precluding certain surgical procedures, mandating surgical venue, or excluding certain practitioners in favor of others. Service fulfillment is an important part of practice success, so all proposed or current third-party health care insurance contracts should be listed here. A danger sign is when any entity encompasses more than 15%–25% of a practice's revenues.
- **Switching Costs:** Notable emotional switching costs include the turmoil caused by uprooting a trusted medical provider relationship and the tangible monetary constraints of fees, deductibles, and copayments. These switching costs serve to either retain patients already in the practice or retard new patients from entering it.
- **Integration Level:** The practitioner must decide early on whether or not his or her practice will be vertically or horizontally integrated. For example, a provider may horizontally integrate as a solo practitioner, while a larger group practice may prefer vertical integration in a bigger medical healthcare complex.
- **Profitability:** When a third-party administrator (TPA) earns a low profit and a specific specialty is an important part of costs, more aggressive bargaining is likely to take place with individual MDs or with their associated networks. Explanations must be made for such unpleasant contingencies.
- **Service Importance:** When a purchased service such as healthcare is provided, the buyer's bargaining power is diminished if the service recipient (patient) is not actually or perceptually pleased. Increasingly, HMOs do not often strive to delight their clients and may be responsible for the beginning backlash and changing sentiments these entities are starting to experience. In medicine, as in any business, the power is in the marketplace. Thus, always do your best.

Threat of New Entrants

Many authorities argue that medical schools produce more graduates than needed, inducing a supply-side provider shock. In additional, some of these graduates receive less than adequate postgraduate training.

Therefore, astute practitioners realize that this dilemma must be mitigated, either macroeconomically in the long term through national organizations, or micro-economically in the short run by individual choice; the latter being a practical, albeit slow, way for most MDs. This is accomplished by practicing in rural or remote locations, away from managed care entities, or in areas with under-served populations.

Current or Existing Competition

In addition to intra-professional competition, heightened interprofessional competition within the entire industry has induced allopathic and osteopathic physicians to increase the intensity and volume of certain medical or ancillary services they provide, and referrals may be correspondingly withheld. Rivalry occurs because a competitors act to improve their standing within the marketplace or to protect their position by reacting to moves made by other specialists. Thus, physicians are mutually dependent, and what one practices does impact on other practices, and vice-versa. Therefore, increased existing competition from nonphysicians and alternate healers must be considered in any well-executed business plan.

Substitutions

Professional substitutes are alternate nonprofessionals that are not branded and perform essentially the same function as a professional. Examples include nurse practitioners for physicians, surgical technicians for operating-room nurses, hygienists for dentists, physical therapists for psychiatrists, and foot-care extenders for podiatrists. Aggregate competition will be particularly acute for generalists, while specialty competition will be increased for subspecialists. Any strategy to ameliorate these conditions will augment the successful business practice plan.

Power of Suppliers

The bargaining power of physician suppliers has weakened markedly in the last decade. Reasons include demographics, technology, and a lack of business acumen. However, physicians will again assume their role as leaders of healthcare if they acquire and update the business skills needed to compete in today's marketplace. Business education produces more potential for the medical practice.

Advertising Channel Methodology

Advertising is often a heuristic activity that generally describes those methods of practice promotion, or channel of information distribution, that are nonspecific in nature, that can be done by anyone, but that incur costs to the practice. However, a well-defined advertising plan should be visually stimulating and include several more rational considerations, as in the following list:

- **Goals and Objectives:** The goals and objectives of any advertising plan should be reasonable and quantifiable. For example, a new advertising scheme will not likely generate 250 new patients a month, but it may add additional weekly patients, or some incremental revenue increase; multiplied by some moderate degree for the first 1–2 years. The Law of Diminishing Returns then becomes apparent as results subside. Moreover, the office should have a brief but specific mission statement that addresses the purpose of the practice; targets patient market or audience, and sets goals for every doctor-patient interaction.
- For example, the mission statement of a physiatrist, osteopath, or sports minded chiropractor might be, *"our goal is to conservatively treat athletic patients with cost effective manual and technological remedies in order to reduce pain and return them to activity as soon as possible."* Of course, proper execution must be the desire of every effective mission statement if it is to become a credo of the practice rather than a mere incantation.

- **Communications and Media Channels:** Typical channels of advertising include print: (coupons, office brochures, newsletter, bill stuffers, billboards, signs), audio (radio), and telecommunications (message "hold" buttons, beepers and pagers). The yellow-page ad is a key to success with these and other media. Eventually, potential patients will have to call and make an appointment with you. Whether directed by other media, or happenstance, it is important that your ad be conspicuous. Do not scrimp with it, and plan to lay it out carefully. Or consult a graphic artist. Denote your specialty in plain English, and include your name, address, location, credentials, insurance affiliations, special skills, and the common conditions you treat. Stick with the same colors or design every year, and include a portrait for self-recognition. Quarter- or half-page ads are not unreasonable. Include your e-mail and/or Web-site address.

- If you believe that video (television) advertising is important but feel you can not afford it, then look into your local public broadcasting station. Often, they do not consider anything they broadcast as advertising but, rather, categorize it as *underwriting*. Your dollars will support local public broadcast programs and therefore quality as a personal tax deduction. These benefits play a dual role by saving you money and providing video exposure for your practice.

- Sometimes, even the media becomes the message, as is the case of the World Wide Web (WWW) and Internet. Certainly, the use of telemedicine in the next decade will increase as the promise and security of quality healthcare, at any time and in any place, becomes a reality. For now, the most commonly used telemedicine clinical applications occur in such specialties as: cardiology, correctional care, dermatology, fetal ultrasounds, home health care agencies, neurology, orthopedics, otorhinolaryngology, pathology, pediatrics, psychiatry, radiology, emergency care, and traumatology. Types of transmission lines currently available include the wideband Internet, dial-up ISDN/switches @ 56 bpm, and dedicated T-1 lines. To find out more about what telemedicine will become, contact *Vidimedix (The Telemedicine Specialists)* @ 888-450-8091 or at www.futureoftelemedicine.com).

- Other basic ways to channel new patients into your sphere of medical influence include: healthcare screenings, service, civic (YMCA, YWCA, PTA) or religious organization involvement, seminars and speaking engagements, hospital auxiliaries and neighborhood welcome wagons, writing and publication in local or community newspapers, and simply having a friendly personality. More specific referral patterns can be cultivated by certain individuals such as: the clergy, nurses, pharmaceutical representatives, bankers, realtors, and accountants, as well as a host of nontraditional healthcare advisors, such as chiropractors, physical therapists, holistic, nutritionists, homeopathic practitioners, and health food devotees. Increasingly, keeping primary-care (gatekeeper) physicians happy is the source of continued referrals, particularly in a managed care environment. This can be accomplished through introductory letters or initial personal meetings; practice mission statement, subspecialty interests or advantages; and follow-up telephone calls and letters outlining the diagnosis and treatment plan for all referred patients.

- Perhaps the most effective way to motivate existing patients is through effective communications. Such techniques include proper body language, attire, eye contact, appropriate facial expressions and verbal acknowledgments, mirroring and paraphrasing; or just spending time with the patient to listen to his or her concerns.
- **Message and Credibility:** The advertising message must be delivered in such a way as to build, change, or reinforce patient and payer attitudes. Advertising has shown that the more honest, fair, and unbiased the audience perceives the source to be, the more credible the message-and the more likely the attitudes will shift toward the source's position.
- **Reinforcement and Repetitions:** An advertisement must be repeated for several reasons: to emphasize the message, keep the audience from forgetting the message and save the costs of producing more messages (print 3–5 times and TV 8–12 times). Exposure time (15–60 seconds) must also be considered. Over-learning occurs when the audience becomes fatigued and further expenditures are wasted on needless advertising. However, the medical advantage may be fleeting if the message is content poor. Intended effects begin with the hierarchy of patient consciousness; progressing to patient awareness, comprehension, and conviction; and ending with the designed behavior on the part of the client or payer.
- **Feedback and Evaluation:** Any advertising campaign must be continuously monitored for efficacy. Methods to evaluate successes include memory tests, practice surveys, recall tests, and, ultimately, revenue effects. In fact, many experts feel that no advertising campaign is better than a poorly monitored one, merely because it is economically unwise.

- **Public Relations:** Generally, public relations is deemed to be much more credible than marketing or advertising endeavors. Media coverage is probably most synonymous with the concept of public relations, since reporters or editors will cover your story if it seems newsworthy, timely, or important to their constituency. If this tool is chosen, it is important to be systematically aggressive (proactive) in design. For example:

  - Target your media audience (reporters, editors, program directors, TV, newspaper and radio editors, etc.).
  - Send your targeted media audience a letter of introduction and offer to tell a personal, or patient based, success story about your medical specialty and practice. Include an office brochure, business card, and brief curriculum vitae.
  - Be available when a reporter calls. Some PR professionals suggest that you always take a media call, and offer to call back at a set time, based on the reporter's deadline. This gives you time to think about the topic and set up your key message. Meet the deadline and always call back to encourage repeat media appearances.
  - If you are fortunate enough to be interviewed directly, keep your message short and supply additional written information to the reporter.
  - Follow-up with a thank-you letter and synopsis of your response. Offer to keep the media representative informed of current updates in your specialty or practice.

- Of course, for larger practices, a professional public relations agent might be useful—at an additional salary of 20–30 thousand dollars per year to your office budget; but true public relations is without expense. Public relations activities include: letters to the editor and op-ed pieces; media coverage and infomercials; by-lined articles and speaking engagements. Public relations are subtle and somewhat uncontrolled. Advertising, on the other hand, is more blunt and controlled. The advantage of true PR is that it is free when "unsponsored." However, since PR agents need to accomplish something to justify their existence, be prepared for even more advertising expenses. Monitor them carefully. Good PR agents should more than justify their costs; if not, replace them or use your imagination and do it yourself.

Remember, it is always more believable when someone else says something good about your practice than when you say something good about it yourself.

- **Crisis Management:** If you remain in practice long enough, something adverse is sure to happen that will negatively affect your business. A patient may die, your hospital may close, the surgery center you frequent may lose accreditation, a trusted employee may be caught embezzling, or a patient may *go ballistic* (i.e., "postal") and injure your staff or yourself. When, not if, this scenario occurs, you must have a crisis management business plan in place to deal swiftly and successfully with the matter. Most management experts suggest the following course of actions when tragedy strikes:

  - Stay calm and relaxed but act immediately.
  - Release detrimental, but accurate, information as soon as possible. Stay neutral.
  - First, educate your employees and staff about the crisis, then your local community.
  - Implement and fix the problem or find an alternate solution to minimize recurrence and routine disruption.
  - Continually release information about the crisis if it is ongoing.
  - Monitor and report the results of your strategy to all affected, or potentially affected, people (patients, managed care plans, community, etc.), both in the short and long run.
  - Thank everyone concerned for their support, and turn a negative story into a positive one through good public relations. You will grow personally and professionally from the experience.
  - Remember, speed and proactivity are the keys to adverse public relations fallout. Do you want to be another Perrier, which never fully recovered from the adverse publicity of finding trace amounts of benzene in its bottle water in 1990; or Johnson & Johnson, which recovered beautifully from the Tylenol-R tragedy a few years ago and not only recovered lost profits but trust in the marketplace, as well? The choice is yours.

Defined Budget: Advertising is an expense that should be controlled. Typically, it is a semifixed, or variable, cost, that is increasingly but often erroneously becoming a greater portion of medical-practice expenses. We suggest that start-up practices devote more scarce resources (5%–7% or even 10% of gross revenues) toward advertising, while more mature practices may devote less than (3%–5%) resources to marketing and branding endeavors.

HUMAN RESOURCES

The name, address, age, prior business experience, educational background, residency training, board certification status, salary requirements, benefit/perquisites, retirement plans, special skills, personal financial statement, number, and caliber of current investors, and any other pertinent information about the current or future physician owner. A resume of the chief-executive medical officer (executive practitioner) must be included in this section. Strengths and weakness of the doctor, manager, or management advisory team should be noted.

Professional organization membership, and a list of firms providing profession services to the practice, such as accountant, public relations firm or advertising agency, financial planner, banker, stock-broker, insurance agent, and professional management consultants should be listed. Payroll processing, worker's compensation, employee recruitment, independent contractor status, and employer liability coverage should also be included, with proper Patriot Act (PA) and Health Insurance Portability and Accountability Act (HIPAA) business-associate agreements. Obviously, some of this information will be sketchy for the beginning practice, but it should be much more detailed for the established one. An organizational chart that reflects management hierarchy is a nice visual addition to the practice management presentation.

An often-neglected portion of the practice management business plan is the acquisition and retention of office employees. A receptionist, billing clerk, back-office assistant, and office manager are important hires relative to the ongoing-concern nature, or goodwill, of the business. Hiring, training, orientation, empowerment, motivation, salary and benefit packages, performance reviews, and continuing education must all be addressed. Insurance and fidelity bonding must also be secured. A reproducible method to accomplish these tasks is through the use of an office, Clinical Laboratory Improvement Act (CLIA), Health Insurance Portability and Accountability Act (HIPAA), Employee Retirement Income Security Act (ERISA), Material Safety Data Sheet (MSDS), employee and/or OSHA compliance *manual.* These manuals may be individually prepared (time consuming and expensive) or purchased (quick and less costly) and then modified for practice specific use. Many employees find such documentation helpful in maintaining the orderliness of the medical office.

BUSINESS OPERATIONS PHILOSOPHY

Some pundits believe that a general medical or even a broad-specialty practice will have limited appeal to patients and buyers of healthcare services in the future. In its place, the doctor must philosophically decide if she or he is to become either a discount, service, or value provider, and then aggressively pursue this business operational strategy. This decision can be presented as an expansion of the practice mission statement or a declaration of practice culture and then outlined in this section of the business plan.

Discount Provider Operations

A discount provider is one who has made a conscious effort to practice low cost but high volume medicine. Unfortunately, this is easier said than done, and this section of the business plan must persuade the reader of the doctor's commitment to this moral and business philosophy through estimated cost-volume analysis projections.

For example, discount providers must depend on economics of scale to purchase bulk supplies, since this model is ideal for multidoctor practices. Otherwise, several practitioners must establish a network, or synergy, to create a virtual organization to do so. In this manner, malpractice insurance, major equipment, and other recurring purchases (especially variable cost-based supplies) can be negotiated for the best price. Another major commitment must be made to management information systems (MIS) and computerized office automation devices. By necessity, discount medical provider offices are small, neat and sparsely furnished, but with functional and utilitarian assets. Most all managed care contracts just be aggressively sought, since patient flow and volume is the key to success in this organizational type.

Make no mistake about it, a low cost philosophy is not evil as it satisfies a real niche in the medical marketplace for basic care. It should not, however, be the operational plan of default (i.e., when all else fails) because low fees, high patient volume, and high office overhead costs may be a formula for grossing (top-line revenues) the practice to death. In other words, low fees are often thought by physicians to be a significant advantage in attracting new patients. And for the short term, they are. The long-term reality, however, is that regardless of how low fees get, there will always be a more deeply discounted competitor willing to do what you do, at a lower fee.

Service Provider Operations

A provider committed to a service philosophy must be willing to do whatever it takes to satisfy the patient. For example, this may mean providing wcckcnd, wccknight, or holiday office hours, instead of a routine 9–5 schedule. House calls, hospital visits, prison calls, and nursing home rounds would be included in this operational model. Children, elderly patients, or those with mental, physical, or chemically induced challenges, are all fertile niches of a core-service philosophy. Charge them for what you do based on your time and expertise, and, especially, the venue. It makes no sense to provide excellent service and charge for mediocre service.

Value-Added Provider

A value-added medical provider is committed to practicing at the highest and riskiest levels of medical and surgical care and has the credentials and personality to do so. Value differentiation is based on such factors as board certification, hospital privileges, subspecialty identification, or other unique attributes such as fluency in a second language or acceptance into an ethnocentric locale. Now, make no mistake about this philosophy, because a certain amount of self-aggrandizement is needed to develop a brand image; and charge for it. In other words, it is just not enough to truly be an expert you must also develop the gravitational pull of a singular public image. This brand identification must be enunciated in your business plan as you answer the question: What can I offer that no one else can? Put less delicately, you have to have a unique practice proposition. Shy personality types might avoid this operational archetype.

A word to reduce complaints about fees in this model is *transparency*—inform your patients about your fees. More medical providers are harmed by fees that are too low than hurt by fees that are too high. Remember, if you never get complaints about fees, it means either that you are providing first-rate care and your patients think it is worth every penny; or you are undercharging them.

FINANCIAL STATEMENTS

Since a start-up medical practice has no historical financial information, simplified pro forma production logs, or statements, are forecasted for three years, along with a projected *practice break-even analysis*. They demonstrate the best care, worst case, and most likely financial scenarios. Computerized spreadsheets are ideal for this task. Other relevant financial information may be included as needed.

Pro Forma (Production Log) Statement

A simple daily production log is shown below, with variance recordings. It may be used on a pro-forma estimated, or ongoing concern, basis.

	A		B	C			D
				Ahead			
Daily	Month-to Today's		(Behind) Ytd	Ytd (Behind)			
Date	Target	Target	Charges	(A − B)	Goal	Charges	(D − C) Frwrd
1	1,600	1,600	1,200	(400)	1,600	1,600	(400)
2	1,600	3,200	1,500	(100)	3,400	2,700	(500)

However, the more sophisticated profit and loss (P&L) statement is a better measure of office performance than is the log (for a given period of time).

Pro Forma Net-Income (Profit & Loss) Statement

By allocating a practice's profit or loss into operating groups, the investor can isolate profitable revenue centers and isolate unprofitable costs drivers. These are then identified in the net income statement (NIS). In certain managed care contracts, an analysis to identify unit or per dollar revenues and gross profits and/or gross margins is vital. Certain noncash expenses (i.e., depreciation, amortization, and deferred taxes) are then deducted from revenues to determine overall net income.

Pro Forma Cash-Flow Statement

The *statement of cash flow (SCF)* is the lifeblood of any medical practice. It projects estimated cash flows by month, quarter, and year, along with the anticipated timing of cash receipts and disbursements. The office's bills and obligations are paid out of cash flow, not net income. It is very important for accrual-based accounting practices, especially in terms of Medicare, Medicaid, MCOs, PPOs, and HMOs that are producing insurance-payment time delays, and other aged-accounting methodologies. Cash flow reflects the internal generation of fund available to investors.

Pro Forma Balance Sheet

The *Balance Sheet (BS)* forecasts the financial condition of an office at a singular point in time. It projects the ability to meet financial obligation and the capacity to absorb financial setbacks without becoming insolvent.

Finally, there are other miscellaneous considerations when estimating financial statements. For example:

- Are business and service revenues seasonal?
- What percentages of revenues come from Medicare, Medicaid, MCOs, HMOs, PPOs, or traditional indemnity insurance plans?
- What are the revenue and cost positions relative to your peers? The industry?
- What are the potential costs or paid-up expenses possible in the future?
- What credit analysis is used to screen potential-private patients?

Break-Even Analysis

Break-even analysis (BEA) is a method of assessing a practices profit potential and down-side risk. It represents the minimum percentage of productive capacity the office must utilize, the minimum patient volume it must generate, and the minimum market share it must obtain to break even. At this production (i.e., revenue) volume, the doctor experiences neither a profit nor a loss. Thus, a comparison can be made between estimated unit services and the number of services that must be produced to break even.

For example, if the office projects sales of 300 new patients during the first year, but only requires the revenue of 150 to break even, then the office has only to attain 50% of its projected volume to break even.

To perform this analysis, the practice's expenses should be divided into fixed costs that do not fluctuate with volume and remain constant as volume increases (i.e., rent, utilities, insurance, interest, and minimal doctor living expenses), and variable costs that are uniform per unit of output (e.g., labor, materials, and equipment) and fluctuate in direct proportion to volume. The break-even point in patient units (BEPIU) and dollars (BEPID) is then calculated with the following formulas:

BEPIU: Fixed Costs / (Revenue Price Per Patient
Unit – Variable Cost Per Patient Unit)

BEPID: (BEP in Patient Units) × (Revenue Price Per Patient Unit)

ASSESSMENT

Professor Gregory I. Kravitt, managing director of a Chicago based investment banking firm, lists six principles as providing a solid foundation for any effective business plan. We have modified them, as listed below, for embryonic physicians as they begin private practice:

- An effective business plan is a detailed, consistent, and factually supported document that persuades bankers and other decision makers to support your medical practice plan. Avoid superlatives and use specific methods to quantify your goals.
- Address your audience, avoid medial jargon, and do not be a slave to minutia. Remember the reader's background (bankers-relatives-financier). Anticipate questions and remember the journalistic five W's (who, what, where, when, and why). This later interrogative is most important since *why* you decide to pursue a certain course of action is usually more important than *how* you pursue it.
- A detailed marketing and competitive analysis is a vital factor to raising cash for a practice. Understanding your own strengths and weaknesses, as well as performing a patient population analysis, is the key to recruiting and maintaining new patients for your practice.
- Define and understand the major problems associated with starting a new medical practice and evaluate possible solutions and contingency plans when launching the business.
- Use Gant, critical path method (CPM), or program evaluation and review technique (PERT) flow charts and Paretto diagrams to illustrate thoughts and reinforce your message. Computerized project management (PM) software, such as *MS-Project Manager-R,* is a sophisticated method to highlight an organizational timetable.
- The quality of management (i.e., the doctor) is the most important element in any business. You must hook the reader with your education, training, or other method of service differentiation that fills the market need and adds an element of excitement to your future practice and business.

BUSINESS FRIENDLY STATES

Do not allow the need for a formal business plan to dissuade you from your dream of starting a medical practice. But, realize that some states are more business friendly than others. A ranking of states friendly to new and existing businesses, including medical practices, is contained in the *2003: Small Business Survival Index.*

Rank	State	SBSI Score	Rank	State	SBSI Score
1	Nevada	27.060	27	Maryland	46.310
2	South Dakota	28.250	28	Oklahoma	46.920

3	Washington	32.010	29	Delaware	46.950
4	Wyoming	32.150	30	Wisconsin	47.380
5	Florida	33.180	31	Nebraska	48.430
6	Texas	34.250	32	Kentucky	48.610
7	New Hampshire	36.250	33	Connecticut	48.830
8	Alabama	36.830	34	Utah	49.242
9	Mississippi	38.160	35	North Carolina	49.590
10	Tennessee	39.540	36	Oregon	50.010
11	Colorado	39.870	37	New Jersey	50.360
12	Michigan	40.205	38	Montana	50.979
13	Illinois	40.290	39	Iowa	51.073
14	Alaska	40.880	40	Ohio	52.870
15	Virginia	41.310	41	West Virginia	53.120
16	Indiana	41.820	42	Vermont	53.514
17	Missouri	42.213	43	New York	54.005
18	South Carolina	42.520	44	California	54.860
19	Louisiana	43.304	45	New Mexico	55.410
20	Arizona	44.178	46	Minnesota	55.890
21	Massachusetts	44.755	47	Kansas	55.980
22	Pennsylvania	44.880	48	Maine	56.150
23	Georgia	45.350	49	Hawaii	57.235
24	North Dakota	45.379	50	Rhode Island	59.011
25	Arkansas	45.420	51	District of Columbia	65.335
26	Idaho	45.590			

CONCLUSION

Writing a medical office business plan is a daunting effort, but it is not nearly as difficult as starting or expanding a practice without one. The writing process methodically forces you, the future or current chief executive, to test assumptions, research markets, analyze competition, and evaluate the viability of your start-up, expansion, or revitalization efforts. It is also time consuming and emotionally challenging, but more often than not, the process leads to an increased likelihood of success and procurement of needed capital. You may even learn something about yourself and whether or not you wish to be a corporate-employed physician or an owner-employer physician. It is a decidedly positive endeavor and well worth the conscientious industry it requires.

CHAPTER 3

Medical Practice Strategic Operating Plan

David Edward Marcinko, Hope Rachel Hetico, and Rachel Pentin-Maki

> Once your medical practice (company) is up and running, convert the business plan to an operating plan, and then religiously keep it updated, using it as a guide on a continuing basis. The operating plan keeps you (the doctor), management, and staff focused on the tasks at hand. This is a working-plan tool that has to be long on detail but may be short on presentation. You can afford a high degree of candor and informality when preparing a strategic operating plan.
>
> —Rick Van Ness, *CEO: www.GrowthConncetion.com*

O nce start-up capital is secured with the help of a well executed medical business plan, the most common avenue to establishing a medical office has been to select a location and start solo practice. Given the initial cost of opening an office in today's competitive climate, this may not be the most practical method to pursue. Fortunately, there are other options available to the health care provider, which include the following:

- Purchase the practice of a retiring practitioner.
- Associate with a group practice with an option to purchase partnership interest.
- Associate with a multidiscipline practice.
- Become a salaried employee of an established delivery system (VA, MCOs, HMOs, military, etc.).

Nevertheless, new or existing office success may be increased by creating a strategic-operating plan that considers some of the following features.

LOCATION

Of primary importance in locating a practice is to work where you enjoy living and then calculate the ratio of specialists in your area of interest. The ideal location should have as many of the following features as possible: (1) central area, (2) accessibility and visibility, (3) demographics, and (4) proximity to personal residence, hospital facilities, and general medical community.

Office Design and Layout

The office reflects its practitioner and the quality of medical practice. Although location is a prime factor in attracting patients, the layout and appearance of the office is vital in keeping patient in the practice. The aim is to establish an environment that is warm, cheerful, professionally competent, and nonintimidating. This effect can be achieved through the proper integration of space, light color, texture, and sound.

- *Design Considerations:* One of the most effect methods to achieve even flow is to establish zones within the office. The primary zones are reception, business, staff, laboratory, radiology, lavatory, storage, and doctor's office.
- *Size Considerations:* Ideally, one should practice in the largest affordable office. One thousand square feet is considered the minimum, although small offices can be efficient and adequate. Allow for future expansion.
- *Interior Decorations:* Wall coverings should be durable and washable, such as commercial-grade vinyl wallpaper. Painting is less expensive initially but needs to be repainted every 2–3 years. Good wallpaper will last up to 10 years.

Floor coverings should be made of durable vinyl sheeting. In hallways, reception, or business areas, carpeting is suggested. It produces warmth and is easy to care for. In treatment areas, a combination of carpet and tile or linoleum can create an effective visual appeal while allowing ease of maintenance.

Hallways should be a minimum of four feet wide to accommodate patient flow. Doorways should be oversized to allow easy access for walkers and wheelchairs. Handrails should be available for the elderly.

Treatment rooms should be a minimum of 8 × 10 feet long. The entrance door should be in the center to allow ease of access. Equipment should be placed according to individual preference, with considerations as to whether the doctor works standing or sitting. This will affect cabinet height placement. Coat hooks and side chairs should be included in the design to allow easier removal of hose, shoes and clothes, as needed.

The reception room should be tastefully decorated according to basic rules:

- Use warm, soothing color schemes.
- Have adequate lighting, and consider the use of lamps and/or indirect lighting.
- Unless florescent, ceiling lights alone do not provide enough light for reading.
- Chairs should have arms high enough to allow the patient ease of entry and exit. To prevent chairs from scraping the wall, chair rails may be used to keep the chairs off the walls.
- Have a closet or coat/umbrella stand available with mirror.
- Maintain all live plants, and periodically freshen artificial ones.

BUSINESS AND PROFESSIONAL INSURANCE

1. Malpractice Liability Insurance

The *Capitation Liability Theory* of malpractice views liability management and premium costs in light of the managed-care revolution. For example, although the indemnity reimbursement model was the bedrock of health care financing, the incidence of litigation is believed to be the most frequent in this system. Similarly, errors of commission, which may be more likely in a fee-based system, are easier to prove than errors of omission in a fixed system. Conversely, a capitated reimbursement system suggests the level of malpractice risk—and associated litigation—decreases as the volume of capitated care increases.

Therefore, since the future is unknown, choose a malpractice insurance company rated A or better by A.M. Best (*www.ambest.com*). True indications of a strong company are often reflected in the firm's net premium to surplus ratio, wherein a lower ratio is better and the industry average is about .81; net liability to surplus ratio, which the industry average is 4.1; net average ratio, where the industry average is 4.9; and reserve-to-surplus ratio, in which the industry average is about 3.6–4.1 (Physicians Insurers Association of America).

2. Fire, Theft, and Liability Insurance

Fire and theft insurance is used to cover office equipment and contents, while *leasehold insurance* protects against loss due to the termination of a favorable lease caused by the insured perils.

3. Worker's Compensation Insurance

Worker's compensation is mandatory to cover a loss of income, medical expenses, and rehabilitation. Most states also have established *second-injury funds,* which are designed to compensate employees who suffer a second disability injury and thus shield the employer/physician from the increased costs associated with a second injury.

4. Business Interruption/Loss of Income Protection Insurance

This covers the ongoing medical offices expenses and income loss following office damage, and it continues during the *Period of Restoration.* Most business interruption is written on an indemnity basis and consists of two broad types: *Business income coverage form (add extra expense)* and *business income coverage form (without extra expense).* Either type requires coinsurance, and both require a choice of three income coverage forms: (1) business income including rental value, (2) business income excluding rental value, and (3) rental value only. Consideration should also be made for man/woman insurance and accounts receivable insurance.

5. Dishonesty Insurance

A *Fidelity Insurance Bond* protects the doctor employer against employee dishonesty and covers the loss of money, securities, or other property resulting from acts by the bonded person. In a *Surety bond*, one party (surety) agrees to be responsible to a second party (obligee), for the obligations of a third party (the principal). In medicine, surety bonds are used in situations in which one of the parties insists on a guarantee of indemnity if the second party fails to perform a specific act. Such a requirement may arise in connection with professional medical employment contracts or other situations in which there may be doubt concerning the ability to perform medical or office related business tasks.

6. Billing Errors & Omissions Insurance

This coverage protects you against liability for unintentional billing errors when you bill a third party, including Medicare/Medicaid or MCOs. This is usually a separate policy that provides limits of liability from $100,000/$100,000, up to $1 million/$1 million to cover both defense and indemnity costs. Others endorsements may also be obtained to pay civil fines, penalties, judgments and settlements, or increased limits of liability, up to $1 million/$1 million. All terms, conditions, and limitations are outlined in the actual policy form (*www.promutual.com*).

OFFICE MANUALS

One of the key management tools of a new, or existing, practice is the office manual. The manual is a book that contains the guidelines to operate the office. If not presently used, start one immediately. It takes some effort to develop an office manual, but once established, it will become a permanent addition to the business portion of the practice.

The manual itself should consist of a loose-leaf binder to which additions or deletions can be made. Section dividers may be used to separate the manual into appropriate areas. The function of the manual is to describe in detail the various operational functions of the office. It will also serve as an instructional tool for new employees as well as a reference source for the doctor and office staff. It should include the following items:

- *Employee section.* Dress code, job descriptions, employee benefits, smoking policy, employment hours, and staff meeting schedules.
- *Office policy.* Telephone priorities, fee schedules, third party insurance carriers, instrument pack list, and a list of suppliers and vendors.
- *Correspondence forms.* Sample letters, patient information, referrals (patient and physician), collection agencies, paperwork, consent forms, assignment of benefit forms, insurance forms, postoperative instructions, and medical-information release forms.
- *Employment benefits.* Sick days, vacation time, holidays, personal leave days, salary, raises, bonuses, health insurance, life insurance, pension plans, retirement, and profit sharing plans.

- *Staff meeting policy.* Improvements, suggestions, complaints, grievances, information exchange, and new office polices.
- *Office Maintenance.* It is very disconcerting for the doctor to be out of town and return to find the office is inoperable because the heating or air-conditioning system is faulty. Therefore, proper maintenance is important. The names and phone numbers of the appropriate personnel should be accessible to keep the office functional.

The key to office efficiency is an organized routine. Its real meaning will allow the doctor to work at full capacity during office hours. Efficiency means everyone will work smarter, not harder. Office organization might consist of the following manuals or checklist items:

- Doctor and assistant chart check and review with treatment plan decisions, materials needed, radiographs, casting, injections, blood tests, or special treatments. Salient comments attached to patient charts on disposable slips of paper.
- Laboratory reports (bacterial, pregnancy or blood tests) available prior to patient treatment.
- Time allotment for phone messages, follow-up calls, and physician consultation/referral.

Other Manuals

In the current legal and medical environment, numerous office manuals are necessary. Some of them are discussed in the following section.

Blood Borne Pathogen Standard Manual

OSHA requires that each medical facility maintain a manual that spell out the employers written *Blood Borne Pathogen Standard* policy for AIDS, tuberculosis, hepatitis, VD, and, or a host of other pathogens. Although not blood borne, SARS may also be a concern with some specialists.

Physicians must also realize that due to an overturned January 2000 response letter from the US Labor Secretary, doctors who are employers may still become responsible for some employees injured while working at home. This might include, for example, transcriptionists, typists, and other off-site workers. To protect themselves, experts suggest medical offices put their policies on home safety in their handbook and provide ergonomic equipment for home workers (*www.thedeltagroup.com*).

Hazardous Communication Standard Manual

Not only does OSHA require each medical facility to maintain a manual corresponding to the *Blood Borne Pathogen Standard,* there is also a requirement that a manual be maintained concerning the employer's written *Hazardous Communication Standard.* The manual should delineate the items in the office that pose a threat to the employees and the protocol to be followed in the event of an exposure incident.

Material Safety Data-Sheet Manual

A separate manual should be kept organizing manufacturer's *Material Data Safety Sheets*. Obtaining, maintaining, and making available the Material Data Safety Sheets is one of the requirements under OSHA's Hazardous Communication Standard. It is often best to keep the Material Data Safety Sheets in a separate and convenient manual (*www.safetydirector.com*).

Discrimination and Sexual Harassment Policy Manual

Since approximately 25% of all new cases filed in Federal District Court pertain to causes of action dealing with discrimination (e.g., racial discrimination, sexual discrimination, age discrimination, and handicap discrimination) and with sexual harassment, the prudent employer will also maintain a Discrimination and Sexual Harassment Policy Manual. Such a manual should delineate the employer's policy against discrimination and harassment and it should contain a reporting and investigative procedure. Above all else, once implemented, the polices-procedures delineated in the manual should be followed!

Workplace Violence Prevention Manual or Policy

The cornerstone of any medical practice violence prevention policy should be prevention, with the ultimate goal of zero incidents. In addition, the policy should make the concept of treating people in a respectful manner and maintaining their dignity a central theme that is integrated into its communication (*www.innovations-training.com*).

Illustrative of a good workplace violence policy statement is the US Department of Transportation's Workplace Violence Policy:

> A safe working environment for all employees, free from violence or any threat of violence, is one goal of the U.S. Department of Transportation. Violence and threatening behaviors in any form are unacceptable and will not be tolerated. . . . The cooperation of (doctors) supervisors, managers, and employees is necessary to implement this policy and maintain a safe working environment. . . . Supervisors and managers are expected to take immediate action to investigate reported threats or violence and any suspicious items or activities, and with the assistance of appropriate officials, reduce or eliminate the risk of workplace violence.

Note that practices are also starting to incorporate directly into their workplace violence prevention policies statements that make it clear that bullying behaviors are considered threatening behaviors because they cause emotional abuse and can lead to situations that create a hostile environment and also create hostile feelings between employees and patients.

- Establish a process for record keeping to be able to track actual threats, incidents, close calls, escalating conflicts, and so forth for trends or patterns. Also evaluate interventions and programmatic efforts to evaluate their success and to maintain continuous improvement.
- Assess your practice's conflict-resolution process and bolster to ensure it is an effective tool for fairly addressing employee concerns and conflicts and for

resolving problems. Usage of this process should be tracked (keep in mind that high usage is not necessarily a bad indicator; it may indicate that people trust your process) and periodically assessed to determine how employees feel about it.

Health Insurance Portability and Accountability Act Manual

This manual describes office policy regarding electronic (1) connectivity, (2) transmission, (3) storage/retrieval, and (4) confidentiality of all health care information (*www.ahima.org* and *www.superiorconsultant.com*).

Medicare Compliance Manual

The Department of Justice has identified health care fraud as its number two priority, behind drug law violations. Because health care fraud has been targeted by federal authorities and because of the proliferation of health care fraud legislation, even ethical practitioners may be engulfed by the dragnet of law enforcement. For that reason, the prudent practitioner will have a manual that details the policies and procedures that the office employs to (1) avoid health care fraud, (2) detect any instances of health care fraud, and (3) correct any instances of health care fraud that are brought to light.

Individual Managed Care Organization Manuals

Even with the proliferation of mergers by health care insurers, there is still a multitude of managed care plans in the marketplace. Each plan has its own policies and procedures. Each plan sends out periodic notices delineating highlights and plan changes. The modern physician office almost needs a full-time librarian to keep track of all of the paperwork received from plans by health care providers. Nonetheless, the practitioner should keep a manual for each and every contracted health care plan. Such a manual can be easily reviewed to assist in patient needs. More important, the manual can be a source of information when appealing adverse plan decisions.

Office Emergency Kit

Every office should have (1) an emergency kit; (2) written emergency protocol; (3) trained staff; and (4) emergency drills. Basic emergency kits include an oxygen tank and a drug kit. More advanced emergency kits will include defibrillators and other advanced cardiac life-support systems.

The oxygen tank should be filled and should be evaluated regularly. It should contain an intact hose and a mask, and it should be accompanied by an *Ambu-Bag.* The drug kit should include items such as IV needles, tourniquet, tongue depressor, tracheotomy needle, various syringes and needles, and drugs, such as epinephrine, nitroglycerin, diazepam, atropine, benadryl, and smelling salts.

RECORD KEEPING AND COLLECTIONS

The rationale for good medical record keeping includes collection success, protection against lawsuits, and business efficiency value of the practice. Patient charts should be organized for the input and storage of information in a systematic way. Charts should include patient information material, progress notes, laboratory reports, correspondences, consultation reports, insurance forms, operative reports, and telephone messages. Radiographs may be stored with the chart or separately. Active medical records should be maintained for three years, while inactive charts should be maintained for seven to ten years.

Unfortunately, repeal of the Glass-Steagall Act contains zero privacy standards, and a bank or insurance company could possibly check your health history before granting credit or underwriting an insurance policy.

Collections

Just as location is a critical element in locating a medical practice, collecting your accounts receivable (AR) is an important critical element in maintaining the financial health of your medical practice. Your practice is not a bank, and an effective billing system should be complemented by an efficient collection system. A policy that is too conservative may result in poor collection rates, while an aggressive policy may be counterproductive and increase liability. Have collectors call early and often. Waiting encourages patients to pay late. Use the 80/20 rule and concentrate on your biggest accounts first. Get nonperforming receivables off the books. Accounts over about 120 day should be turned over to third party agents (*www.access-health.com*).

Out-sourcing to collection agencies varies significantly in terms of quality and results. Most charge from 30% to 50% of what they collect (*www.per-se.com*).

According to John Broderick, an executive staffing consultant from New York, the following should be considered when selecting a collection agency or using in-house personnel:

- *Assertiveness and Analytical Skills.* Collectors should be able to break a billing problem into component parts and aggressively pursue each part without being unduly tactless.
- *Creativeness and Curiosity.* Collectors should keep abreast of new computer and software technology and pursue innovative philosophies related to the billing process.
- *Empathy and Communicativeness.* Collectors should be able to communicate with both patients and doctors, yet still be able to put themselves in others' shoes to view problems from each perspective.
- *Perspective and Stability.* Collectors should be able to see the patients entire economic picture and maintain an emotionally objective and neutral attitude toward the collection process.
- *Integrity and Tenacity.* Collectors should have steadfast attitude and still earn the trust of clients, relatives, and the doctor/employer. Collections should begin immediately, since waiting frustrates patients and decreases receivables receipt.
- *Salary.* An entry-level full-time office billing collector should be familiar with most state laws regarding the collection process and be paid in the low 20s of thousands of dollars per annum. If not, after a while, he or she may take their experience and training to another office for considerably more compensation.

Receptionist Management Planning Tip:

The median number of full-time-equivalent (FTE) medical receptionists in multispecialty groups increased between 1999 and 2000, from .91 to .98.

Source: Aventis Managed Care Digest Series, 2003.

Remember, small claims court is the last avenue for payment. Often a decision has to be made whether to forgive or "write off" a patient's balance if indemnity insurance coverage is maintained, and this decision is best made on an individual basis. Unfortunately, malpractice claims have resulted by pursuing past-due accounts too aggressively. This is especially true with surgical patients, and it is best to pursue payment diplomatically, gently, and—often—forgivingly.

You could be losing money if your practice is still using a traditional checking account for its daily cash activities. One way to make your cash work more effectively is to open a cash management account with a brokerage firm. This will ensure that your practice's money is earning a much higher rate of interest.

Pro Bono Care

A survey several years ago suggested that more than 40% of the country's doctors are now doing less pro bono work due to managed care. However, the organization Volunteers in Health care (VIH) offers a free computerized patient-record system to track the care given to the uninsured. The VIH software allows you to track and store information on patients, visits, providers, clinics, referrals, and more. It is menu driven, with canned reports that provide summary statistics on patients and providers (*www.volunteersinhealth care.org*).

HUMAN RESOURCES

The first step in hiring personnel is to determine the number of employees needed and their office functions. Most practitioners choose to screen personnel independently. Disqualifying characteristics include poor communication skills, abrasive personalities, transportation difficulties, or a lack of other specific qualifications. Miscellaneous recruitment sources include college placement offices, medical assistance schools, secretarial schools, and local state unemployment offices. Professional employment agencies are often good sources of potential employees for a busy practice, but expect to pay a premium for the service. References and background checks may be performed though services such as: *www.references-etc.com.*

Interviewing an Office Candidate

A list of interview questions for job candidates may prove useful to established and new practitioners as they attempt to avoid the legal complications often intrinsic to the hiring process. Further information should be obtained from a competent civil-rights expert or local small business association (SBA).

1. **Birthday or age of applicant.**
   A three decade long federal ban on age discrimination and many state age-bias laws, preclude asking about birthdays. Related inquiries about high school or college graduation dates are also fraught with similar danger. In some states, questions regarding smoking and sexual orientation are also prohibited.

2. **Where were you born?**
   Questions regarding place of birth may pose a problem because of Federal National Origin Laws, described earlier. Do not ask it.

3. **If hired, what accommodations would be required for your wheelchair?**
   According to the Americans with Disabilities Act (ADA) of 1990, any questions about disability accommodations are permissible if the problem is overt or voluntarily disclosed. If a disability is not obvious, do not ask the question, since a major goal of the act is to remove employment barriers confronting people with disabilities. You may refuse to hire someone only if a disability prevents performance of essential functions of the job. However, the ADA generally requires you make reasonable accommodations to enable a disabled employee to perform required duties. Similarly, a medical examination may be requested, but only after a conditional job offer has been tendered.

4. **Have you ever filed a Worker's Compensation claim with another employer?**
   Until a conditional job offer has been made, this question is barred under the ADA.

5. **Have you ever been convicted of a crime?**
   Questions about criminal convictions are allowable but should be followed be a general statement that a conviction is not necessarily a bar to employment. Questions concerning arrests are not advisable.

6. **Can you arrange your child-care schedule in order to work late hours?**
   Asking only women applicants about child-care arrangements might be problematic under current sex discrimination laws. However, asking this question of all applicants is permitted, especially if working late is an essential job requirement.

7. **Do you own a home or rent an apartment?**
   This question may discriminate against minorities who statistically may have a lower rate of home ownership. It is not appropriate to ask.

8. **What is your native language?**
   Again, laws barring discrimination on the basis of national origin could preclude this question.

9. **Are you legally eligible to work in the United States?**
   Although no specific documentation is mandated, employers must require proof of legal eligibility after an applicant has been hired to work, but not before.

10. **Our office is open on both Saturdays and Sundays. Can you work on these days and satisfy this requirement?**
    Although this requirement may pose a religious conflict ("undue hardship") for some applicants, this question is allowable if working weekends is a key

job function. If the office is closed, however, the question is moot and is not permitted.

Legalities not withstanding, most physicians asked the question, "What are your strengths and weaknesses?" However, interviews are often short on this type of probing question and focus too much on the information listed in the applicant's résumé. Here are some additional questions that can be used for eliciting information behind the facts.

- Where do you see yourself in five years?
- What motivates you and what will the references on your résumé say when called?
- Why are you in the job market and what professional accomplishments are you most proud of?
- What is your biggest professional mistake, and how did you overcome it?
- What is your management style, and how do you solve disputes?
- Have you ever been fired, and why?
- What is your ideal work environment?

The general rule for any inquiry is this: *Is the question job related?* If not, there is no reason to let it enter into the conversation. Further free information guidelines addressing the issue of preemployment questioning may be obtained from U.S. Equal Employment Opportunity Commission, Office of Communications and Legislative Affairs, 1801 L Street, N.W., Washington DC, 20507.

Human Resource Costs

Some medical offices are labor intensive and cognitively orientated; while others using the latest equipment, technology and gadgets may be very capital intensive. Although these differences may reflect the doctor's personality, office culture, and medical specialty, they may also affect his bottom line in terms of over- or under-applied HR costs.

HR Management Planning Tip:

Between 1999 and 2000, multispecialty group practices increased the median number of FTE registered nurses (RNs) and licensed practical nurses (LPNs) per FTE physicians. The median number of RNs per FTE doctor for all groups rose 6.5%, in 1999, while the overall median number of LPNs edged up 4.5%.

Source: Aventis Managed Care Digest Series, 2003.

Human Resource Costs

Typically, labor or related human resources make up a large portion of any medical office overhead costs. Several nonspecific labor costs are reviewed in the following section.

Idle time represents the cost of an office employee (direct office labor) who is unable to perform his or her assignments due to power failures, who has nothing to do because of slack time, and the like.

Let's suppose a full-time employee is idle for four hours during the week due to the doctor's unavailability while in surgery. If the employee is paid $20 per hour and works a normal 40-hour week, the labor cost would be allocated, as depicted below, between direct labor and office overhead.

Direct Labor Cost ($ 20 × 36) $720
Office Overhead ($ 20 × 4) 80
Total Costs for Week 800

Overtime Premium Costs

The overtime premium paid to all office workers (direct and indirect labor) is considered part of the general office overhead. Let's assume that an employee is paid time and a half for overtime. During a given week, this employee works 46 hours and has no idle time. Direct labor costs would be allocated as depicted below:

Direct Labor Cost ($ 20 × 46 Hours) 920
Office Overhead ($ 10 × 6 Hours)...60
Total Cost Week 980

Fringe Benefit Costs

Labor fringe-benefit costs are typically made up of employment related costs paid by the office. These costs may be handled in two different ways: as indirect labor added to general overhead costs or as fringe benefits added to direct labor costs.

Just-in-time labor (JITL) means that employees are acquired, or outsourced, just in time to report to the medical office for work. In JITL, human resources are "pulled" through the office flow process as needed. This approach is contrasted to the "push" approach used in conventional medical offices. In the push system, labor is on site, with little regard to when it is actually needed. In the JITL pull system, the overriding concern is to keep all employees busy to reduce direct labor costs. The key elements of a JITL include four parts:

- A few dependable employees willing to work with little advanced notice.
- A work force that is cross-trained in many different service settings.
- Improved treatment room layout to reduce patient and employee travel distance.
- Use of a total quality control system to delight patients through inter-active skills.

Office Efficiency

Much of what is done in JITL is aimed at reducing the doctor's wait time, the patient's time, move time, and quality time; which results in an increase of actual patient-doctor service/treatment time.

Only the patient's treatment time (doctor-patient interaction) adds value to the medical service. All other time is nonvalue added and should be eliminated through appropriate delegation of tasks. When correctly applied, JITL may be expected to yield the following benefits:

- Greater doctor and employee productivity.
- The potential to see more patients, or the same number, with less time urgency.
- Patient quality and services rendered in a cost-effective and value-added manner.

Staff Planning Tip:

Multispecialty groups with 10 or fewer FTE physicians had a median support staff ratio per FTE physician of 5.21 in 2000, up 3.8% from 5.02 in 1999. This marked the fifth straight year the FTE support staff-to-physician ratio increased.

Source: Aventis Managed Care Digest Series, 2003.

Full-Time-Equivalent to Doctor Ratio

The FTE-to-doctor (provider) ratio of an office is often more useful to know than the total amount of staff salary expense, according to Dr. Jon Hultman, MBA, since comparable salaries have a wide geographic variance. Since payroll is the largest singe expense driver of most practices, an optimal staffing ratio must be determined for every practice, considering quality, productivity, and patient satisfaction at the lowest possible cost. Reducing the FTE ratio, and hence overhead salary expenses, is desirable only when it does not lower productivity, quality or patient satisfaction. Most FTE ratios are significantly high, with no corresponding benefit, and the typical medical practice, if there is such an entity, establishes an environment which, at any given point, idle time is about 30%, and redundant or unnecessary task time is about 25%. The fact is that smaller FTE ratios may be consistent with higher levels of productivity, while lower FTE ratios may actually be consistent with lower levels of productivity, lower quality, and higher costs, all other things being equal.

The 2002 Statistical Report of the National Association of Health care Consultants (NAHC) is shown below, and it may be more reliable than other surveys because the numbers were reported by accountants, not doctors. As famed investor Warren Buffett said, "There is a right staff size for any business operation. For every dollar of sales (professional service income), there is an appropriate level of expense."

Specialty FTE-to-Physician Ratio

Specialty	FTE Ratio
Ophthalmology	5.19
OB/GYN	4.35
Dermatology	4.30
Otolaryngology	4.22
Hematology	4.19

Oncology	4.19
Family Practice	4.18
Orthopedic Surgery	4.12
Pediatrics	3.79
Gastroenterology	3.75
Internal Medicine	3.51
Dentistry	3.00
Urology	2.94
Podiatry	2.94
Neurology	2.70
General Surgery	2.50

Capital- Versus Labor-Intensive Office Costs

Now that we understand something about human resource costs, we can compare two offices that produce medical services for the same markets. But beware—even the acceptance or rejection of capitation contracts may affect these costs. One of the offices has chosen to be a procedure orientated health care provider (office surgery-*capital intensive*), while the other has chosen to rely more on human resource inputs (internist-*labor intensive*).

The following table sums up a cost comparison of the two office types:

Parameter	Capital Intense	Labor Intense
Cont. Margin Ratio:	High	Low
Operate Leverage:	High	Low
Increasing Rev:	Rapidly	Slowly
Decreasing Rev:	Rapidly	Slowly
Volatility (Net Income):	Greater	Less
B.E.Point:	Higher	Lower
Margin Safety:	Lower	Higher
Management Latitude:	Less	Greater
Medical Practice Risk:	**Greater**	**Less**

Employee Dismissal

The *Fair Labor Standards Act (FLSA)* demands care when dismissing an office employee. Ideally, a dismissed employee should depart on a friendly or at least neutral basis. Explain the rationale for termination and end the interview on a positive note. Suggest an alternative type of employment and wish the former employee good luck in future endeavors Take care that retaliation can take place in the form of vandalism, theft, breaches of confidentiality, or the alteration of medical records. Have the severance pay, accumulated compensation, and letter of reference prepared in advance. Remember, some day a dismissed employee may be needed to testify in a malpractice lawsuit.

TECHNOLOGY BUSINESS ISSUES

Influence of the Internet

The Internet is having a substantial impact on physician practices, and its level of influence will only continue, according to a study from the Boston Consulting Group (BCG). "While health care prognosticators have been conducting post-mortems of failed e-health start-ups, and speculating about the impediments to e-health, doctors have been steadily adding the Internet to their medical bag of tools." So, this technology must be continually addressed in your strategic operating plan.

However, this has occurred only for the busiest of practices and not yet for the rank-and-file practitioner. Fully two-thirds of physicians who spend at least 65 hours per week seeing patients, say they seek medical information on-line, vs. 54% among those who devoted 20–34 hours a week to patient care. About 34% of respondents in the study reported that on-line information had a "major impact" on their clinical knowledge of new treatments, while 13% said the Internet has had the same effect on their drug-prescribing habits. "These doctors may well represent the first wave of e-health practitioners," the report summary in *Modern Physician* (December 2002) concluded.

Health Care Internet Technology Adoption

Moreover, doctors are notoriously slow adopters of even basic information technology advances, despite the HIPAA enactments of October 2003. Such health care IT adjuncts include electronic prescription writing. In fact, according to Deloitte Consulting,

- 94% of physicians are not currently prescribing electronically.
- 40% express a future interest in electronic prescribing, a noticeable increase from 2000.
- 20% of the market will likely use e-prescribing by 2005.

Unfortunately, physicians, nurses, and other hospital staff now spend at least 30 minutes on administrative paperwork for every hour of care provided to the typical Medicare patient. To help mitigate these inefficiencies, the Microsoft Health Care Users Group (MS-HUG) developed a manual called the *Medical Practice Management Technology Solutions Guide,* available from the American Academy of Family Physicians. And, Bill Joy Chief Scientist and Cofounder of Sun Microsystems, predicts a telecommunications-driven future for health care delivery that includes the following:

- An array of Advanced Digital Cellular networks, allowing mobile phones to act as wireless data terminals, complete with high-speed Internet access and medical text messaging.

- A variety of Smart Antennas that broadcast directly to individual physicians, hospitals, or clinics, alerting them of emergencies and needed clinical, administrative, or office tasks.
- A number of medical information portals, with ultra-wideband (UWB) radio frequencies, allowing object pass-through and secure log-on for information consolidation from a variety of sources and vendors.

ASPs in Health Care

An Application Service Provider (ASP) enables health care organizations to run complex software programs, or applications, on remote servers that can be accessed from numerous sites and by numerous devices. By installing and maintaining central, instead of on-site servers, ASPs reduce the complexity, time, resources, and cost involved in application management. Upgrades are quickly deployed, and health care organizations or medical offices can experience affordable and secure (*www.comtrust.com* and *www.verisign.com*) business critical applications (*www.citrix.com*). Even e-mail messages can be electronically encrypted for privacy by such firms as www.zixmail.com or www.securedelivery.com.

And the following companies offer other useful billing and electronic medical record management systems:

(*www.globaltelemedix.com*).

(*www.vidimedix.com*)

(*www.speachmachines.com*)

Reverse ASPs in Health Care

Healthblocks (*www.healthblocks.com*) coined the term "reverse ASP" to signify that, as an ASP, it provides unique solutions through its enSite e-Health Foundation Enabler-TM, which is tailored toward the situations and circumstances that face health care organizations and care givers on a daily basis. More formally, a reverse ASP deploys, hosts, and manages access to a packaged application and to a single party from its own health care facility. The applications are delivered over networks on a subscription basis, and the reverse ASP remotely manages the packaged application over a network.

Medical Record Websites

Medical Record Institute:
www.medrecinst.com

Coding Institute
www.medville.com

Electronic Medical Record Software Vendors

- Noteworthy Medical Systems (Cleveland, Ohio).
- Medscape (New York, New York).
- Cerner Corporation (Kansas City, Mo).
- Pediatric Software International (Piscataway, New Jersey).
- Jobscience, Inc. (Oakland, California).
- Superior Consultant Company (SUPC-NASD) Southfield, Michigan

Computer Firewall and Security Services

- Internet Security Systems, Inc. (*www.iss.com*)
- WatchGuard Technologies Inc. (*www.watchguard.com*)
- Check Point Software (*www.checkpoint.com*)
- Secure Computing, Inc. (*www.securecomputing.com*)
- SonicWALL, Inc. (*www.sonicwall.com*)

PROFESSIONAL RELATIONS

Establishing Rapport Within Your Medical Community

The following are useful "tips and pearls" to enhance your awareness among known and unknown physician colleagues in your strategic operating geographic locale:

- Send office announcements to all health professionals in the community. Include pharmacies, pediatricians, family practitioners, nursing, and convalescent facilities. All are potential sources of patient referrals.
- Meet other health professionals personally and establish a one-to-one relationship with them. This will serve to educate them to your abilities and practice.
- Send written reports to all practitioners who refer patients.
- Do not hesitate to refer patients for consultations when appropriate. This is not only good business sense but good medicine.
- Use novel business cards, such as the new CD-ROMs cut into the size of a standard business card by One Voice Technologies (located in San Diego). For about a dollar, depending upon quantity, you can order a labeled disc with all the business information of a standard card, which also functions as a CD-ROM that can contain up to 100 megabytes of multimedia data about your practice.

Increasing Referrals from the Alternative Medical Community

Recent medical marketing surveys indicate that almost one-third of managed-care patients use some form of complementary medicine and that one-third more are considering these new, yet often ancient, techniques. Nationally, it is estimated that Americans spend over $20 billion per year, including 600 million visits annually, on complementary and alternative medicine. These figures will increase in the future (*www.medcareers.com*).

What Is Alternative Medicine?

Complementary medicine covers a broad range of topics, philosophies, and approaches, such as: herbal formulas, acupuncture, chiropractors, massage therapy, mind-body techniques, neurofeedback, nutritional therapy, and traditional Chinese medicine.

What Are Common Conditions Treated by Alternative Care Practitioners?

The following symptoms have shown treatment success when conventional medicine has not produced the results that both patients and physicians desire:

- allergies
- anxiety
- back pain
- cluster headaches
- depression
- digestive problems
- headaches
- sprains and strains

How Legitimate Is Complementary Medicine?

More than 50 U.S. medical schools now teach some sort of alternative medicine as part of their standard medical curriculum. MCOs, such as Oxford Health Plans, in Norwalk, Connecticut, Health care Plan, in Buffalo, New York, HealthEast, in St. Paul, Minnesota, and Prepaid Health Plan of Syracuse, New York, all have panels of non-traditional health care providers.

As a Traditional Medical Practitioner, Should You Learn More About These Concepts?

Yes, but only if you want your practice to flourish, as cultivating these referral sources is now a mandatory addition to your strategic operating plan.

CONCLUSION

Writing a strategic medical office business plan is important, but executing the plan is vital for practice success. It forces you to continually test office operations and to allocate or withdraw resource from their respective operating segments. Like all continual quality improvement initiatives, it is an endeavor that never ceases.

CHAPTER 4

Establishing Healthy Medical Partner Relationships

Kriss Barlow and Carolyn Merriman

> If they are analytical, give them data. If they like to read, give them articles. If they need testimonials, have them meet your other partners.
>
> —Steve Moeller
> The Business of Advice

Building successful and lasting relationships among medical partners and colleagues is the best way to weather the storms of change and challenge in healthcare today. The key to working more efficiently, effectively, and happily depends increasingly on how well physicians create and nurture key business and professional relationships. Though some might consider it an art, relationship building is a process that, managed well, will reap huge rewards in professional and personal satisfaction and, ultimately, financial security.

The patient relationship has always been a top priority for physicians. They learn to focus on clinical care, and rightly so, in medical school and residency, where they develop skills as clinicians and diagnosticians. But in the dynamics of daily practice life, physicians are thrust into a number of different relationships—with colleagues, office staff and hospital administrators—that demand time, energy, focus and, in many cases, different skills than those taught in their formative academic years. Adding dollars into the mix only intensifies the fray. Practice ownership, practice management, and joint ventures have forced new relationships. Many of these partnerships are purely business deals and may not spring initially from mutual respect or trust. Indeed, physicians carrying huge debt loads may decide to partner with an individual or join a group practice based solely on their desire and need to ink the best financial arrangement. They assume the relationship will work well without always giving enough thought, or devoting enough energy, to life after the contract.

The good news is that learning to live together by creating mutually productive and satisfying relationships, while certainly essential, is also very achievable.

Relationship Basics 101

What do physicians expect from their business and working relationships? Like anyone, they want a positive environment where they can succeed. They want a culture that is committed, passionate, and dedicated. They want to be able to practice successfully—that is, spend quality time with patients—that depends in large part on their ability to pick, choose, and advance professional and long-lasting relationships.

There are a number of common elements that characterize healthy connections:

- *Avoiding Assumptions*. Physicians in sound relationships avoid making assumptions. They never assume that "no news is good news" or that issues will resolve themselves. People who relate well to one another do not presume to understand what others want and need without actually having had a conversation, because they understand that disconnects over assumptions and innuendos can crumble relationships.
- *Sharing Information*. One of the best ways to build a trusting relationship is to share timely information on such important matters as patient care philosophy, practice expectations, and personal goals.
- *Creating Connections*. Successful relationships are built on purposeful connections, not happenstance encounters. Seeking out and sitting down with colleagues is a basic need, not a luxury. Relationships thrive and survive, even as life gets complex, when physicians pay close attention to the continuity of communication. Regularly planned and managed connections keep working and business relationships humming harmoniously.
- *Offering Validation*. Secure relationships spring from confirmation, appreciation, consideration, and respect for one another as medical partners and professional colleagues.

Understanding that there are common threads that run though every relationship, what are some specific strategies that physicians can use to create and sustain a more positive working connection with partners and referral colleagues? Equally important, how can physicians enhance day-to-day living staffing the office and at the hospital?

Practice Partnerships: A Business Marriage

In small practices and large, partnerships are every bit a marriage, with revenue expectations and demands more often than not topping the list. Ideally, physicians are committed to the partnership for a very long period, and they should respect and like one another enough and have enough similar interest, so they can be independent yet have a relationship together.

However, not all physicians evaluate business partnerships from the perspective of how comfortably people might fit or work together. When adding partners, they tend to consider only the candidate's specialty, academics, and interest in joining. While these attributes are surely significant in a practice partnership, physicians who are looking to expand their practice would do well to weigh some of the additional components that make a partnership mesh before adding someone new.

Obviously, an individual's personal and business style play a key role in a successful partnership. Beyond personality fit, the culture, work environment, lifestyle approach, and practice development capabilities also drive the importance of the match. It is wise to look for a partner who complements existing personalities and practice styles to make for a smooth working environment.

Determine Must-Haves

With baseline clinical capabilities a given, what process can physicians follow to evaluate a would-be partner's overall fit within the practice? The first step is for the partners to determine a set of criteria—"must-haves" versus "nice-to-haves"—that a new physician would need to bring to the practice. And because every partner is likely to have different needs, the list should be ranked and value-weighted so that everyone agrees about priorities and emphasis. For example, the list of must-haves could include special clinical expertise, second language capability, or an outgoing personality for a highly visible community practice. A criteria-based value-weighted process helps avoid gut decisions and keeps all of the partners heading down the same path.

Does the Shoe Fit?

If there are several partners within the group, each one could assess a specific criterion to be sure all the bases are covered. For example, one partner could evaluate the candidate's clinical capabilities, technique in the operating room, and ability to work with the nursing staff. Another could explore how the prospect views working in the office environment and the rules and expectations he or she might have as it relates to decision making and interacting with the staff. If the group is very community oriented, then someone needs to take on that piece as well and weigh the candidate's interest and willingness to make a contribution in this area.

When it comes time to decide on hiring, partners can share information and impressions based on their prioritized agreed-upon criteria, and in this way, they can make a better informed decision about which candidate would be the best overall fit.

Mentoring

Once the decision is made and the new candidate has arrived, a strong mentoring relationship and plan will safeguard the investment the practice has made to bring the new doctor on board. The mentor should have appointments with the new physician. Regular conversations—weekly, monthly, and eventually quarterly—can address and resolve any issues that might arise.

A mentoring plan, detailing the kinds of orientation and training activities that need to be accomplished and when, helps ensure a nurturing environment. The new physicians understand how they can fit in and who they can count on to help them with some of the nuances of practice style, practice politics, office routines, and lifestyle issues.

Partners can use the same hiring model to mentor the new recruit to be sure he or she is succeeding in each specific area such as clinical, office, and community relationships. In private meetings, partners should also find time to discuss and evaluate the new hire to be sure the relationship is off to a smooth start.

Living Happily Ever After

Recognizing that in a business relationship, just like a marriage, there is no perfect partner, what is the physician's role in making new relationships work? The magic salve is flexibility. When physicians are flexible, available, open, and amenable to helping one another, they can learn together and succeed.

Obviously, it's important to try very hard to make new partnerships work because of all the time, energy, and dollars that are invested. When issues do arise, and they certainly will as new people settle into a practice, the physicians involved might consider options that can be changed and adapted and issues that are amenable to compromise so that both parties can meet halfway. Negotiation skills are key here; they are essential to relationship building—and yet, these skills are not the kind of expertise physicians typically draw upon in the world of clinical care. However, being flexible enough to negotiate what will work for all—instead of decreeing this is the way the practice has always operated or handled a particular issue—will go a long way toward advancing relationships and embracing innovation, change, and improvement.

Other steps for moving relationships forward include deciding on and evaluating ways to measure success. It could be as simple as one partner's saying to another, "Let's review charts together to see if that works better," or "Let's agree to meet next month to revisit the issue and assess how we feel." Identifying areas for improvement and eyeing each with a figurative measuring yardstick is another opportunity for a positive connection, a chance to share information, and a surefire way to build trust and respect.

Make It Work

In the spirit of "Let's make it work," it's helpful if physicians keep in mind that there is no one right way to address issues or connect with partners or colleagues. Unlike clinical protocols, where there are standards of care to follow, relationship building comes down to personal style and a desire to get to the other side with direct communication instead of assumptions. It involves a commitment to managing the relationship and negotiating ways to continue to move forward together.

If, after all manner of steps and processes and options have been exhausted, including outside consultant help if necessary, and both the practice and new partner just can't find middle ground, then parting company may be the best option for all parties concerned. But even ending a relationship can be accomplished from a win-win perspective, using a plan, process, and dialogue. Just talking with one another instead of pointing fingers may uncover some room to close gaps in expectations and performance.

Steering the new hire to outside consultants can also help each party find another person or situation that is a better fit.

Creating and Managing the Referral Relationship

How can physicians breathe life into the referral relationship?

Developing and cultivating a steady stream of referrals involves good planning, an investment of time and energy in the referral relationship, and a keen understanding of referring physicians' needs and priorities. Enhancing the referral relationship is a step-by-step process, not unlike the clinical process, that begins by identifying target physicians and their needs, prioritizing the list of referral contacts, and then determining the best way to reach them. The case study at the end of this chapter reviews one large academic medical center's approach to ramping up referral relationships for a wave of newly arrived surgeons. Once again, there are many ways to create and maintain the relationship. Doctors should choose the approach that works best for them, put together a plan, and stay consistent.

The Golden Rule

It really comes down to the age-old rule of doing unto others as you would want them to do unto you. Not surprisingly, referral relationships are built on mutual respect, trust, and courtesy. Focusing on the needs of the referring physician is the best way for both relationships to thrive.

Communication is especially important in not only nurturing the referral relationship, but in also improving the quality of care. A recent study that examines the attitudes primary care physicians have regarding communication with hospitalists[1] found that just barely half of primary care physicians are satisfied with the communication they receive from hospitalists and that information about discharge is very often delayed. The study suggests that improving the communication between the primary care doctor and hospitalist, especially pertaining to matters of hospitalization and discharge orders, could enhance quality of care. The survey also notes that it is possible to tailor communication to individual primary-care doctors according to their preferences.

Indeed, the most responsive specialists ask the referring physician how best to stay in touch, because one size does not fit all. Some physicians prefer face-to-face contact; others prefer phone or facsimile; and still others prefer e-mail. Primary-care doctors want to work with specialists who recognize their role in treating the patient. Many want frequent communication about the plan of care and status. At the very least, tertiary specialists should always pay the courtesy of discharge communication—a phone call, timely letter, or fax when they return patients to the community physician. The specialist should include the diagnosis, any issues that he or she may have identified, any changes in treatment and medication, follow-up recommendations, and a phone or pager number if the referring physician has questions or concerns. Paying close attention to these relationship basics builds trust and respect among colleagues and improves care to patients.

Systems Can Help

Some specialists have put systems in place for timely follow up and thorough communication. A cardiac surgeon in the Northeast with a very busy practice dictates immediately following each case, and then at the end of the day calls to update the referring physician even if he just leaves a voice mail with his pager number. The

---

[1]Steven Z. Pantilat, M.D., et al., "Primary care physician attitudes regarding communication with hospitalists," *American Journal of Medicine,* 21 Dec. 2001, 111: 15S–20S.

referring physician has 24/7 access to the cardiac surgeon, who, two weeks later, has his practice administrator send a thank-you note for the referral. Said he to a conference of specialists, questioning their own ability to commit to this level of time, "How can you *not* afford to pay attention to this part of your practice?"

Acknowledge the Referral

Thanking the referring physician with a note or a telephone call is a great way to advance the relationship. Some specialists return the favor by doing a continuing medical education (CME) seminar or inviting the referring physician into a Grand Rounds. Other specialists offer telephone access to talk about patient care even when there is no specific referral involved. Easy access to a specialist for informal discussions about treatment is a very positive byproduct of a healthy and dynamic relationship. In this way the specialist continues to create still more loyalty and a deeper connection with the referring physician.

Who's Your Doctor?

What about the patient who wanders into the specialist's office without a referral? Here is another opportunity to strike up a connection. The specialist should ask the patient for the primary care doctor's name, note it on the patient's chart, and follow up with the primary-care physician to begin a new relationship. Equally important, the specialist should tell the patient why by acknowledging "I am so glad you came to see me today. I want to keep in touch with your primary doctor just so she is aware of all your needs. Please tell me your doctor's name so that I can follow up with her?" Again, this kind of relationship building makes a big impact on the quality of the patient's overall health care, letting the patient know how important teamwork is in the process and clearly pointing to the specialist's desire to strike up a relationship that benefits the patient.

Professional Courtesy

One potential disconnect in referral relationship harmony is when doctors disagree on plan of care. Still, handled right, differences of opinion do not have to sink the relationship. It's healthy to disagree, as there are many different treatment modalities, but how physicians inform one another involves the delicate art of professional courtesy. Doctors who disagree with plans of care should call one another to discuss the patient in question. They should respect one another enough to pick up the telephone and have the discussion. Often, it can be a learning opportunity. Clearly, though, if one doctor has genuine concern about another colleague's medical ethics or competence, then he or she should contact medical leadership and work through appropriate channels to safeguard patient care.

The bottom line in the referral relationship is for physicians to extend to others the same professional consideration and courtesy that they would demand for themselves.

Promoting Relationship Harmony in the Office

What do physicians want their role to be as it relates to office staff? How should they interact with nonphysician office members to ensure the most beneficial working relationships?

Set the Tone

The physician's responsibility is to set the overall tone and culture in the practice and the baseline expectations for how the relationship is going to function. Physicians should continue to put out the messages and their belief system about the value and rights of patients. But physicians are, first and foremost, diagnosticians. So while they preach the mantra that everybody in the office should value the patient, they can generally entrust their office manager or practice administrator to marshal the necessary forces to deliver on a customer service and business management strategy.

Lead the Team

As leader, physicians need to identify who on the office support team is accountable and responsible for which day-to-day activities. In small practices, it is easier to get the message out and manage. But as practices grow and expand and get busy, and they start adding physicians and/or support staff, relationships can get more complicated. It is imperative, then, for physicians to establish how the office team should work together, especially when there may be a multiplicity of functions within the office. The physician's role in the relationship is to cross boundaries, clearly articulate expectations, and then coordinate from the top—or appoint someone to do so—to be sure people are working smartly and smoothly together.

Reward Positive Behavior

Apart from setting tone and expectations and assigning accountability as team leader, part of the physician's relationship with staff is to reward positive behavior. They can do this by recognizing and thanking people for their efforts, offering to provide a birthday cake for a staff-person's birthday and/or acknowledging longevity of service. The office manager may need to prompt the process, but it is the physician's job to offer the positive strokes. Sometimes unplanned recognition is the best—pizza for lunch at the end of an especially grueling workweek, for example. Appreciating outstanding performance goes a long way toward solidifying positive working relationships.

Hire Right

Staff embody, and are an extension of, the physician's customer-service culture and policies. So physicians really need to hire the right people, at the front desk and in the exam rooms, who can represent their philosophies regarding customer relations. Recruiting the best people mirrors the physician-hiring process: deciding on criteria and ranking "must-haves" in order of importance. Some practices are highly innovative, and they will need staff who are creative thinkers and open to change. Other practices may need people who have more clinical expertise so that they can be charged with making some of the calls back to patients. Still others just need a competent and organized person who can confidently manage the day-to-day basics of the clinic. The practice must be able to acknowledge where the gaps are and then hire to fill them. Using a prioritized list of criteria makes the decision process more objective and ensures the likelihood that the practice will find the person who is the best fit for the job.

Again, personality can drive the match, because teamwork is critical, especially in a smaller work environment. Hiring the right team and encouraging positive relationships helps avoid the costs associated with high staff turnover, poor service, decreased morale and lower productivity.

Physicians do need to pay close attention to high turnover because it could signal a red flag that relationships are not working. It may be time to reassess staff, roles, and responsibilities. If the group cannot come to consensus, getting some outside help for guidance on how to hire the right people and how to promote teamwork can be a worthwhile investment.

Once on board, physicians do need to allow staff the freedom to do their job. Certainly, part of the physician's relationship with staff is to be responsive and offer help, guidance, and direction when asked. Incentives such as customer service training or conferences for personal and professional development make staff feel a part of the practice and vested and committed to its success. When the practice takes steps to keep the office environment healthy, by paying close attention to all manner of relationships, medical and office staff thrive and patients benefit from continuity of care and an organization that is in tip-top shape.

Strengthening Physician-Hospital Relationships

Professionals who have spent their careers in healthcare are familiar with the tensions within physician-hospital relationships. Business initiatives are very often at the core of those relationship issues. Physicians are the first to assert, for example, that the hospital should not get involved in decisions of patient care. Conversely, hospital wisdom believes that the physicians should leave the business decisions to the "suits." To the outsider, it must seem strange that the groups work together, yet may not partner well.

Certainly, from the physician's perspective, a better relationship with hospital leaders and hospital staff makes life infinitely easier. They do, after all, share a common denominator—the patient. Like the physician, the hospital is equally interested in providing patients with the very best quality and service possible.

What steps, then, can physicians take to enhance the well-being of their relationships with hospital leaders and staff? They can

Share expectations. Physicians have a responsibility to share with hospital administrators what works best for them in terms of services and communication. Physicians must understand, though, that because the hospital serves many, many customers—other physicians and patients, too—they may not always get everything they want. Being reasonable is the order of the day. Is it fair for a physician to demand that he or she be able to review medical records on a palm pilot when the hospital does not yet have the technical wherewithal to do so? However, it is fair for the doctor to request that medical records information be available within a certain amount of time.

Speak out. It's no surprise that hospitals can sink into tunnel vision, focusing only on their needs, their bottom line, agenda or concerns. The physician needs to be a spokesperson in the relationship, continually reminding the hospital administrative team that although they may have two different agendas, it is in everybody's best interests to be mutually supportive. And both parties should approach their relationship with the patient in mind.

Drop the gloves. Ninety-nine percent of the time, hospitals do not purposely set out to harm the relationship with physicians or patients. Physicians who have a good working relationship with hospitals understand that broken systems in a bureaucracy can take time. They try to give administrators the benefit of the doubt. In this way, interaction is not a "we versus they" confrontation, but a workable win-win approach. Often, hospital leaders just don't understand or haven't thought about a particular issue from the physician's point of view. Again, physicians can help facilitate any necessary change by voicing their concerns and being open to reasonable compromise.

Understand the challenges. Hospitals are under relentless competitive assault from all sides and there are certain limitations as to what they can and cannot do for physicians on staff. It helps further the relationship if physicians can give hospital leaders some room about business strategies. Quality notwithstanding, there are many different ways to manage a product, to organize patient flow, to staff the operating room, or handle scheduling, and physicians' preferences cannot always match hospital policy.

Join in. If there are issues around policies and procedures, or broken systems that need a boost, physicians help everyone, especially themselves, when they speak up and get involved. People handle constructive criticism better when it comes with offers of help and support. Physicians can collaborate with hospital administrators about steps for improvement and offer to sit on a committee or chair a task force to address an issue. A strong relationship is built when people work together to forge solutions.

Smooth Sailing

Sometimes hospitals think they are doing busy physicians a favor by not bothering them and by presenting them, instead, with a finished product, be it a new service, system, or policy. Physicians who want to improve their relationship with hospital leadership should seek out key administrators early in the process, voice their interest in the project at hand, and ask if they can play a role.

There may be times when hospitals simply can't meet physicians' expectations and physicians are not able to compromise without impacting their list of "must-have's" that are imperative if the practice is to succeed financially or continue to provide a certain level of patient care. In this case, physicians do have options. They can look to do more within their own practices, develop a joint venture or different relationship arrangement with the hospital in order to meet personal and professional goals, or seek a new hospital that may be a better fit for the kind of services the physicians wish to provide.

Today's medical environment demands so much more of hospitals and physicians alike. Connections with one another become all important as partners build practices, work with office staff to streamline services, collaborate with specialists to provide advanced care, and align with hospitals to tap into sophisticated treatment and diagnostic resources. So much more can be accomplished and offered, and the complexities of business and professional life simplified, when relationships are cultivated, maintained, and appreciated.

CASE STUDY

Establishing Referral Relationships

When a tertiary academic medical center in a large metropolitan community decided to expand the breadth of its surgical base—by simultaneously recruiting a number of high-end specialists—it created a pressing need for a sound referral strategy. Senior leaders were eager to facilitate as quickly as possible new long-term relationships with primary and specialty service referrals. They recognized how critical these relationships would be to the medical center's overall financial success.

Although specific for newly hired surgeons, the steps this hospital's leadership took for implementing an outreach plan can apply to any medical organization or private practice that wishes to enhance its referral relationships.

Identify the target market. First, department leaders researched and created a matrix, pinpointing by name the referring physicians, their practice group, and community hospitals that were important to the medical center and to each specific specialty surgeon—most of whom were new to the community.

Move on from low-hanging fruit. With matrix in hand, the staff assisted in prioritizing the list, choosing first to connect with those physicians who already had managed care contracting relationships or clinical affiliations with the medical center. From there, they enlarged the market, taking into consideration that many of the new tertiary specialists needed a very broad referral base throughout the region.

Select the best vehicle. What's the best way to get as many surgeons in front of key referring audiences as quickly as possible? Working the phones, the staff booked surgeons—sometimes individually or in small groups—as CME presenters at area hospitals, guest lecturers at Grand Rounds, and dinner speakers at department meetings. In some cases, the surgeons prepared a one-page outline highlighting their backgrounds and areas of expertise.

Share strategies for success. At a one-time custom-designed training session, the new surgeons met as a group to discuss ideas and strategies for boosting a referral base. The coaching program provided by consultants emphasized a solution-driven attitude and the use of personal style and clinical expertise to proceed effectively and naturally through the referral development process. Throughout the discussion-based format, seasoned surgeons shared many of their own experiences with new specialists fresh out of fellowships.

Focus on the referring doctor's needs. The training program hammered home the maxim that conversation should always revolve around the needs of the prospective referring physician. Surgeons were encouraged to go forth and ask questions: What kinds of cases do referring physicians see? What resources do referring doctors need when presented with those patients? What do they want from specialists in terms of responsive and timely communication?

The medical center and its staff of new surgeons recognized early on the significance of the referral relationship to long-term financial health, strategic positioning, and program expansion. The specialty surgeons and senior medical center leaders followed a step-by-step process to create and sustain referral relationships and to advance the overall mission of the medical center itself.

CHAPTER 5

Compliance Programs for Medical Practice Health

Patricia A. Trites

Physicians and (medical) directors need to be warned that absent an effective compliance program, including one that addresses board conflicts, they may not be insured against the normal risks of being a director. You need a policy with an appropriate trigger point. You should have a structured, step-by-step process in place by which, at a certain point, you decide whether or not an incident of misconduct is serious or likely to be true.

—Mark J. Pastin, PhD, Council of Ethical Organizations

Many physicians equate the term "compliance" with "governmental intrusion." This is not an accurate comparison. The word compliance, as defined by Webster's Dictionary,[1] means "(1) The act of complying (to act in conformity; consent; obey), yielding, or acting in accord (2) The disposition or willingness to please." This presents a dilemma. most people are willing to please, but, at the same time, they usually don't like being told what they may and may not do. Most people don't have problems with the term compliance when it applies to driving rules, banking and investment regulation, immunization criteria, or medication and treatment protocols. Corporate compliance is a fundamental business objective and should be viewed as a standard for good business practice. *http://oig.hhs.gov/fraud/docs/complianceguidance/040203CorpRespRsceGuide.pdf.*

Regulatory compliance is abundant in all industries. Health care has not been singled out for over-regulation. Occupational Safety & Health Administration(OSHA), and the Employee Retirement Income Security Act (ERISA) compliance applies to all employers, The Clinical Laboratory Improvement Act (CLIA) compliance applies to all facilities performing laboratory tests, Limited English Proficiency (LEP) compliance applies to all entities that receive Federal funding/assistance, and privacy and security laws apply to the majority of industry. The Health Insurance Portability and Accountability Act of 1996 (HIPAA) happens to be the name of the health care industry's specific law.

If one takes the position that compliance is a means to validate both a willingness to please and to comply with the rules, it can more accurately be substituted with a term all health care entities are more comfortable with: *documentation.* Just as a physician documents the medical record with the patient's current and past problems and care plan, the health care entity must document the practice's current and past problems and issues as well as the business's plan of action. There are two forms of compliance documentation. The first form consists of the actual policies and procedures that a health care provider or entity provides for the provider's own business functions, including training of the staff. The second is the documentation that demonstrates that the provider is compliant.

CORPORATE COMPLIANCE

A corporate compliance program is the *process* each practice implements to achieve the stated goals of the organization. The program should encompass all areas of regulation applicable to the medical practice. Because each practice is unique, each compliance program should be developed to enhance and protect the individual practice. That is why a "canned" or "off the shelf" product is not considered an appropriate solution to developing or maintaining a compliance program.

Any compliance program (or any of the elements of a compliance program) that is developed and then not followed and maintained is far more hazardous than not having any compliance program in place at all. If a practice or organization knows what they are supposed to do and then decides, either consciously or unconsciously, to ignore these rules, they have the potential to be accused of "knowing and willful" intent or violation. That is not to indicate that a practice should not bother with a formal, written compliance program, because compliance programs enhance employee stability and morale and most often create a more efficient, effective, and profitable business entity.

The Office of Inspector General (OIG) was given the responsibility to create compliance guidance for effectively all areas of health care. *The Final Guidance for Individual and Small Group Physician Practices* was published in September 2000. This is a document that outlines what is expected of all health care providers and practices as it applies to following the established federal and state laws and Federal Health Care Program regulations. It is based upon the Corporate Integrity Agreements that have been put in place by the OIG when billing and reimbursement problems have been found in practices. It contains explanations and areas of risk that most medical practices should address and insure are being followed within their organization. **Exhibit 2** (see the end of this chapter for Exhibits) outlines the areas that are specifically addressed within this guidance. The entire document can be obtained from: *http://oig.hhs.gov/authorities/docs/physician.pdf.* This is the blueprint any practice can use to address the specific areas of billing and reimbursement compliance.

It should be emphasized that compliance is not just a set of documents, although documentation is the foundation. Compliance is truly a behavior that permeates an organization. It becomes a source of pride among the staff and management of the practice. There are very few people who purposefully break laws or rules, and fewer still who will hire a person who has this goal in mind. It is inherent in the health care industry to provide exceptional care and comfort to patients. The concept of corporate compliance is an extension of this mindset, but it focuses on the health and welfare of the business functions of the organization. Staff and management who understand not only what needs to be accomplished, but also how the tasks are to be accomplished, will have a willingness to provide this same level of exceptional care in their day-to-day work-practices. Never underestimate the power of content and confident people.

As long as a provider is not under a government mandated corporate integrity agreement, there is no federal law that states that a physician practice must have a corporate compliance program. There are laws and regulations to follow, some are mandatory and others are just "strong suggestions." It makes sense that an organization's intention is to follow all of the rules and regulations, so documenting them in a formal manner is just the next step in conveying the organizations mission and goals of providing good medical care in a safe and law-abiding environment.

This chapter is actually a guide to many areas of compliance. It provides compliance information that is of importance to the physician and his/her staff. Taken as a whole, this is a basis for a corporate compliance program. Other areas of compliance that should be addressed by every practice include OSHA, LEP, HIPAA, and CLIA (if there is any laboratory testing performed). It will also provide additional information to help the physician provide a "compliant" practice and workplace. It is not an all-inclusive guide but should give the physician an understanding of many of the issues that must be addressed and expanded upon within their practice.

OSHA COMPLIANCE

OSHA was created to oversee the safety of all employees. Many states and territories (approximately 25) have their own OSHA agencies or departments. The state agencies are responsible for administering both the Federal and State OSHA Standards and Regulations. Those states or territories that do not have separate state agencies are overseen by the federal OSHA agency, which is a component of the U.S. Department of Labor.

OSHA's most important mandate involves training employees about the potential hazards and safer working habits involved in their individual jobs. Training is an annual requirement, and depending on the employee's position, involves many topics. If the employees have reasonable anticipation of occupational exposure to bloodborne pathogens, they must be instructed on such items as work practice controls, personal protective equipment, and what to do if an exposure occurs. This is also the standard that requires the employer to offer the hepatitis B vaccine to employees. The *Hazard Communication Standard* mandates that training be provided to all employees about any hazardous materials they may come into contact with in their employment capacity. This is also the standard that requires the compilation and retention of *Material Data Safety Sheets* (MSDS) for hazardous chemicals and materials. Employees should be informed and trained annually in other areas as they apply to employment, including tuberculosis, violence in the workplace, fire safety, and, in some states, ergonomics.

The original *Bloodborne Pathogen Standard* became effective in 1992 and has significantly reduced the number of HIV and hepatitis infections contracted by health care workers. It is the intention of OHSA to continue to protect health care employees from these life-threatening diseases. The *Bloodborne Pathogen Standard* was revised in 2000. It provided new regulations regarding needlestick injuries, safer needle (sharps) devices, safe needle committees, and increased hepatitis B requirements for the employers. Since 2002–2003, this is a regulation that both federal and state OSHA agencies have committed to increase inspection and enforcement of this revised standard.

LIMITED ENGLISH PROFICIENCY COMPLIANCE

There is nothing new about LEP compliance. It became law in 1964 with the enactment of the Civil Rights Act (Title VI). This law provides equal access without discrimination based upon race, religion, place of origin, and so forth for all persons in facilities or businesses that receive federal assistance. This includes health care. The Health Insurance Portability and Accountability Act of 1996 required the Department of Health and Human Services to produce and publish compliance guidance for the health care industry. (Even the government agencies are told what to do!) This was published and can be found on the Internet at: *http://www.hhs.gov/ocr/lep/ guide.html.* The guidance provides information regarding the obligation of "covered entities" (as defined by this law and not to be confused with the definition of covered entity in the HIPAA legislation) to provide free language assistance to LEP patients. This includes competent oral language translation and in some cases written translation of some or all of the practices written materials.

CLIA COMPLIANCE

Many health care providers incorrectly consider CLIA to be only a billing and reimbursement requirement. The Clinical Laboratory Improvement Act was passed in 1988 and became effective in 1992. It established quality standards for all laboratory testing to ensure the accuracy, reliability and timeliness of patient test results, regardless of where the test was performed. Any provider, practice or facility that performs ANY laboratory test is subject to the CLIA regulations, regardless of whether or not they bill for the service.

There are three basic levels of CLIA registration: waived complexity, moderate complexity, and high complexity. The classification Provider Performed Microscopy, is a sublevel of moderate complexity. CLIA specifies quality standards for proficiency testing (PT), patient test management, quality control, personnel qualifications, and quality assurance, as applicable. There are additional requirements for cytology laboratories. Every laboratory (each location) that performs tests must register and obtain a CLIA certificate. The only exception is a mobile laboratory, which may utilize the CLIA certificate of the home-base lab.

Physician office laboratories (POL) that are performing waived tests only, may apply and obtain a certificate of waiver. The criteria for waived tests are for those tests that are cleared by the U.S. Food and Drug Administration (FDA) for home use, employ methodologies that are so simple and accurate as to render the likelihood of erroneous results negligible, or to pose no reasonable risk of harm to the patient if the test is performed incorrectly. The list of laboratory tests that are classified as waived is available at: *www.fda.gov/cdrh/CLIA/index.html.* This information is updated monthly. Waived laboratories have no personnel standards or proficiency testing requirements (except those that are part of the testing kit.) However, labs performing waived tests are expected to follow good laboratory practices, such as following manufacturer's instructions. Also, tests listed as waived by CLIA on a federal level may not be recognized as waived tests by every state.

Physician office laboratories (POL) that are performing provider-performed and/ or other moderate tests have increased standards to follow, including the requirement to have a laboratory director. Moderate complexity labs must establish and follow written quality control procedures for monitoring and evaluating the quality of the analytical testing process of each testing method to assure the accuracy and reliability of patient test results and reports. Each laboratory must have a written procedural manual for the performance of all analytical methods used by the laboratory, and the manual must be readily available and followed by laboratory personnel. An important element that is often overlooked is that the procedures, as well as each change in any procedure, must be approved, signed, and dated by the director.

High-complexity laboratories have even higher standards to document and follow. There are also increased inspection and survey requirements. Many laboratories that perform this level of testing contract with consultants that specialize in CLIA compliance. The misconception that CLIA is driven by the billing and reimbursement systems is due to a 1997 requirement from the Centers for Medicare and Medicaid Services (formally the Health Care Financing Administration [HCFA]).

To enable HCFA, the Medicare carriers, and Medicaid State Agencies (MSAs) to accurately identify all physicians who perform or directly supervise laboratory tests in a shared laboratory, all claims for laboratory services performed in a physician's office must include the laboratory's CLIA number on the HCFA-1500 as a condition for payment. Claims for diagnostic laboratory services without CLIA numbers for physician office laboratories will be returned as incomplete claims.[2]

This mandate allows the governmental payors to monitor providers who are billing for laboratory tests that are "outside" or "above" their current certificate.

CLIA compliance has recently been increasing. A two-state pilot study, which expanded to a nine-state study found significant noncompliance in laboratories. There are ongoing studies planned and it is expected that there be will increased inspection and compliance initiatives in the future. (See **Exhibit 1** for results of the nine-state study)[3]

HEALTH INSURANCE PORTABILITY AND ACCOUNTABILITY ACT

The Health Insurance Portability and Accountability Act (HIPAA) of 1996 has received more than it's share of publicity and has produced an inordinate number of myths and misconceptions. HIPAA provides expanded powers to the government in the areas of health care fraud and abuse in both the public and private (nongovernmental) domain. This law also provides increased funding for searching out and prosecuting suspected fraud and abuse. This law provides incentives (bounties) for informants and increased penalties for those convicted of violations, including exclusion from participation in federally funded health care programs. HIPAA enacted a new category of "federal health care offenses," which include health care fraud, theft, and embezzlement; making false statements, obstruction of criminal investigations, and money laundering. These criminal offenses apply to federally funded and private health care programs.

The majority of hype pertains to the Administrative Simplification provisions of this legislation. The health care industry asked for a more simplified, standardized way to submit claim data. This was accomplished through this legislation; but, in order to pass this section of the law, there had to be assurances that the privacy and security of the transactions were also addressed. "This regulation has three major purposes: (1) to protect and enhance the rights of consumers by providing them access to their health information and controlling the inappropriate use of that information; (2) to improve the quality of health care in the U.S. by restoring trust in the health care system among consumers, health care professionals, and the multitude of organizations and individuals committed to the delivery of care; and (3) to improve the efficiency and effectiveness of health care delivery by creating a national framework for health privacy protection that builds on efforts by states, health systems, and individual organizations and individuals."[4]

Although the Standardized Transaction and Code Set Rule was first to be passed, it was allowed an implementation extension to October 2003. The Privacy Rule has since reached the implementation date and should be implemented and in force in every "covered entity," including most medical practices. The Security Rule has been passed in final form, but the implementation date was April 2005. This does not mean that practices can ignore the provisions of the Security Rule, because there are security provisions (Mini Security Rule) in the Privacy Rule.

THE STANDARDIZED TRANSACTION AND CODE SET RULE

Part of the hype that has been heard and published pertains to the cost to implement the Administrative Simplification Rules. It is the Standardized Transaction and Code Set Rule that will, over the long run, provide significant savings and improved cash flow to the medical practice. There are some noteworthy, positive aspects to this legislation.[5]

First, the ability to transmit billing and claims information in one standard format will save both providers and payers a significant amount of money. There will eventually be one set of forms that will be submitted and received electronically that will streamline the billing and payment systems. These forms to date are health claims, health plan eligibility, enrollment and disenrollment, payments for care, health insurance premiums, claims status, first report of injury, coordination of benefits, and other related transactions.

There will no longer be the need to submit paper for secondary claims, and there will be no need to attach explanation of benefits (EOBs) forms to paper claims, because the transmission will include detailed coordination of benefits (COB) information such as, the previous payer's payment, adjustments, etc. More information will be able to be transmitted at one time such as, up to eight diagnosis codes, 19 different dates at the claim level and 15 at the service line level, as many as 8 different providers and additional information for ambulance, chiropractic, home health, durable medical equipment (DME), and so forth.

Many providers have not taken advantage of automatic posting of payments and electronic deposits of funds, but if and when they do, their organizations will be able to post payments automatically, take write-offs and roll responsibility to the next payer or to the patient and save time and money because there will probably be a significant decrease in posting errors. This equates to the staff's being able to perform more important duties, such as patient care.

Other time and money saving advantages to this "one system" is that payers will have to clearly explain any bundling and unbundling in the remittance advice. They will be required to perform complete reversals of incorrectly paid claims, that is, no partial adjustments will ensure that your accounts receivable system can post accurately. This will also allow the organization a faster and more accurate way to monitor outstanding claims and control accounts receivable (AR).

Organizations will be able to send a claims status inquiry a minimum of twice a month; either as a batch or real time, and receive a uniform response to the status inquiry. The payer will send a response to your request and will use a standard set of codes to explain the status of the claim. Although not mandated, a payer can also send a claim response when the provider has not sent a request, such as when there is missing data or when the patient is not a member, etc. According to one study, 30–40% of all claims rejected are due to incorrect or missing Member ID's—and half of these are never resubmitted.

The cost savings available because a provider has the ability to verify insurance information, either in a batch the night before or on the spot when the patient arrives in the office, can be great. If the payor's system has the ability to send additional specific information, the savings could be even more. Some of the information that will be available includes the following:

- policy limits
- in-plan vs. out-of-plan benefits
- deductibles, copays, and coinsurance, including remaining deductible and/or patient responsibility amounts
- COB information
- procedure coverage dates and limits
- coverage limitations
- noncovered services and amounts
- Primary care provider (PCP)

Another example of this cost savings is verification of eligibility. A California Medical Association (CMA) study estimated that there is a 30-minute average call time just for eligibility information. With the referrals and authorizations transactions you will be able to request

- specific provider and services
- authorizations for service by a specific specialty rather than a specific provider
- multiple providers and services (surgeon, hospital, and procedures)
- up to 12 specific procedures on each request
- specific numbers of services or frequency
- precertification of hospital admission
- approval of referrals for specialist care
- authorization of specific health care services
- concurrent review for inpatient days/services
- appeal of care management decisions

- notification of health care events (admission, discharge, and certification changes)
- unsolicited notice of service review (PCP notifies specialist of referral of patient)

CMA estimates manual referrals cost $20 for specialists and $40 for primary care doctors. This amount will add up quickly to offset any hardware or software upgrades necessary to perform these standardized transactions.

There is no doubt that this system will be superior to the current procedures that are being performed each day throughout the country, but it will take time and effort to ensure that the systems are functioning correctly and to institute the necessary changes in technology and training. As with any major change, this too will have a rocky-road to overcome, but it appears that the results will be well worth the trouble.

Most providers believe that their billing/AR software provider is responsible for complying with this portion of the law. This is not quite accurate. Although it will be imperative to work with the software provider, it is the responsibility of each provider to insure that their practices are in compliance with the implementation standards. The actual data sets and implementation standards can be found and downloaded from the Internet (See **Exhibit 3**.)

THE PRIVACY RULE

The enactment of the Privacy and Security Rules were necessary because Protected Health Information (PHI) is stored and sent in electronic form. Most of the rules that have been promulgated could be considered common sense.

Most organizations have an understanding of privacy and security, although they do not always practice these concepts, as they know they should. It should be understood that organizations are not required to guarantee the safety of protected health information against all threats, in fact, the theft of PHI may not be a violation if there are reasonable polices and procedures in place. It is necessary to understand the rules, to formulate these policies and procedures, and to then train the staff regarding the policies and procedures adopted by the organization.

This privacy rule allows for the transfer of protected health information (PHI) for the purposes of treatment, payment, or health care operations (TPO) without specific authorization from the patient. Except as otherwise allowed by law,* or for the health and safety of the public, patients must specifically authorize any other release or disclosure of their protected health information. (A list of elements considered to be protected health information is seen in **Exhibit 4**.)

Required by law means a mandate contained in law that compels a covered entity to make a use or disclosure of protected health information and that is enforceable in a court of law. *Required by law* includes, but is not limited to, court orders and court-ordered warrants; subpoenas or summons issued by a court, grand jury, a governmental or tribal inspector general, or an administrative body authorized to require the production of information; a civil or an authorized investigative demand; Medicare conditions of participation with respect to health care providers participating in the program; and statutes or regulations that require the production of information, including statutes or regulations that require such information if payment is sought under a government program providing public benefits.

When the Privacy Rule was published in proposed form, the myths and misconceptions began. There are still many of these being promulgated, so it is advisable that all providers have some education on the privacy rule and, more important, know where to look for accurate information.

First, when one provider is treating a patient and asks another provider to consult or comanage a patient's care, then the disclosure and/or transfer of protected health information is allowed. Second, patient sign in sheets, the patient's name used in the office and reception area, and charts or records at the bedside or on the door of the patient's treatment room are also allowed. Most patients understand that they will see other patients in the physician's office. Most patients understand that the office must have some way of documenting when a patient arrives in the office. Most patients understand that they may hear or see glimpses of information while they are being cared for in the office or hospital setting. These are all allowed disclosures because they are incidental to the treatment, payment and health care operations of the practice.

What is important is to train the staff (including any volunteers and/or students in the workplace) of the need to be discreet and to be aware of who is around them when they are speaking about or to a patient. It is also important to train the staff on the necessity of keeping paper and electronic protected health information away from areas that someone may have an opportunity to have more than an incidental exposure to the information.

For example, the following practices are permissible under the Privacy Rule,[6] if reasonable precautions are taken to minimize the chance of incidental disclosures to others who may be nearby:

- Health care staff may orally coordinate services at hospital nursing stations.
- Nurses or other health care professionals may discuss a patient's condition over the phone with the patient, a provider, or a family member.
- A health care professional may discuss lab test results with a patient or other provider in a joint treatment area.
- A physician may discuss a patients' condition or treatment regimen in the patient's semiprivate room.
- Health care professionals may discuss a patient's condition during training rounds in an academic or training institution.
- A pharmacist may discuss a prescription with a patient over the pharmacy counter or with a physician or the patient over the phone.
- In these circumstances, reasonable precautions could include using lowered voices or talking apart from others when sharing protected health information. However, in an emergency situation, in a loud emergency room, or where a patient is hearing impaired, such precautions may not be practicable. Covered entities are free to engage in communications as required for quick, effective, and high quality health care.

Third, physician practices and other health care organizations do not have to redesign and reengineer the physical structure of their office space. There does not have to be soundproof glass, doors, and walls. The medical records need to be secure, not locked up so tightly that the staff, who need them, have restricted access. The purpose of the Privacy Rule is not to inhibit access to health care, although the original legislation and interpretations did have the probability of restricting access.

Fourth, only those persons, outside the practice who have access to protected health information and who are not other health care practitioners must sign a business-associate agreement. Employees do not have to sign business-associate agreements, nor do those people who may have only "incidental" exposure to PHI, such as janitors or building maintenance personnel.

A business associate agreement is a form of contract, or an addendum to a contract, that simply states that the business associate will follow the requirements of the Privacy Rule as it pertains to them and the information they receive from the practice in the normal course of business. The Department of Health and Human Services developed and published *Sample Business Associate Contract Provisions*. This can be retrieved at: *http://www.hhs.gov/ocr/hipaa/contractprov.html.*

Fifth, patients do not have to sign a HIPAA consent form to allow the physician to treat and bill for the services. The consent provision that was in the original Privacy Rule did mandate this, but it was modified when it became apparent that this would be a barrier to health care access. Consent was not totally removed from the rule, but it became Nonmandatory. The Privacy Rule does require the "covered entity" to obtain, if possible, an "acknowledgement of receipt" from patients when they are given a copy of the practice's Notice of Privacy Practices. If the patient is unable or refuses to sign this acknowledgement, then the staff member who gave the patient the Notice of Privacy Practices should document this on the acknowledgement form. The patient may still be treated and the practice may still use the patient's protected health information for treatment, payment, and health care operations.

The Notice of Privacy Practices is the form or booklet a practice delivers (usually in person when the patient is seen in the office) to each patient. This material explains how protected health information will be used and disclosed and also contains the patient's rights as they pertain to protected health information. This is not an optional task. Each patient must physically receive a copy of the practice's Notice of Privacy Practices. The practice must also display a copy of the notice in their office(s) where the patients will have easy access to it to read it. Many practices have posted the notice in frames on the wall of the reception area, while others have made multiple copies, laminated them, and placed them in notebooks in the reception area and/or examining rooms. If the practice has a website, the notice should also be posted on the home page. The notice only has to be delivered one time to the patient, unless the practice makes changes to the document. At the time of the patient's next visit, the revised notice should be distributed, and another acknowledgment should be obtained.

The myths and misinterpretations of this legislation are many, but an understanding that the privacy rule is basically common sense and that most practices are operating in compliance will help in fulfilling the requirements that have been published. The areas that are necessary (but in most practices need to be developed) are the written policies and procedures, the training, and the documentation showing that the requirements have been met. An excellent source of information as to the interpretation of the Privacy Rule was published by the Office of Civil Rights, the governmental agency that has been charged with oversight of the Privacy Rule. This guidance document can be found at: *http://www.hhs.gov/ocr/hipaa/.*

Training is the key to all areas of compliance and is a requirement of this legislation. Members of the physician's workforce must receive training relevant to the functions they perform with respect to protected health information. Initial privacy training was to be provided by April 14, 2003. Privacy training must be provided to each new member within a reasonable period of time after the person joins the workforce. The practice must also insure that members of the workforce, whose job functions are affected by a material change to the policies or practices required by the privacy rule, are retrained within a reasonable period of time after such material change.

Essential elements of privacy training include the following requirements of the Privacy Rule:

- the rights of individuals
- duties and responsibilities of a covered entity
- duties and responsibilities of business associates
- the specific impact this rule has on each employee's day-to-day work environment, including specific policies and procedures, and sanctions/discipline for violation

Another basic principle that may help in the training and subsequent understanding of the Privacy Rule is to emphasize that any and all information that is collected, maintained, and possibly distributed by a practice "belongs to a person." To further emphasize the concept, have the staff consider that the information is not just their work product, but their own personal health information or the health information of a family member. The primary question to ask is, "How would you like this information handled, maintained, retained, and disclosed?" This perception will likely help each practice in understanding, implementing, and maintaining the privacy of the protected health information.

The policies and procedures that must be developed, implemented, and maintained can be found in many sources. As was stated in the Corporate Compliance Section, each practice is unique and must tailor these policies and procedures to the needs of the practice. The HIPAA legislation pertains to the entire health care industry, so many of the items that are delineated in the Privacy Rule may not apply to most physician practices.

Documentation of all an organization's compliance efforts should become second nature to the organization. If any person or entity were to inquire about specific development or implementation areas, this information should be readily available, at any time.

THE SECURITY RULE

The Final Security Rule was published on February 20, 2003. Its implementation date for physician practices, which are covered entities, is April 21, 2005. The final rule significantly reduced the number of mandatory items that must be implemented by a covered entity from the initial or proposed Security Rule.

The final rule contains a matrix (Appendix A of the Final Rule) to show the list of obligations of the covered entity, both those that are required and those that must be addressed. (See Exhibit 5.) This rule covers the security of Electronic Protected Health Information (EPHI), whether transmitted or stored, wherein the Privacy Rule covers all protected health information, in any form. The security provisions in this rule are in addition or an enhancement to the Mini-Security Rule that is found within the regulations of the Privacy Rule.

The final security rule's emphasis is on each covered entity performing a risk analysis or assessment. In this way, the organization can determine which parts of the Security Rule are appropriate for their organization and how to address them. This is actually a more flexible and more common sense approach to development and implementation. As the organization goes through the Security Rule–Appendix A, it will develop policies and procedures to comply with the required components and will either develop policies and procedures for the applicable addressable components or document why they have not/or do not need to comply with the component.

The language in the final Security Rule states that covered entities must, "conduct an accurate and thorough assessment of the potential risks and vulnerabilities to the confidentiality, integrity, and availability of electronic protected health information held by the covered entity." It also states, "The required risk analysis is also a tool to allow flexibility for entities in meeting the requirements of this final rule . . . "[7]

This boils-down to four general requirements: (1) Each covered entity must ensure the confidentiality, integrity, and availability of all electronic protected health information that they create, receive, maintain, or transmit. (2) The organization must protect against any reasonably anticipated threats or hazards to the security or integrity of the information. (3) It must protect against any reasonably anticipated uses or disclosures of such information that are not already permitted or required by the Privacy Rule. (4) The organization/covered entity must ensure compliance of its workforce.

As with all areas of compliance, this is not a one-time risk assessment. Each organization must maintain its compliance program by periodically analyzing or assessing changes in its operations or environment. The organization must identify where EPHI is stored or maintained within their facility/systems, as well as how it is used and disclosed.

Training is also a vital part of the Security Rule. For each of the elements that the practice develops policies and procedures, it must provide training to the workforce about their role in the security plan.

Documentation of the policies and procedures, as well as any documentation of risk assessments, training, violations, and remedies, should be maintained and retained by the practice to demonstrate the organization's compliance with this law.

CONCLUSION

If compliance is viewed as preventive medicine, it may make more sense to the health care organization. Just as physicians recommend preventive medicine for their patients, compliance is the same concept for medical practices. Patients are advised to obtain yearly health maintenance exams, periodic immunizations, and screening (laboratory, radiological, and other tests). This can be compared to an analysis of the practice's current policies and procedures and audits of the organization's current practices. Patients are encouraged to comply with medication or lifestyle changes in order to become or to stay healthy. Medical practices are encouraged to comply with specific billing, personnel, safety, and privacy rules and make modifications to their current procedures in order to stay financially healthy and to increase the morale and efficiency of the workforce. Physicians design protocols for good patient care, and the government agencies have developed protocols for good business practices. When patients need additional care, they may be referred to specialists. When practices needs help with an area of compliance, they may obtain expert advice from consultants. Physicians provide counseling to their patients and should also provide access to training for themselves and for their staff regarding the laws and regulations that are a part of their business's health. Compliance is not a dirty word; it is a term that means preventive medicine for your medical practice!

EXHIBIT 1

Quality Problems in Waived Laboratories

- 32% failed to have current manufacturer's instructions
- 32% did not perform QC as required by manufacturer or CDC
- 16% failed to follow current manufacturer's instructions
- 7% did not perform calibration as required by manufacturer
- Additional Quality Problems in Waived Laboratories
- 23% had certificate issues (i.e., change of name, director, or address)
- 20% cut occult blood cards and urine dipsticks
- 19% had personnel who were neither trained nor evaluated
- 9% did not follow manufacturer's storage and handling instructions
- 6% were using expired reagents/kits

Quality Problems in Policy, Planning and Major Projects (PPMP) Laboratories

- 38% had no policy and procedure training (did not evaluate test accuracy two times a year)
- 36% had no microscope/centrifuge maintenance;
- 28% no director approved as a secure online project manager (SOPM
- 25% did not document personnel competency (Quality Assurance)
- 23% had certificate issues

EXHIBIT 2

- Scope of the Voluntary Compliance Program Guidance
- Benefits of a Voluntary Compliance Program
- Application of Voluntary Compliance Program Guidance
- The Difference Between "Erroneous" and "Fraudulent" Claims to Federal Health Programs
- Developing a Voluntary Compliance Program

  - The Seven Basic Components of a Voluntary Compliance Program
  - Steps For Implementing a Voluntary Compliance Program
  - Auditing and Monitoring

- Standards and Procedures
- Claims Submission Audit

- Establish Practice Standards And Procedures

  - Specific Risk Areas

    - Coding and Billing
    - Reasonable and Necessary Services
    - Documentation

      - Medical Record Documentation
      - HCFA 1500 Form

    - Retention of Records

  - Additional Risk Areas

    - Improper Inducements, Kickbacks, and Self Referrals
    - Reasonable and Necessary Services
    - Local Medical Review Policy
    - Advance Beneficiary Notices
    - Physician Liability for Certifications in the Provision of Medical Equipment and Supplies and Home Health Services
    - Billing for Noncovered Services as if Covered
    - Physician Relationships with Hospitals

      - The Physician's Role in the Emergency Medical Treatment and Active Labor Act (EMTALA)
      - Teaching Physicians
      - Gainsharing Arrangements
      - Civil Monetary Penalties for Hospital Payments to Physicians to Reduce or Limit Services to Beneficiaries
      - Physician Incentive Arrangements

    - Physician Billing Practices

      - Third-Party Billing Services
      - Billing Practices by Nonparticipating Physicians
      - Professional Courtesy

    - Rental of Space in Physician offices by Persons or Entities to which Physicians Refer
    - Unlawful Advertising

- Designation of A Compliance officer/Contact(s)
- Conducting Appropriate Training and Education

  - Compliance Training
  - Coding and Billing Training
  - Format of the Training Program
  - Continuing Education on Compliance Issues

- Responding to Detected offenses and Developing Corrective Action Initiatives
- Developing Open Lines of Communication

- Enforcing Disciplinary Standards Through Well-Publicized Guidelines

- Assessing a Voluntary Compliance Program
- Criminal Statutes

  - Health Care Fraud
  - Theft or Embezzlement in Connection with Health Care
  - False Statements Relating to Health Care Matters
  - Obstruction of Criminal Investigations of Health Care Offenses
  - Mail and Wire Fraud
  - Criminal Penalties for Acts Involving Federal Health Care Programs

- Civil And Administrative Statutes

  - The False Claims Act
  - Civil Monetary Penalties Law
  - Limitations on Certain Physician Referrals ("Stark Laws")
  - Exclusion of Certain Individuals and Entities From Participation in Medicare and Other Federal Health Care Programs

- OIG-HHS Contact Information

  - OIG Hotline Number
  - Provider Self-Disclosure Protocol

- Carrier Contact Information
- Internet Resources

EXHIBIT 3

Provider Taxonomy Codes:
http://www.wpc-edi.com/codes/Codes.asp

Current Dental Terminology Codes:
http://www.ada.org/

Current Procedural Terminology Codes:
http://www.ama-assn.org/

Healthcare Common Procedure Coding System (HCPCS)
http://www.cms.gov/medicare/hcpcs

The non-medical code sets, named in the implementation guides, are available for review and download on the *http://www.wpc-edi.com/*

The National Council for Prescription Drug Programs (NCPDP) website at *www.ncpdp.org* has information on NCPDP implementation guides.

EXHIBIT 4

The following are identifiers of the individual or identifiers of relatives, employers, or household members of the individual. If all of these elements are removed, the information is considered "de-identified" and can be disclosed without specific authorization.

Names

All geographic subdivisions smaller than a state, including street address, city, county, precinct, zip code, and their equivalent geocodes, except for the initial three digits of a zip code *if,* according to the current publicly available data from the Bureau of the Census,

1. The geographic unit formed by combining all zip codes with the same three initial digits contains more than 20,000 people.
2. The initial three digits of a zip code for all such geographic units containing 20,000 or fewer people is changed to 000.

All elements of dates (except year) for dates directly related to an individual, including birth date, admission date, discharge date, date of death; and all ages over 89 and all elements of dates (including year) indicative of such age, except that such ages and elements may be aggregated into a single category of age 90 or older.

Telephone numbers

Fax numbers

Electronic mail addresses

Social security numbers

Medical record numbers

Health plan beneficiary numbers

Account numbers

Certificate/license numbers

Vehicle identifiers and serial numbers, including license plate numbers

Device identifiers and serial numbers

Web Universal Resource Locators (URLs)

Internet Protocol (IP) address numbers

Biometric identifiers, including finger and voice prints

Full-face photographic images and any comparable images

Any other unique identifying number, characteristic, or code and

1. The covered entity does not have actual knowledge that the information could be used alone or in combination with other information to identify an individual who is a subject of the information.

EXHIBIT 5

Final Security Rule Appendix A to Subpart C of Part 164
Security Standards: Matrix

ADMINISTRATIVE SAFEGUARDS

Standards	Sections	Implementation Specifications (R) = Required, (A) = Addressable	
Security Management Process	164.308(a)(1)	Risk Analysis	(R)
		Risk Management	(R)
		Sanction Policy	(R)
		Information System Activity Review	(R)
Assigned Security Responsibility	164.308(a)(2)		(R)
Workforce Security	164.308(a)(3)	Authorization and/or Supervision	(A)
		Workforce Clearance Procedure	(A)
		Termination Procedures	(A)
Information Access Management	164.308(a)(4)	Isolating Health care Clearinghouse Function	(R)
		Access Authorization	(A)
		Access Establishment and Modification	(A)
Security Awareness and Training	164.308(a)(5)	Security Reminders	(A)
		Protection from Malicious Software	(A)
		Log-in Monitoring	(A)
		Password Management	(A)
Security Incident Procedures	164.308(a)(6)	Response and Reporting	(R)
Contingency Plan	164.308(a)(7)	Data Backup Plan	(R)
		Disaster Recovery Plan	(R)
		Emergency Mode Operation Plan	(R)
		Testing and Revision Procedure	(A)
		Applications and Data Criticality Analysis	(A)
Evaluation	164.308(a)(8)		(R)
Business Associate Contracts and Other Arrangement	64.308(b)(1)	Written Contract or Other Arrangement	(R)

PHYSICAL SAFEGUARDS

Standards	Sections	Implementation Specifications (R) = Required, (A) = Addressable	
Facility Access Controls	164.310(a)(1)	Contingency Operations	(A)
		Facility Security Plan	(A)
		Access Control and Validation Procedures	(A)
		Maintenance Records	(A)
Workstation Use	164.310(b)		(R)
Workstation Security	164.310(c)		(R)
Device and Media Controls	164.310(d)(1)	Disposal	(R)
		Media Re-use	(R)
		Accountability	(A)
		Data Backup and Storage	(A)

TECHNICAL SAFEGUARDS (see § 164.312)

Standards	Sections	Implementation Specifications (R) = Required, (A) = Addressable	
Access Control	164.312(a)(1)	Unique User Identification	(R)
		Emergency Access Procedure	(R)
		Automatic Logoff	(A)
		Encryption and Decryption	(A)
Audit Controls	164.312(b)		(R)
Integrity	164.312(c)(1)	Mechanism to Authenticate Electronic Protected Health Information	(A)
Person or Entity Authentication	164.312(d)		(R)
Transmission Security	164.312(e)(1)	Integrity Controls	(A)
		Encryption	(A)

ENDNOTES

1. The New International Webster's Pocket Dictionary, Revised Edition. Trident Press International, 1997.

2. CLIA Alert for Physician Office Labs (POL), Centers for Medicare and Medicaid Services, 1997.

3. CMS CLIA Waived/PPMP Laboratory Project, Centers for Medicare and Medicaid Services, 2001.

4. 45 CFR § 160.101

5. HIPAA Says Software, Version 1.0.7, Health care Compliance Information Systems, 2003.

6. OCR HIPAA Privacy, Standards for Privacy of Individually Identifiable Health Information, December 2002.

7. 45 CFR 164

CHAPTER 6

Insurance Coding Guidelines

Patricia A. Trites

> The balancing act of running a medical practice, providing quality medical care, and getting paid for services has become more and more difficult these days. With ever increasing Medicare and health maintenance organization (HMO) regulations governing what is reimbursable, one could dedicate all of their time just keeping track of it all.
>
> —James Hart, Hart Associates, Inc.

E ffective coding results from an understanding not only of the details found within the pages of various billing guidelines, but also of an appreciation for the overall philosophy of third-party reimbursement. This chapter is designed to assist the health care provider better appreciate the whys and therefores of billing and reimbursement methodology, leading to more accurate and effective coding and subsequent payment for services rendered.

MEDICAL AND SURGICAL FEES

Determining your professional fees may, in fact, be one of the last entrepreneurial acts afforded the physician in the highly regulated health care system in which we practice. In the old days, the physician's fees were based on his or her determination of what they felt the service was worth or valued. In many cases, the evaluation, examination, and management services as well as minor procedures were lumped by primary care physicians under a single office-visit fee. Patients were expected to pay their doctor's fee at the time of service. Third-party payers primarily covered large-ticket major medical items, such as surgery and hospitalization.

Things have changed. Most physicians accept patients whose insurance is supplied by one of the over 200 federal health care programs. This, in essence, makes physicians "Government Contractors". The American people, physicians included, become a little more than slightly aggravated when they hear about government contractors charging ridiculous amounts for hammers and toilet seats. Physicians and other health care providers are now being asked to comply with the government contracting rules regarding documentation of services for appropriate payment. Why do physicians have to follow these complicated and time-consuming rules when they have more important duties to complete? It all boils down to the golden rule. "He who has the gold—makes the rules." This applies to both federal insurance programs and private insurers.

Federally sponsored health insurance is certainly not the only payer, and while private indemnity insurance types still exist, it is endangered and fading away as an option. Over the years, managed care has replaced usual, customary, and reasonable fee for service with a contracted fee schedule. Essentially, under managed care, you can charge just about anything you want, but the managed care organization (MSO) will only reimburse up to its maximum contractual allowance as determined by a set fee schedule. The greater the difference between your charge and the allowable reimbursement, the more you will eventually write off your artificially inflated accounts receivables.

So is it worth your time and effort to determine the procedure and service fees?

Absolutely. Despite changes in insurance models, a health care provider's fees should reflect what the doctor feels his or her services or procedures are worth. The type of insurance that the patient has should not play an influencing factor in either the fee determination or services rendered. Additionally, fees should not vary based on the patient's insurance type, or what the patient's managed care contract determines is the maximum payable allowance.

Determining a professional fee for a given service takes into account many factors including the professional work performed, nonclinical work performed, unusual skills required, time for service, practice expenses (e.g., staff salaries and benefits, disposable items, rent, utilities, etc.), risk, as well as direct (surgical global care) and indirect (communicating with other health professionals, laboratory finding evaluation, review of x-rays, etc.) follow-up care.

In establishing professional fees, the operative phrase is "provider determined." While the input from knowledgeable experienced staff is certainly desirous, the ultimate responsibility for determining fees rests on the shoulders of the health care professional providing the service. Of course, the medical treatment administered, and for which reimbursement is sought, is assumed to be performed on the basis of medical necessity and effectiveness.

So why are reasonable fees and reimbursement for services important? Well, medicine is a business, whether physicians like to admit it or not. Businesses that are not profitable do not remain businesses for long. Today, most health care professionals will admit they are working harder, putting in more hours, and seeing more patients to maintain practice revenues. Even so, in many cases, expense increases are outpacing revenue increases. In an age of managed care, even *Marcus Welby, MD,* would have to work harder.

Medical fees must be reasonable. How is fee reasonableness determined, since physicians are not allowed to sit down and discuss specific fees (collusion, price fixing)? A good rule of thumb is to take the Medicare allowance and multiply it times a million. Just kidding.

Actually, reviewing the annual Medicare rules and regulations found in the year ending Federal Register is a good place to start. That issue printed between November 1 and December 15 of each year lists all the *American Medical Association Physicians' Current Procedural Terminology Manual* (CPT) codes and their Centers for Medicare and Medicaid Services (CMS) (formerly Health Care Financing Administration—HCFA) determined relative value units (RVUs). The RVUs are procedure comparable. You can assume if, for example, a free muscle flap procedure using microvascular techniques is valued at 68.65 total RVUs, it would be a relatively more complicated procedure than a simple repair of a small laceration at a total 4.34 RVUs. You would price your procedure fees accordingly. Generally, if a managed care allowance exceeds what you have billed; your fee is unreasonably low. The true test of reasonableness is your comfort (emotional as well as economic) level in charging the cash patient the same fee. If you feel it is in the "reasonable" range, and you are not consistently writing off 98% of your charges, it probably is reasonable. Under a managed care fee schedule, the service billed amount generally only has significance when the fee charged is less than the contract allowance. In that case, the MCO allowance is reduced to the lesser amount billed. The physician's fees should not be lower than the highest contractual reimbursement rate.

Medical fees must cover the practice overhead. Managed care organizations (MCOs) as a rule prefer "a few good men/women" rather than wholesale acceptance when contracting with health care professionals. Credentialing of providers is one means to limit the number of health care professionals under contract; forming exclusive provider networks is another means of limitation. In populous urban areas, it is not uncommon for health care providers to sign any and all managed care contracts presented to them in order to ensure an adequate volume or pool of patients in the practice—especially in light of expected reduced reimbursement. Unfortunately, many providers fail to read or analyze the MCO contracts they sign. A few practitioners may reason that some managed care money is better than no money at all. But that is not always the case. A careful review of your practice's financial health may determine that you, in fact, may be losing money for each patient seen and treated under some managed care contracts. Not being able to cover your practice overhead is not a good practice and should be avoided. It is advisable that before a provider signs a contract, he or she should review not only the providers list of duties, but the patients' handbook to fully understand the extent of the services he or she is contracting for.

Understand how services or procedures are coded for third-party billing purposes. The only reason the billing codes exist is for use in third-party reimbursement. Providers certainly do not have to bill cash patients using CPT codes. The universality and acceptance of standard third-party billing and coding systems such as the AMA's *Health Care Provider's - Current Procedure Terminology (CPT)*, *HCFA's Health Care Financing Administration Common Procedure Coding System (HCPCS)* for supplies, orthoses, prostheses, and so forth and the *International Classification of Disease 9th Revision Clinical Modification* (ICD-9-CM) have contributed immeasurably to refining the claim submission and adjudication. Not only were codes developed for billing purposes, but each manual contains a wealth of information, rules, and guidelines to aid making the reimbursement process universal—or reasonably so—or somewhat reasonably so.

Unusual circumstances and higher fees. On occasion, a significant modification on the part of the health care provider may be necessary in the performance of a service or procedure. This significant service or procedure, if not defined under another more or less comprehensive service, may warrant an increase or decrease in a "standard" fee for the "standard" service. This valuation variation is commonly coded with a CPT-modifier reflecting the unusual circumstances.

There is no guarantee that a third-party payer will approve additional reimbursement for the provider service or procedure. The medical record or operative report would have to be very clear and detailed in distinguishing a usual and customary modification of a procedure from a significant unusual variation in a service or procedure.

MEDICAL PAYMENT REIMBURSEMENT

First-party reimbursement is defined as the direct financial relationship between the patient and the provider of services. Second-party reimbursement involves a guardian or guarantor of the patient being legally responsible for service payments. Third-party reimbursement removes the obligation for payment of the incurred health care cost payment from the patient to a third party (e.g., an insurance company, government agency, self-insured trust, administrator, etc.). While 75 years ago, first- and second-party reimbursement dominated health care payment in the United States, today, third-party reimbursement is the predominate means of health care cost payment.

Third-party payers determine the cost of the health care insurance (to the employer, to the taxpayer, or to the beneficiary) based on a set benefit package and reimbursement allowance. While some payers, such as managed care organizations, require the health care provider to submit claims for services on the patients' behalf, others give the beneficiary the option of assigning the rights to the payment of the claim directly to the provider. The act of assignment obliges the payer to deal directly with practitioner who is acting on behalf of the patient. Reimbursement generally follows the assignee of the claim.

With third-party reimbursement comes a whole host of rules, regulations, definitions, and restrictions. While some of these are universal, many more vary from third-party payer to third-party payer. Unfortunately, this variation often leaves the health care provider wondering what rules and restrictions apply to the particular patient currently being treated. It is impractical for the provider's office to keep copies of the most current insurance policies their patients have in order to avoid errors in claims submission. Understanding this, each provider's office must develop a standard protocol for capturing practical and available information that is important for managing third-party reimbursement. Much of this information is available on the beneficiary's health insurance card and driver's license—both of which should be copied at the time of the initial office visit. The important information is listed in the following list.

1. A photo and name of the beneficiary (this prevents fraudulent use of health insurance benefits by non-beneficiaries).
2. Current beneficiary address (or an opportunity to update the address by the front office staff).
3. The name of the insurance plan.
4. Policy, group, contract, and/or identification number.
5. Customer service telephone number(s).

6. Possible assigned medical group or primary care physician name and telephone number.
7. Possible assigned hospital.
8. Possible benefit (e.g., prescription benefits) listing.
9. Possible co-payment requirements.
10. Instructions on card use.

The provider of services must keep in mind that possession of an insurance card is not a verification that the health insurance benefits are in effect. A critical function of the front office is to call the customer service number and verify that the insurance is in effect. As long as the office staff has the insurance representative on the telephone, they should ask either if there is list of general benefit limitations or requirements that can be faxed directly to the office, or if the representative can list any specific benefit limitations or requirements of particular interest for that office or specialty (e.g., physical therapy preauthorizations and limitations, MRI preauthorizations and assigned radiology locations, hospital vs. ambulatory surgical center site of service requirements, etc.). If you are fortunate enough to receive a faxed list, make two copies; one for the patient's chart and the other for a folder filed by insurance or payer companies containing similar plan benefit limitations and/or requirements.

Policy benefit limitations or exclusions are absolute and not debatable or appealable. These are plainly issues of plan reimbursement and not medical necessity. Often, the denied benefit—because of policy exclusion—may be medically necessary, but because of the way the original insurance premium was structured and plan benefits were developed, that particular service, item, or procedure was specifically excluded from reimbursement. Payment for that excluded service, item or procedure would be the responsibility of the patient (unless the provider's managed-care contract specifically forbids billing the patient), and not the third-party payer.

The reimbursement allowance is the third-party payer's payment obligation based on the submitted claim for service and tempered by actuarial determinations, negotiated benefit allotments, policies, guidelines, and other influencing factors. The levels of reimbursement can vary from contract to contract and from third-party payer to third-party payer for the same services. Regardless of the insurance model, maximum reimbursement allowances are determined by the third-party payer. Under an indemnity insurance model, fee-for-service reimbursement may seem to be open-ended, but, in fact, it is limited by usual, customary, and reasonable (UCR) allowance profiling. Under most managed care models, a fee schedule limits the allowances per service or procedure. The health care provider, under managed care, agrees to accept a discounted version of usual and customary indemnity reimbursements in exchange for the opportunity to see and treat patients under the managed care contract.

Regardless of the fee schedule limits, health care providers should continue to bill services at consistent fees regardless of the third-party payer type. Obviously, the greater the disparity between the billed amount and the contract allowance, the greater the accounts receivables appear—but the amount may have no basis in reimbursement reality. When the explanation of medical benefit (EOMB or EOB) statement is received, the receivable write-offs may be considerable. Fortunately, most medical computer software automatically adjust differences in office fees and known payer allowances.

Health care providers should also make sure that they are billing the correct services. Many physicians believe that because they are billing a managed-care company, for which they have a capitated contract (a set fee per month for each of the practice's patients in the plan), it doesn't matter which code they use. This can be a very expensive misunderstanding. Physicians are profiled by the insurance companies. This is a statistical analysis that indicates what types of services that are being provided to the plan's patient population. If the provider always reports low level service codes, or does not include additional service codes, then it will appear that he or she only provides "basic" services. If the physician is a specialist, the managed care company may decide that the services reported could be performed by the primary care physician (PCP) or that the contractual rate that has been negotiated for the specialist's services needs to be revised (lower) because he or she is not performing the anticipated and more complicated procedures or services. Physicians should remember to always "document what you do, and then, bill for what you have documented."

Another area in which physician's lose reimbursement dollars is not billing for services outside (over and above) the contractual arrangements. This goes back to having a complete understanding of all of the aspects of their managed care contracts. There may be services that are not included in the capitated or negotiated rates that are billable at the physician's usual and customary fee schedule. A notebook listing these types of services should be developed and kept at the checkout desk to ensure that all additional services are included in the billing. As physician's reimbursement rates decline, it is important to capture all of the services performed and bill them accordingly.

DEDUCTIBLES, COPAYMENTS, AND PATIENT DISINCENTIVES

In order to reduce the prospect of beneficiaries casually seeking medical attention which may generate unnecessary costs especially when the problem is minor or very self-limiting, third-party payers built "first dollar payment" requirements into their health care plans. That is, the patient would be responsible for deductibles and copayments, thus extending some financial responsibility to the patient. In their own way, they allowed the patient to determine the need to seek professional care by creating a financial disincentive for the patient.

The deductible is an annual amount that the patient (or beneficiary family) must first pay out-of-pocket in order to activate third-party reimbursement benefits. The copayment is a similar patient first-dollar contractual obligation, but it occurs with each patient/health care provider encounter in which insurance is utilized for benefit-reimbursement purposes. There may be minimal exceptions to the demand for copayment—depending on the individual insurance policy language—such as instances of multiple encounters with the same provider in a single day or in cases of true emergency services.

Studies have shown that the higher the deductible and copayment amounts, the more reluctant patients are to casually take advantage of their insurance benefits. With these financial disincentives in place, the patient is put in a position of making the initial determination of professional medical necessity: Should they try to treat a cough with over-the-counter (OTC) medications, or should they go directly to the doctor for examination and treatment? One would assume that if the deductible and copayments were high enough, only patients with persistent or truly worrisome health problems would end up in the doctor's office. But reality does not always follow theory. Unfortunately, there are many examples of patient concern over the costs of the deductible or copayment, resulting in delay or failure to seek medically necessary professional care. The results can range from the escalation of a moderately simple problem to a severe—even life threatening—one. One would think that reasonably high deductibles and copayments would be made to order for managed-care cost control, but due to the competitive nature of the business, many managed care organizations have severely reduced or eliminated deductibles or copayments as beneficiary inducements to seek care by contracted health care providers.

Health care providers who routinely waive their patients' deductibles and copayments are contributing to patients' sidestepping mandated insurance policy requirements and could jeopardize their patients' insurance benefits. Without financial disincentives in place, it has been shown that billing abuse and over-utilization of services increase the upward drive of the overall cost of health care. The National Health Care Anti-Fraud Association has stated that in some cases, it may be billing fraud for health care practitioners to routinely forgo the collection of deductibles or copayments. The Office of Inspector General states, in the Special Fraud Alert, "outline waiver of deductibles" and co-payments by charge-based providers, practitioners, or suppliers is unlawful because it results in (1) false claims, (2) violations of the anti-kickback statute, and (3) excessive utilization of items and services paid for by Medicare."[1]

Interestingly, and again for competition reasons, some capitated HMOs have utilized television, radio, and print media advertisements to induce patients to join their plans. Some of the benefits, according to the ads, include no paperwork, no balance billing by doctors, and no deductibles and copayments Because these reimbursement models are based on a capitated scheme (a single amount is paid per member per month to the provider regardless of services utilized), no direct increase in provider costs are generally realized. Yet the capitated providers may see an increase in numbers of patients with seemingly minor complaints and not gain a dime more of compensation. In some providers' offices, the deductible and copayment amounts add up to a sizable amount of money over the year.

MEDICAL CODING DEFINITIONS

The CPT manual is the recognized coding manual used by health care providers to bill third-party payers. No quantitative values are assigned the codes contained within the CPT manual. Each third-party payers determines a value, whether a direct dollar or unit value, for each CPT code. Each CPT code represents a service, procedure, test, or study. The CPT manual attempts to define each of the codes specifically by individual descriptive phrases, generally utilizing guidelines, rules, and definitions related to code groupings: medical, surgical, pathological, and diagnostic services. Third-party payers develop for internal use additional protocols, guidelines, rules, and definitions.

The value assigned to each CPT code is based on a determined amount of work, practice expense, and risk inherently bundled into the service or procedure. Each procedure or service is further defined as a body of work made up of multiple lesser components all valued within the main CPT code. As an example, if the surgical lengthening of a leg tendon is the main procedure to performed, it would be assigned a unique CPT code. Within the tendon lengthening code definition and assigned value would be included (bundled or "packaged") seemingly obvious lesser procedures available to the surgeon in achieving the ultimate goal of the tendon lengthening. These lesser procedures include the incision itself, retraction of vital structures, tying off small vessels, suturing the tendon in a lengthened position, closing the soft tissue in layers, suturing the skin, application of a dressing, and application of a posterior splint. While some surgeons in a particular case may not need to tie off small vessels because no vessels interfered with the surgical exposure, or maybe they had to tie off two more vessels than they usually have to do, or they may elect not to apply a posterior splint, or the procedure takes 20 minutes more because a required instrument falls on the floor and needs to be resterilized, the overall code value of the tendon lengthening procedure does not change. Essentially, with the exception of minor modifications one way or another, the main procedure remains essentially the same. Those minor modifications or variations in technique would be included in what would be called the global surgical description and allowance. Not all potential secondary or minor procedures need to be performed to fully reimburse the primary procedure.

The fragmentation, breakdown or unbundling of the main or primary procedure through the billing of each secondary procedure is billing abuse at best, intentional double billing at worst. Bundling is also addressed in the Correct Coding Initiative issued by the Centers for Medicare and Medicaid Services (CMS). This is a quarterly publication that lists the procedures and/or services that cannot be billed on the same day for the same patient. Health care providers intentionally billing unbundled services may be committing fraud or abuse.

MEDICAL DOCUMENTATION

Most physicians, third-party payers, and legal consultants agree that the medical record represents a real time document evidencing pertaining facts, findings, and observations regarding (1) the nature of the presenting medical problem, (2) a patient's medical history, (3) the clinical examination findings, (4) the doctor's medical decision making considerations, (5) diagnostic impressions, and (6) any resulting physician actions. The medical record chronologically documents the care of the patient. The medical record facilitates the ability of the physician to evaluate and plan the patient's treatment, to monitor the patient's health status over time, to readily access information necessary to communicate to other health care providers involved in the patient's care, and to act as a testament validating medical necessity and evidencing the performance of services.

Medical record legibility, accuracy, and thoroughness are fundamental elements required to validate third-party payer reimbursement. How much information to record seems to be the topic of endless debate. Generally, it is the quality, not the quantity, of the information that is important. The physician, in his or her best judgment, must determine if the patient's medical "story" is adequately documented so that another health care professional could pick up the chart and equally understand the patient's course of medical events. Poor record keeping may have a profoundly negative impact—not only on issues of reimbursement, but on the care of the patient. The quality of the medical record does play a significant role—either positive or negative—in circumstances involving questions of legal liability.

Often, the question arises as to ownership of the medical records: Is it the property of the health care provider or the patient? While the physical record is the sole property of the provider, the medical record content is not. The information contained in the patient's medical record documents medical status, progress, and future actions, some or all of which may be of considerable value, for example, to (1) the patient transferring care—for whatever reason—to another health care provider, (2) doctors covering the practice of a vacationing physician, (3) an insurance company requesting record copies, or (4) a consulting health care specialist. Doctors should have established administrative protocols for allowing release of information from a patient's medical record. While a third-party payer may require direct copies of progress notes for specified dates of service, the patient requesting records to be transferred may, at the election of the doctor, be given either a complete photocopy of the chart or a detailed summary letter containing relevant portions abstracted from the medical record. It would be a breech of patient confidentiality and the Health Insurance Portability and Accountability Act of 1996 (HIPAA) legislation to casually allow protected information to be sent to unauthorized parties. The physician has a paramount obligation to only release patient medical information upon receipt of a written and duly signed authorization from the involved patient or guardian.

While styles of record keeping may differ, there are general principles that must be kept in mind.

Completeness

The medical record should reflect pertinent and essential medical information related to the patient's condition and treatment. Basic data should include subjective, historical, and objective findings; treatment, prescriptions, and diagnostic findings (laboratory, x ray, etc.); and reports. An incomplete medical record may fail to validate the performance of services and/or procedures. Consequently, claimed medical treatment may not be reimbursable or could be selected for refund.

Clarity

The patient record must be organized in a manner to allow for quick review of previous notations. Shortcuts in record keeping, allowing for assumptions on the part of the reader, can be dangerous. Illegible handwriting, use of "personal," not universal, abbreviations, and special codes are not considered to be consistent with the standards of the medical community.

Precision

Inappropriate terminology, misspelled words, and vague conclusions are negative reflections on the "precision" of the chart. The medical record should not be subject to multiple interpretations.

Consistency

The physician has a duty to be consistent in charting the medical record. Clinical workups should follow accepted documentation standards. Objective and subjective findings, test results, and treatment programs should be presented in a logical fashion. Consistency in the transfer of information between the medical record and billing records is also important.

Objectivity

The health care provider has a responsibility to present clinical facts as observed. These facts, when combined with the patient's subjective statements and medical history, should represent, as accurately as possible, a picture of the patient's medical status. The doctor must maintain objectivity throughout the process of gathering and interpreting the facts surrounding a medical case.

Appearance

The medical record should read as though written for a third-party, another health care provider, insurance company, or attorney. The handwriting should be legible not just to the provider who wrote the information, but to anyone who reads the medical record. Typed notes are preferred, although not mandatory. If a mistake in documentation occurs, the error should be struck through one time and initialed. The physician should not erase parts of the record or scratch out or black out sections. The physician should avoid writing in the margins of the chart and/or documenting patient encounters out of chronological order. The chart should appear clean, orderly, and professional.

Medical Necessity

A physician's definition of medical necessity is quite simple:It is what he or she believes is necessary for the health and well being of the patient. Unfortunately, this is not the same definition used by third-party payers. Medical necessity for billing purposes means, Is there sufficient and appropriate documentation to justify the medical services provided? The CPT code defines the service provided and the ICD-9 (diagnosis) code defines why the services were provided. If the diagnosis code(s) are not of sufficient severity to justify the services performed, the physician's office will receive a notice, usually an EOMB, that denies or downcodes the claim.

SUBMITTING REIMBURSABLE "CLEAN" CLAIMS

The service and procedure billing codes and fees are submitted on universal claim forms or on electronic forms. The current standard paper form is known as the CMS (HCFA) 1500. Although this form is accepted by the vast majority of third-party payers including government agencies, there are still some payers that, for whatever reason, choose to mandate use of their unique forms. Fortunately, these third-party payers are few in number. Universal claim forms allow for transmitting essential information in a consistent format. This allows third-party payers to more accurately adjudicate claims, thereby reducing the chances for processing and payment delays. The universal claim form has been widely accepted by both providers and payers because of its ready adaptability to computer-generated billing programs.

Electronic claims submission follow standard protocols requiring special computer access and software. Each claim is electronically checked for accuracy prior to adjudication. The benefits of electronically submitted claims include both an increased processing speed and quicker payment receipt. The advent of the Administrative Simplification Rules of the HIPAA legislation has mandated the use of a standardized universal electronic billing format. This will significantly reduce, if not eventually eliminate, the use of any other billing forms or procedures.

Accuracy is essential when submitting a claim for review. The practitioner should be well advised to include all relevant information requested on the form. As stated above, electronic filing is by far the most efficient form of billing and reimbursement. In the event the provider's office is manually processing the claim, the office staff should consider the following items:

- Forms should be typed for easier adjudication and faster payment.
- Patient information should include the correct birth date, policy numbers, social security numbers, and a listing of any secondary insurance.
- If the condition was the result of employment or accident, the appropriate area on the form should be completed.
- The date that the illness, injury, or first symptom was noted must be filled in the form, along with the date that the patient first consulted the physician for the condition.
- The most specific and descriptive ICD-9 codes should be listed in order of relevancy and linked to their related CPT codes.
- Each service or procedure claimed should be line-item listed individually along with its date of service, place of service, CPT code, and an appropriate modifier.
- Fees should be specifically listed for each independent service or procedure performed.
- Supplementary supportive information (e.g., pathology report or operative report) should be included along with the claim to expedite claim processing and reduce the chances of payment delays.

Superbills. The complexities of medical practice, as well as the need for communication and improved efficiency among the health care provider's office, the patient, and the third-party payer led to the development of the "superbill." Originally, superbills, which were forms containing vital practice, patient, service and diagnostic information, were attached to a minimally completed HCFA 1500 claim form and submitted to third-party payers. Because generally the same information requested on the HCFA 1500 form was contained in the superbill, many insurers agreed to accept their use. Unfortunately, over the past 20 years, submission of multiple varieties (in terms of sizes, fonts, colors, and layouts) of superbills led to increasing payer refusal to process superbill submitted claims. As a result, offices have limited superbill use to that of an internal patient charge ticket. This allows for physician-directed billing information to be accurately submitted to the office insurance staff. The amount of information contained on a completed well designed superbill is generally sufficient to allow the office insurance staff to complete either the CMS 1500 claim form or most electronic billing formats without repeatedly interrupting the health care provider for additional information.

The two most obviously important sections of a superbill are the CPT (service, procedure, supply, etc.) coding area, and the ICD-9 (diagnosis) coding area. Both sections should contain the practitioner's most commonly utilized codes. It is very important to note that not all of the ICD-9 codes can be printed on the suberbill and that if the exact diagnosis, to the ultimate specificity, is not listed, then the diagnosis should be handwritten on the form so that the billing or insurance clerk can choose the correct code. Evaluation and management codes should include the entire range of service levels and not be limited to only the upper levels. If possible, procedure or service fees should not be pre-printed on the superbill. It is a good idea to have the superbills serially numbered to prevent loss of income from lost encounters that do not get billed or are billed inappropriately.

GLOBAL SURGICAL SERVICES AND MULTIPLE-FEE RULES

Surgeons commonly perform multiple independent surgical procedures during a single surgical session. As a consequence, over the years, third-party payers have developed multiple fee rules that allow reimbursement of the primary procedure at 100% but may discount or reduce the value of any lesser or secondarily procedures performed. This reduction in secondary procedure allowance is reasonable because there does exist an overlap of global services—work, practice expense, and malpractice—among procedures performed during a single surgical session. As an example, if hand surgery was performed on the left hand that included a carpal tunnel release and a trigger finger correction, and both of these independent procedures have 90-day follow-up periods (under the Medicare program), the post surgical visit follow-up care for both of these procedures shares dressing changes, staff time (e.g., scheduling the patient, bringing the patient into and out of the examination room, cleaning the room and preparing it for the next patient, etc.), the doctor's time to grossly examine the surgical sites, supplies, and so forth. This sharing of work and practice expense during a single global period obviously reduces the overall value of the procedures compared to a hypothetical situation separating their performance by one year.

Two examples of commonly used multiple fee rules:

- 100% for the first procedure, 50% for all subsequent procedures
- 100% for the first procedure, 50% for the next 5 procedures, 25% for all subsequent procedures

Actual multiple fee rule discounts vary from third-party payer to third-party payer—and sometimes from insurance policy to insurance policy. Physicians, when submitting claims, are often confused as to what the particular third-party payer requires of them, what the ultimate reimbursement may be, or, in the case of an indemnity plan, exactly what is the patient's eventual financial responsibility. The most expensive procedure should always be listed first on the billing form and then subsequent procedures should be listed according to their values. This way, the physician receives the most benefit from the discounted multiple procedures performed.

The use of CPT modifiers is essential in avoiding misunderstandings over billed fee amounts between the doctor and the patient, or the doctor and the third-party payer. Once the provider determines which procedure is the primary or highest valued procedure, it is recommended that the modifier "–51" be attached to the end of the five-digit CPT procedure code, signifying that the procedure is (1) a separate procedure from others performed and billed, (2) a secondary or lesser procedure in terms of value to the primary procedure, (3) that regardless of the billed amount for that procedure, the provider is aware and understands that the procedure will be subject to the payer's multiple fee rule, and (4) the third-party payer is to apply their unique multiple-fee rule to the billed amount for that procedure code. In order to optimize legitimate reimbursement, it is suggested that each service and/or procedure be billed at 100% of its value. The 100% value when coupled with the procedure code modified with "–51" lets the third-party payer know that the provider, while understanding that an allowance reduction may occur under the payer's multiple-fee rule, the doctor is unwilling to second guess the third-party payer regarding the amount of that reduction. Simply put, it is impractical for health care providers to have complete knowledge of every third-party payer's internal multiple fee rules, and since each third-party payer reimburses according to its own set rules and fee schedules, the payer will automatically apply its multiple-fee rule reduction and pay at a reduced rate. If the doctor, fearful of being perceived as an abusive biller, reduces on billing the value of the secondary or lesser procedure, that provider may find that (1) the procedure he or she thought was the secondary procedure (and reduced in value) was actually valued by a particular payer as the primary procedure—but now at a lesser amount thanks to the inappropriate value reduction by the provider—and that (2) the payer may, without giving it a second thought, automatically reduce what in reality is the already provider reduced secondary procedure fee. These errors in billing and adjudication are not uncommon and can significantly affect a practice's financial position.

Billing additional codes are the exception to using the –51 modifier rules. Additional codes are those that are noted in the CPT manual as payable as separate services. An example is "Code 22612: Arthrodesis, Posterior Or Posterolateral Technique, Single Level; Lumbar (With Or Without Lateral Transverse Technique), and Code 22614: Arthrodesis, Posterior Or Posterolateral Technique, Single Level; Each Additional Vertebral Segment (List Separately In Addition To Code For Primary Procedure)"[2]

The global surgical services are defining components inherent to each procedure. Ultimately, procedure value is based on these components. Generally, they include the following:

Preoperative Component is made up of the immediate preoperative visit (usually within 24 hours of the procedure), performance, and documentation of the elective surgical history and physical, reviewing ordered test or diagnostic findings, discussions with relevant health care professionals—nursing, anesthesia, primary or specialty care, and so forth, and consent preparation along with its discussion with the patient.

Intraoperative Component is made up of the surgical examination of the patient, performance of the integral parts of the surgical procedure itself, procedure related flushes and injections—antibiotic, local anesthetic, and dressing applications.

Postoperative Component is made up of preparing the postsurgical medical record, discussing and dispensing patient instructions, discharging the elective patient from the facility, doing follow-up visits, and performing uncomplicated tasks that the postoperative patient needs (concomitantly supplying basic, usual, and customary materials such as gauze and dressings) for a specified period of time (i.e., the global follow-up period).

BILLING PROCEDURES FOR EVALUATION AND MANAGEMENT SERVICES

Unlike coding and billing for multiple procedures, when an evaluation and management service is performed during the same patient encounter that a procedure is performed, several factors must be considered.

First, if this is an initial office visit, significant weight is given to the patient's initial evaluation, decision, and considerations to manage the problems encountered as well as preparing the patient's record from scratch. It is usual and customary, therefore, to bill and be reimbursed for the initial evaluation and management service. If a minor procedure is also performed during the initial patient encounter—assuming it is both a policy benefit and medically necessary and not considered a bundled service—it, too, should be reimbursed. Modifier "–25" (significantly, separately identifiable evaluation and management service by the same physician on the day of a procedure) is generally required to be attached to the five-digit initial evaluation and management code. Obviously, the medical record must be complete and sufficient to validate the level of evaluation and management as well as the medical necessity and performance of the procedure billed.

Second, if this is an initial patient encounter, such as a consultation, requiring an immediate or same day major surgical procedure to be done, the appropriate evaluation and management service would be billed with a modifier "–57" (decision for surgery) attached to indicate that a decision to perform major surgery (defined under Medicare as a procedure assigned a 90-day global follow-up period) was made. The "–57" modifier is an indicator to the third-party payer that a major procedure should be expected for adjudication bearing the same date of service as the evaluation and management service.

Third, if this is an established patient encounter for follow-up procedure outside a global follow-up period, for example, a second cortisone injection in the left knee joint for an acute flare up of arthritic symptoms, and the patient asks the doctor about a red swollen right hand, the evaluation work-up and initiation of management for the "Oh by the way" right-hand problem deserves reimbursement separate from the injection of the left knee, which is a known condition having follow-up treatment. In order to properly communicate to the third-party payer that the evaluation and management service and procedures should be independently reimbursed, the health care provider must attach to the five-digit evaluation and management CPT code the modifier "–25." Modifier "–25" indicates that the service and procedures were separately identifiable services. In a recent clarification, modifier "–25" was also approved to be used if the diagnosis was established, but the evaluation and management service was a significantly medically necessary re-evaluation of a known condition also receiving procedural treatment. It is very important that the documentation clearly supports the independence and medical necessity of the condition(s) and the procedure(s). It is also important that the CMS claim form or electronic submission specify which diagnosis code is linked to which procedure or evaluation and management code.

Fourth, if an established patient is returning the office for an appointed, procedural treatment, whether a new treatment or a follow-up treatment, and the service rendered is primarily procedural, no evaluation and management allowance is independently reimbursed—only the procedure allowance is reimbursed. For example: The patient is appointed and seen for the removal of a planter's wart or for a bone-density test. The point generally made is that every procedure, by global definition, has *some* level of evaluation and management in it. Unfortunately, no one has sufficiently clarified the "some level" consideration, so the rules of "usual and customary" and "reasonableness" hold.

THE STANDARDS OF MEDICAL BILLING

No one will argue that health care providers deserve a fair reimbursement for the time, efforts, and service they render their patients. The classic problem results when what health care providers feel is fair and what third-party payers feel is fair are in conflict. Provider must realize that insurers (1) are obligated to the beneficiary, and (2) reimburse based on the limits of the policy and internal guidelines. Third-party payers must keep in mind that a lack of written guidelines, little to no peer review, and consistently ignoring standards of billing and review practices open them to charges of bad faith and litigation. Both providers and payers must be fully aware of and speak the same language of reimbursement.

Standards of Billing Practice

Standards of billing practice have been developed over the years to cover appropriate treatment and care rendered patients. These standards are determined by third-party payers, physician organizations, and specialty associations/societies. As third-party medicine evolved, it was necessary to develop a universal set of guidelines and systems to ensure that the health care provider and third-party payer had similar understandings of the protocols necessary for claim reimbursement.

In the 1950s, the *California Relative Value Scale* (CRVS) was published. It contains a universal coding nomenclature and definitions for specific medical services and procedures; in addition, it assigns values to those services. As the CRVS was revised in 1964, 1969, and 1974, services and procedures were added, and the guidelines were expanded and refined. The code values were maintained, upgraded, or downgraded with each subsequent CRVS revision.

The CPT manual developed parallel to the CRVS and was its ultimate successor. CPT is universally accepted, willingly or reluctantly, as the preeminent guide to reimbursement management by health care providers and third-party payers. While practitioners establish medical service and procedure fees by using the code descriptors and their respective guidelines within CPT, third-party payers likewise use similar protocols and definitions to assign values and allowances to the same service and procedure codes.

BILLING GUIDELINES

The following suggested guidelines are important for physicians treating patients and submitting claims to third-party payers:

TERMINOLOGY

The New Patient

The new patient is defined as one who has not received professional treatment or care (defined as face-to-face care or encounter) by an individual provider within a three year period. This definition is extended to include any provider of the same specialty within a single group. A new patient would usually require the practice to establish both medical and administrative records.

The Established Patient

The established patient is defined as having received professional treatment or care (defined as face-to-face care or encounter) by an individual provider within a three-year period. This definition is extended to include any provider of the same specialty within a single group. An established patient would usually have existing medical and administrative records. It is important to note, though, that a physician who leaves one group or solo practice and joins with a new group, with a new employer Identification Number, who sees/treats his/her former patients, is still treating established patients even though a new set of medical and administrative records may have to be created.

Referral

A referral is an actual transfer of partial or total independent patient care from one health care provider to another—generally of a different specialty or in a different geographic area. There must be an understanding between the provider transferring the patient and the provider receiving the patient that a transfer of care is intended. From the *Medicare Carrier's Manual,* "A transfer of care occurs when the referring physician transfers the responsibility for the patient's complete care to the receiving physician at the time of referral, and the receiving physician documents approval of care in advance."[3]

Consultation

A consultation is defined as, a type of service provided by a physician whose *opinion or advice* regarding evaluation and/or management of a specific problem is requested by another physician or other appropriate source. In order to bill appropriately for a consultation, consulting physicians must meet three requirements. First, they must have a request for a consultation from an appropriate source and the need (reason) for consultation must be documented in the patient's medical record. In the case of a primary care physician's (PCP) office making a telephone request for a consultation, the consulting physician's office could fax a short note to the PCP's office confirming the request and information (see Exhibit 1, p. 124). Second, all of the components of the Consultation Evaluation and Management Service, as defined by the appropriate CPT code, must be completed and documented in the patient's record. Third, the consultant's opinion and any services that were ordered or rendered must also be documented in the patient's medical record and communicated to the requesting physician or other appropriate source in writing.

Setting Straight the Myriad of Consultation Myths

A physician consultant may initiate diagnostic and/or therapeutic services at an initial or subsequent visit. Subsequent visits (not performed to complete the initial consultation) to manage a portion or all of the patient's condition should be reported as established patient office visit or subsequent hospital care, depending on the setting. An exception to this is during a confirmatory consultation. The consulting physician may provide diagnostic services but may not provide treatment, as only an opinion has been sought.

It is acceptable and payable if one physician in a group practice requests a consultation from another physician in the same group practice, as long as all of the requirements for use of the CPT consultation codes are met.

It is acceptable and payable to bill for a consultation code for a preoperative consultation for a new or established patient performed by any physician at the request of a surgeon, as long as all of the requirements for billing the consultation codes are met. But, if subsequent to the completion of a preoperative consultation in the office or hospital, the consultant assumes responsibility for the management of a portion or all of the patient's condition(s) during the postoperative period, the consultation codes should not be used.

A physician (primary care or specialist) who performs a postoperative evaluation of a new or established patient at the request of the surgeon may bill the appropriate consultation code for evaluation and management services furnished during the postoperative period following surgery as long as all of the criteria for the use of the consultation codes are met and that same physician has not already performed a preoperative consultation.

If the surgeon asks a physician who had not seen the patient for a preoperative consultation to take responsibility for the management of an aspect of the patient's condition during the postoperative period, the physician may not bill a consultation, because the surgeon is not asking the physician's opinion or advice for the surgeon's use in treating the patient. The physician's services would constitute concurrent care and should be billed using the appropriate level visit codes.

Following the initial consultation, if an additional request for an opinion or advice is received regarding the same or a new problem from the attending physician and documented in the medical record, the office consultation codes may be used again. However, if the patient were only returning as a follow-up at the consulting physician's request, the visit would be coded as an established patient visit.

Inpatient follow-up consultations are not the same as ongoing treatment of a patient that a physician has provided an initial inpatient consultation service to. Follow-up consultations are visits to complete the initial consultation or subsequent consultative visits requested by the attending physician. Follow-up consultations include monitoring progress, recommending management modifications, or advising on a new plan of care in response to changes in the patient's status and the primary physician's request for additional opinions. If the physician consultant has initiated treatment at the initial consultation and participates thereafter in the patient's management, the codes for subsequent hospital care should be used.

Provider self-initiated conferences, discussions, admissions, or presurgical workups of established patients do not fall within the definition of a consultation.

Second Opinions

Second opinions are confirmatory consultations soliciting only another opinion or advice from another health care provider. A consultation report containing the second opinion findings must be sent to the requesting doctor. Treatment or ongoing care is not part of the second opinion evaluation and management service.

Patients are prudent to seek a second opinion when they are concerned about current or future medical treatment and/or existing, persistent, or suspected medical conditions. If the second opinion is requested by the patient, the consultant provider has a primary responsibility to relate his or her findings back to the patient. The patient may request in writing that the second opinion be transmitted to a previous health care provider or other person.

On occasion, a second opinion is requested by a third-party payer. After examination, the consultant is expected to render an opinion regarding the presenting current and future medical condition and an opinion regarding the medical necessity of the current or proposed treatment. Upon conclusion of the evaluation, a consultation report should be sent to the requesting third-party payer. When billing for a third-party payer-mandated second opinion, the consultant should qualify the five digit confirmatory consultation CPT code with a "–32" modifier.

It is unethical for the consultant to solicit patients seeking a second opinion. If the patient insists on the consultant taking over their care, the health care provider, if he or she feels comfortable with that request, may do so without breaching medical ethics. The provider would be wise to note the circumstances of the patient request to take over their care.

Postoperative Complications

Postoperative complications involve conditions that are not usual and customary, unexpected, or not normal considerations within a post-surgical follow-up period. Immediate postoperative pain, edema, joint stiffness, local superficial infection, minor wound dehiscence, and skin discoloration are some of the more common and expected findings following the performance of surgical procedures. Cellulitis, total wound dehiscence, severe prolonged pain or edema, and joint stiffness one month postsurgical are some unexpected, significant complications that would warrant independent reimbursement for evaluation and treatment inside a global surgical follow-up period. Each instance of complication should be thoroughly documented in the medical record to substantiate the severity of the problem. When a significant post surgical complication occurs, the five digit evaluation and management CPT code should be qualified with a "–24" modifier (unrelated evaluation and management service by the same physician during a postoperative period.) If surgical management of a complication is required, the five digit procedure CPT code is qualified with a "–78" modifier (return to the operating room for a related procedure during the postoperative period). Both of these modifiers communicate to the third-party payer that a service or procedure was independently performed during an existing global surgical follow-up period.

Evaluation and Management Services

The level of evaluation and management service performed should be commensurate with the complaint, history, examination, diagnosis, treatment consideration, and medical decision(s) made. The level of evaluation and management service billed should be commensurate with the supporting documentation contained within the medical record. Each evaluation and management service level has established sets of criteria that must be documented as having been met in order to qualify the service for reimbursement.

The levels of service are established through the documentation of key evaluation and management components: history, examination and medical decision making. Other contributing, but not key, components, include time spent providing counseling and/or coordination of care.

Evaluation and Management services constitute approximately 75% of all services billed, subsequently; the billing and documentation guidelines must be understood and followed by the health care profession.

There are a lot of written materials, training, and tools to help the physician choose the correct evaluation and management code in the outpatient setting. Inpatient evaluation and management coding has not received as much educational attention. The basic components of history, exam, and complexity of medical decision making are also involved in this type of service code, but there are some additional components of the CPT descriptors for these codes that may help the physician in selecting the correct code for the service performed.

Most inpatient evaluation and management coding (with the exception of inpatient consultations) have three levels. Example: Initial Hospital Care: 99221, 99222, 99223, or Subsequent Nursing Facility Care: 99311, 99312 and 99313. For most of these services, the descriptions in the CPT publication include the requirements for history, exam, and medical decision making plus the following:

- Level 1: Usually, the patient is stable, recovering or improving.
- Level 2: Usually, the patient is responding inadequately to therapy or has developed a minor complication.
- Level 3: Usually, the patient has developed a significant complication or a significant new problem.

Diagnosis Coding

Some of the most common reasons for claims not being paid are related to the diagnosis code that was sent on the billing form. According to a 2002 audit of

Medicare claims by the Office of the Inspector General (OIG), the Medicare fee-for-service payments that did not comply with all of the Medicare laws and regulations was $13.3 billion in both fiscal years 2001 and 2002. Improper payments in 2002 occurred mostly in three areas: medically unnecessary services (57.1%), documentation deficiencies (28.6%) and miscoding (14.3%). How do you prevent or reduce denials or reduction of payment when claims are adjudicated as "not medically necessary"? Begin by following the diagnosis coding documentation guidelines. These are

(1) *Code to the ultimate specificity.* There is a significant difference between 716.90, Arthritis, Type and Site Not Otherwise Specified, and 716.39, Menopausal Arthritis, Multiple Sites-Joints.

(2) *"Use Additional Codes" and "Underlying Disease Codes."* Many conditions require, by medical record coding rules, that you use two ICD-9 codes and that these codes are put in the appropriate order. An example is 533.30 Peptic Ulcer-Acute and Without Obstruction, and 041.86, Due to Helicobacter Pylori Infection.

(3) *Use Multiple Codes To Fully Describe The Encounter.* This includes coding any additional comorbidities and/or signs and symptoms that impact the patient's current encounter.

(4) *Choose The Appropriate Principal Diagnosis and Properly Sequence Secondary Codes.* List first the ICD-9-CM code for the diagnosis, condition, problem, or other reason for encounter/visit shown in the medical record to be chiefly responsible for the services provided. Then list additional codes that describe any coexisting conditions or symptoms.

(5) *Avoid using .8 And .9 "Catch-All" Codes.* In the ICD-9 system, descriptions and digits are provided for times when a physician does not have information as to a patient's exact condition or diagnosis. These codes commonly end in .8 or .9 and are commonly referred to as "catch-all" codes. Under Medicare coding guidelines, these codes should only be used when the specific information required to code correctly is "unknown or unattainable."

"Incident To" Services

Almost every day, a physician's ancillary staff members perform health care services for patients in the office. These include taking vital signs, administering injections, and so forth. In some cases, the physician may have nonphysician practitioners performing services such as follow-up visits or diagnostic testing. In these instances, the physician may still bill Medicare for the service as if he or she performed it. Medicare will pay for services that meet all of the following four requirements. The service(s) (1) are an integral part of the physician's diagnosis or treatment of an injury or illness; (2) must be provided under the "direct supervision" of a physician; (3) are performed by an individual who is acting under the supervision of a physician regardless of whether the individual is an employee, leased employee, or independent contractor of the physician or of the same entity that employs or contracts with the physician; and (4) must be ordinarily done in a physician's office or clinic (in a noninstitutional setting to noninstitutional patients).

Direct supervision (as referenced in (2) above) means that the supervising physician must be in the office suite *and, not or,* immediately available.

The service does not have to be incident to a specific physician action; it can be part of the normal course of treatment that the physician has specified. It is important to remember that the physician must institute the initial course of treatment; in other words, the physician must see the new patient. Although this is not specifically addressed in the Medicare Carrier Manual, it is also strongly recommended that the physician see any new problems that an established patient may report; as the "incident to" service must be an integral part of the physician's diagnosis and treatment. The physician must also periodically see the patient to reflect his or her participation and management of the patient's treatment plan.

Same-Day Surgery

With the exception of emergent, urgent, or very minor surgical procedures, it is considered the standard of care to allow a patient a reasonable time to reflect on surgical information and possibly discuss the information with family and friends prior to committing to undergo the procedure. It would be unreasonable to think that a patient could fully comprehend all the ramifications and treatment options available for a moderate or major elective surgery when there is a push to perform that surgery on the same day it is initially recommended. Some examples of relatively minor surgical procedures that could be performed on the same day are small-site superficial biopsies, destruction of benign skin lesions, or injection therapies.

The Assistant Surgeon

The ultimate medical necessity to utilize the services of an assistant surgeon is based on the surgeon's judgment. This decision should not be linked to whether the third-party payer will reimburse the assistant surgeon for services performed. Each third-party payer has an internal guideline that defines the payer's determination of medical necessity and the contractual obligation to pay for that necessity. Certain procedures fail to meet the test of medical necessity, and consequently are routinely denied reimbursement by third-party payers. The site of service, whether inpatient hospital, ambulatory surgical center, or office operating room, should not alter the assistant surgeon medical necessity; neither should performing multiple minor procedures versus a single minor procedure change the medical necessity.

The assistant surgeon should be reimbursed for all surgical procedures performed during the surgical session if at least one of the procedures is assistant-surgeon-qualified for reimbursement. It is unreasonable to think the assistant surgeon should step back and not assist the surgeon during the "nonapproved" assistant surgeon codes, then step back to the surgical field to resume assisting on the remaining approved procedures. Medicare is the only payer of significance that pays the assistant surgeon only for the qualified Medicare procedures.

Operative Reports

An operative report is a detailed record of the events surrounding and describing the surgical procedure(s) performed. The operative report must include the date of the surgery, the patient's name, the surgeon's name, the name of any assistant surgeon present, the anesthesiologist/anesthetist's name, the type of anesthesia administered (if a local anesthetic is used, the name, dosage and location of administration should be noted), the preoperative diagnoses, the postoperative diagnoses, a detailed narrative of the procedure(s) actually performed, any unusual findings, and the surgeon's signature attesting to the validity of the record.

Operative reports are medical-legal documents that should be both exact and complete. Preprinted operative reports are held to the same standards as any other type of operative report. Operative reports should be typed or legibly handwritten. A description of incision length, suture type, fixation devices utilized, and injectables administered are essential for reporting accuracy.

Once an operative report is completed and returned to the surgeon, it should be carefully read. If no errors are noted, the report should be signed by the surgeon.

Surgical Follow-Up

As previously discussed, the global surgical service definition includes a bundled payment—prepaid, if you will—for postoperative care for uncomplicated usual and customary encountered findings or conditions. The global follow-up period is predetermined by the third-party payer, based on the type of surgery performed. This is a very important point. The surgeon should never assume that a non-Medicare payer uses Medicare guidelines for the length of the global follow-up period. In a significant number of cases, by having the office insurance staff contact the third-party payer just prior to or following the performance of the procedures, they may be surprised to find what Medicare lists as having a 90-day follow-up period has, for example, a 45- or 30-day follow-up period. This difference allows the surgeon to begin billing medically necessary services, in the example, after the 45th or 30th day. And that can mean a better overall reimbursement.

There are several guidelines governing the surgical follow-up period: (1) multiple surgical procedures are not cumulative but are based on the procedure with the greatest number of follow-up days; (2) certain services, procedures, and diagnostic evaluations are not included in the global surgical follow-up period (e.g., radiology services, cast application, fiberglass casting material, and unrelated evaluation and management services and unrelated procedures); and (3) only when there is clearly identified and significant complications—not usual or customary as expected in the global surgical follow-up period—is the surgeon permitted to bill for independent services or procedures related to the previous surgery.

Significant complications can include, but are not limited to, cellulitis, total wound dehiscence, severe prolonged pain or edema, and joint stiffness one month after surgery (postsurgical, etc.). When they do occur, the surgeon may bill, as in the following examples:

- The evaluation and management services using modified "–24" signifying the service was performed during a global postoperative period, and/or . . .
- the physician may need to indicate that a procedure or service was repeated subsequent to the original service. This circumstance may be reported by adding the modifier "–76" to the repeated service.

- The physician may need to indicate that a basic procedure performed by another physician had to be repeated. This situation may be reported by adding modifier "–77" to the repeated service.
- The surgical procedures necessary to resolve the complication using modifier "–78," signifying a medical necessity existed to perform another procedure on the same or related surgical site in order to resolve the problem. The value of a surgical procedure modified with "–78" is subject to the multiple-fee rule of the original operation.

Complications should not be a routine occurrence for any practice.

Discontinued Services

There are times when the physician or surgeon must stop a procedure. This can occur for many reasons. Again, Medicare has given the physician a way to explain the unusual circumstances through the use of modifiers.

- Discontinued Procedure: Under certain circumstances, the physician may elect to terminate a surgical or diagnostic procedure. Due to extenuating circumstances or those that threaten the well being of the patient, it may be necessary to indicate that a surgical or diagnostic procedure was started but discontinued. This circumstance may be reported by adding the modifier "–53".
- Discontinued Out-Patient Hospital/Ambulatory Surgery Center (ASC) Procedure Prior to the Administration of Anesthesia: Due to extenuating circumstances or those that threaten the well being of the patient, the physician may cancel a surgical or diagnostic procedure subsequent to the patient's surgical preparation (including sedation when provided and being taken to the room where the procedure is to be performed), but prior to the administration of anesthesia (local, regional block(s), or general). Under these circumstances, the intended service that is prepared for but cancelled can be reported by its usual procedure number and the addition of the modifier "–73".
- Discontinued Out-Patient Hospital/Ambulatory Surgery Center (ASC) procedure after administration of anesthesia: Due to extenuating circumstances or those that threaten the well being of the patient, the physician may terminate a surgical or diagnostic procedure after the administration of anesthesia (local, regional block(s), general) or after the procedure was started (incision made, intubation started, scope inserted, etc.). Under these circumstances, the procedure that was started but terminated can be reported by its usual procedure number and the addition of the modifier "–74".
(*Note:* The elective cancellation of a service prior to the administration of anesthesia and/or surgical preparation of the patient should not be reported.)

Office Surgical Suites

The high costs of hospital-based operating facilities and freestanding outpatient ambulatory surgical centers have prompted a number of surgeons to develop surgical suites within their office settings. An in-office surgical suite is convenient for both the patient and the surgeon; it reduces the overall direct and indirect costs of surgery and procedures in this environment have a historically low rate of infection and complication.

Although there is a substantial cost associated with developing, equipping, and maintaining a quality surgical suite, the profitability of such a facility is also substantial in an age of reduced surgeon's allowances. Reimbursements from office-based surgical suites can vary considerably depending on the certification or lack of certification that the facility maintains. It is safe to say that third-party payers do not recognize noncertified in-office surgical suites for reimbursement at the same percentage as they do for certified facilities. Certification is recognized by the Joint Commission on Accreditation of Health care Organizations (JCAHO) and the American Association of Accreditation of Ambulatory Surgical Facilities (AAAASF).

Avoiding the expense of accreditation, many surgeons elect to perform their procedures in their office operating rooms. Many times the only reimbursement—other than that negotiated on a managed care contract by managed care contract basis—is a single bulk payment for the facility, sterile trays, equipment, instrumentation, personnel, and supplies used. The Healthcare Common Procedure Coding System (**HCPCS**) supply code number used generally is A4550 ("sterile tray") with the CMS 1500 claim form description reading "Surgical Facility/Supplies/Tray." While an itemized listing of the items used may be included, the actual allowance will be determined by the third-party payer based on (1) a maximum rate based on the overall classification of the procedures performed (e.g., minor, soft tissue; major, bone; major, bone with power equipment), (2) a percent of the total surgeon's allowance, or (3) an item rate schedule. Medicare does not reimburse noncertified in-office surgical suites but will reimburse a very low allowance for supplies for a handful of procedures.

It is the responsibility of the surgeon using an in-office surgical suite to ensure the quality of care, health, and safety of the patient. The surgical suite should be used for no other purpose other than surgery. The assistants should be trained, not only in sterile technique and assisting, but in emergency procedures should a medical problem arise. The surgical suite should be equipped with the appropriate resuscitation equipment and emergency supplies. Performing surgery in an office setting does not exempt the physician from the maintaining the standards of care. Prior to each case, any medically necessary work-ups, examination, laboratory tests, consultations, and so forth should be performed to help ensure that the highest quality of care is delivered.

Requests for Medical Records and Reports

The physician is the guardian of the original patient medical record. As such, from time to time, requests will be received to release all or portions of the record. This release can be requested by other health care providers, third-party payers, or the patient. All requests must be in writing, with the patient's signature clearly evident. Under no circumstances should the original copy of the medical record be released. The physician must assume that once the medical record leaves the office it will never return. When a request for medical records is received, either a photocopy is made and released or a written summary is provided, depending on the nature of the request. Most third-party payers will not accept summaries of events or services for reimbursement purposes.

If the records are unusually long and detailed, a reasonable administrative charge may be charged to cover transcription, copying, and mailing costs. When a third-party payer requests a specific date of service be copied from the medical record and submitted for review, the issue is generally the health care provider's reimbursement. Prior to demanding a set fee for the release of records to the third-party payer—some will pay a reasonable fee, others will not pay any fee—it is in the provider's office best interest to check to see if the third-party payer's policies allow for the payment of any clerical fees. If the answer is no and the physician refuses to send the requested records, the third-party payer will simply not reimburse the providers medical claim based on a lack of supporting medical records. If the third-party payer is Medicare or Medicaid, the provider would be in violation of his or her participation agreement and will most likely encounter either an in-person audit of multiple records or a subpoena for medical records. He or she also could be subsequently excluded from participating in these and/or other government programs.

A request for x-rays is not unusual, but it is more controversial, since once they are lost they cannot be reproduced. Patients requesting x rays often demand them on the basis that they own them because they paid for them. Patients do not, in fact, own their x rays. They are entitled to a copy of the x-ray findings. Only copies of radiographs should leave the office. If an office has x-ray copying equipment, they can be done on the spot. If an office does not have the capabilities to copy x rays, the local hospital radiology department, for a fee, can. The expenses for copied radiographs should be borne by the party requesting the films.

When a third-party payer is requesting a complete copy of the medical records covering a certain interval of time, the provider should be careful to include all relevant material that is part of the record—progress notes, laboratory findings, radiology reports, consultation letters, studies and tests—to support the reimbursement claimed. Sending partial medical records only increases the chances of inappropriately lower reimbursement. All submitted material should not only be complete but also clear and concise. In some cases, prospective submission of certain studies or reports (e.g., pathology findings, operative reports, laboratory test results) with the claim can expedite reimbursement.

Telephone Calls to Patients

If you telephone a patient (rather than a family member) in order to discuss results of diagnostic testing, coordinate medical management, evaluate and discuss new information, or initiate a treatment plan; the call may be coded with one of the following three CPT codes:

- *99371:* Telephone call by physician to patient or for medical management or consultation, or for coordinating with other health professional (simple or brief).
- *99372:* same as above (intermediate).
- *99393:* same as above (complex or lengthy).

Note: Medicare considers these codes bundled with evaluation and management codes/services, and they are not payable codes/services.

CONCLUSION

This chapter presented a broad overview of coding and billing definitions, guidelines, and rules. Within the chapter content were a number of pearls of wisdom designed to help the health care provider better understand effective insurance billing while improving the chances of getting paid appropriately and fairly for his or her services. **Note:** One reference source for determining which medical/surgical procedure has the highest value is the *Federal Register*. The issue containing HCFA rule changes for 2004 has CPT tables and each code's relative unit value.

EXHIBIT 1

Sample Letter for Confirmation of Consultations

Dear Dr. _____,
It is our understanding that you have requested Dr. _____ to perform a consultation on your patient, _____, for the following condition, symptoms or problem: _____. We have appointed this patient on (date and time) _____. Please forward any necessary medical records to our office that you believe is pertinent for the evaluation of this patient's condition.

If our information is incorrect, please notify us as soon as possible so that we may make the necessary changes. Dr. _____ will forward you his/her opinion regarding this patient as soon as possible following the appointment.

Thank you,

ACKNOWLEDGMENTS

The author of this chapter for the first edition was Dr. Harry Goldsmith.

REFERENCES

EM Check™ and E & M Software: Evaluation and management documentation tools for Windows 95/98/2000 and NT. (281) 491–9789.
Physician Practice Compliance Report. MGMA and Opus Communications. Vol.1, No.7, 2003 (800) 650–6787.
Medicare Carrier Manual. Publication 14, Part 3: Claims Process (Publication 14-3).

ENDNOTES

1. Federal Register: December 19, 1994, Department of Health and Human Services Publication of OIG Special Fraud Alerts, Special Fraud Alert: Routine

Waiver of Copayments or Deductibles Under Medicare Part B (Issued May 1991)
2. Alpha II for Windows, Unicor Medical, Inc.
3. Medicare Carrier Manual 14-3 §15506
4. Medical Office Compliance Program Guide, © 2003.

CHAPTER 7

A Six Sigma Primer for Health Care Providers

Daniel L. Gee

Six Sigma is more than simply allocating resources to correct a problem—it's a proven methodology designed to uncover, isolate, understand, and remedy the root causes of problems.

—P. Daryl Brown, Source Medical, Inc.

The key to winning in sports is to gain a competitive edge. Athletes must train harder and seek out new training methods and new ideas for physical or mental conditioning just to stay ahead. Likewise, in health care, gaining and maintaining a competitive edge, or even surviving, in today's health care environment will demand strong managerial skills and an organizational culture devoted to cutting-edge thinking.

All stakeholders in health care, from physicians to hospital board members, are searching for ways to deliver quality and service for greater patient satisfaction at affordable costs. They want to improve reimbursements, operational efficiencies, retention of labor, medical and pharmaceutical error reduction, and, above all, minimize expenditures. Achieving these lofty goals requires looking beyond the borders of one's own industry for management initiatives that drive both quality and low cost while serving the customer in his or her own best interest. The health care industry's holy grail of providing quality, while minimizing cost is often thought of as extremely difficult to attain—until now.

What is happening in the manufacturing and outside service industries is a valuable lesson for health care managers and providers in how to stay competitive. The hottest management improvement initiative sweeping many industries is the one approach with the most visible success above all improvement methods so far. It is not a hot new fad or passing fancy but, rather, a flexible system built on the best of past management ideas and proven practices of the business world's most successful companies. It is a philosophy designed to markedly improve an organization's performance and its management leadership.

Six Sigma methodologies, made famous by Jack Welch, the former CEO of General Electric Corporation (GE), have attained widespread appeal in all business industries because of its wholesome concept of data-driven process improvement to drive quality and minimize costs. When problems and solutions are quantified, the numbers don't lie. Decisions are made from a more concrete and tangible viewpoint. Welch even calls Six Sigma the "code that changes corporate DNA." The Six Sigma approach to a process-improvement problem reveals the underlying "physics" of the process. There are no assumptions or innuendos about whether things get better or not—it is about how much and in which direction.

Health care providers are beginning to incorporate this culture changing philosophy of Six Sigma to improve upon or even replace current quality initiatives they already have in place.

The goal of this chapter is to help the health care executive to better understand what Six Sigma is, how it can help to improve performance, and why the provider needs to take a closer look at its potential benefits to an organization, particularly in comparison to previous process improvement programs.

THE STORY OF SIX SIGMA

The concepts of process improvement and total quality management emerged after WWII, when the Japanese auto and electronics industries, in a quest to capture the U.S. marketplace, virtually transformed the term "made in Japan" from a worldwide mark of inferiority to a mark of quality and endurance. Toyota Motor Company soon became the ideal model to emulate by U.S. companies such as Ford, Motorola, and, later, General Electric. The Deming model and subsequent total quality improvement/continuous improvement management initiatives, copied from Japan, evolved with a passion when brought to America. The search for best practices led to the popularity of accolades such as the Malcolm Baldridge Quality Award; an award that became Olympic gold to a company's marketing campaign.

The quality envelope was pushed further in the 80s when Motorola Corporation augmented traditional improvement tools with a systematic problem solving method based on rigorous statistical analysis. This evolution of a process-oriented problem solving approach soon became the genesis of what is now known as the Six Sigma Methodology. The ultimate goal of the Six Sigma model is to find the root causes of variation in a processes of a business, find the problems that created the variations, determine ways to measure them, and control (or eliminate) the process variations; with the intent of process improvement that has long-term sustainability. The achievement of quality to its greatest extent would be a measured in a quantifiable metric of "sigma." The greater the sigma level reached, the more efficient the process.

In reaching the Six Sigma level, there is almost no variation from the most desired and efficient way of doing things. Is this ultimate goal of perfection too ambitious a goal for health care? Perhaps. For service industries and the health care industry, the goal of virtual perfection may be impossible by virtue of the significant number of variables involved. But, one must consider the implications of a less than almost perfect system, as illustrated in Figure 7.1.

The term "sigma" is from the 18th letter of the Greek alphabet and represents the statistical symbol for standard deviation. In statistics, when a standard bell-shaped normal population distribution is used, one sigma represents a certain percentage of variation from the mean two-sigmas represents an even greater variance, and so on.

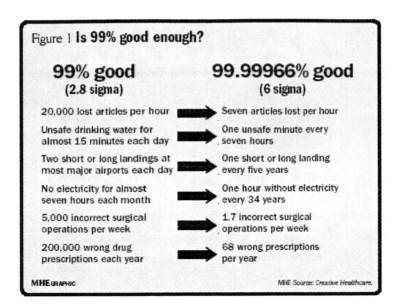

FIGURE 7.1   Is 99% good enough? (From Keith Butler, MD, and Ian Lazarus, Fellow American College of Healthcare Executives, "The Promise of Six Sigma," in Managed Healthcare Executives, October, 2001, p. 2.)

In Six Sigma vernacular, the bell-shaped curve becomes a representation of variation itself; in other words, achieving a Six Sigma process means virtual perfection in the upper standard limits of being 99.99966% good, as shown in Figure 7.2.

Cost of Quality

The cost of quality actually goes up when the variation and error rate of a process goes up. For example, the costs of pharmaceutical errors alone, in terms of lives and money, are huge. Consider the legal implications of incorrect procedures to an institution. Coding errors that lead to variability in reimbursements costs physicians and other providers lost revenue. Think also of the cost of additional safeguards, such as inspectors, that must be put into place to oversee defective processes. When a process is improved, the cost of quality goes down. There are fewer costs due to redundancy, lost time, and lost labor.

The concept of looking at variations in a process is analogous to the process of teaching a child to ride a bicycle for the first time. The child will be wobbly when he or she gets on the bicycle at first and may even fall several times. As long as you are watching closely and help the child back on the bicycle, help steer a little, and provide encouragement, the child soon learns to ride smoothly, and it all appears so natural. The child soon learns to balance from the feedback gained from you and the internal feedback from the brain. After studying the learning process closer, you may find the child to be more successful learning on a set of training wheels or on a bicycle a little smaller in size. Regardless, the closed-loop feedback, analysis,

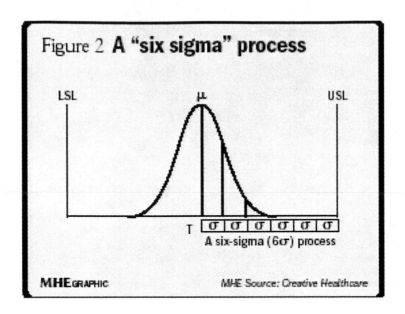

FIGURE 7.2   A Six Sigma Process. (From Keith Butler, MD, and Ian Lazarus, FACHE, "The Promise of Six Sigma," in *Managed Health Care Executives*, October 2001, p. 2.)

and monitoring by a teacher or "process champion" keeps the child from wobbling too much and helps him or her stay on a straight and narrow course.

Businesses wobble, too, in their processes and, in Six Sigma terminology, this wobbling is the variation that needs continual feedback to help correct and stabilize. Unlike riding a bike, wherein once learned, it becomes natural and smooth going, businesses continue to wobble in their processes and may fall and not be able to get back up. The institution of Six Sigma methodology is a closed feedback loop to prevent instability in processes.

Virtual perfection may not be as easily attainable in a service industry as computer chips coming off an assembly line, and the health care industry certainly has its share of "wobbliness." It is, nonetheless, this desire to constantly improve operations, to perfect the way business is done, and to tune in to what the customer needs that separates this improvement method from those that have come before. Moreover, the benefits of setting high performance goals is a strategic decision to accelerate improvement, promote continual learning, and sustain efforts to succeed. It is a cultural change in mind-set to attain quality at its highest level.

Example of the Variation in Process Concept in a Health Care Institution

The radiology department at the University of Texas M.D. Anderson Cancer Center in Houston, Texas, had goals of increasing its capacity, reduce patient waiting time, eliminate wasted errors, and improve morale in the department. At first glance, when expansion efforts have previously failed, the tendency is to address the needs by hiring more staff, minimizing hardware limitations by adding more CT scanners, and adding more physical space. In essence, this is duplicating the current process to meet demands.

Six Sigma consultants, hired by MDACC, looked at the entire process of patient CT throughput (or CT cycle time) at the Anderson Center, and, using Six Sigma tools, identified where the greatest variations occurred. They found the greatest variation and the greatest opportunities in improvement were in the handling of patients and maximization of the radiologist's time, not the scanning speed or number of CT scanners. In fact, the rate-limiting factors for CT cycle time results were found to be in the interpretation, transcription, and interpretation of CT films. Innovations in time-saving opportunities meant hiring facilitators in handling clinician phone calls and people to match and hang up current radiology studies with previous studies so that the radiologist can complete interpretations faster while maximizing time. Future MDACC changes will involve voice recognition technology to improve transcription cycle time.

The cultural lexicon of Six Sigma defines quality as measures in the reduction in variations or "defects" in the process per million opportunities of occurrence. Each incremental increase in sigma-level achieved represents significant reduction in defects, as shown in Figure 7.3.

Many companies, including those in health care, are said to operate at a sigma level of 3, which means about 5,000 nationwide incorrect surgical procedures each week—hardly an acceptable number.

The Six Sigma movement gained its greatest notoriety and acceptance by major industry in the 90s, when Jack Welch of GE wanted to empower his employees and challenge them to participate in the decision-making process. The company had reached a plateau of growth, and Welch knew that staying there meant death by stagnation. He wanted GE to constantly change and improve, becoming an even more dynamic organization. Welch elicited the advice of Honeywell's CEO Larry Bossidy, and soon the largest, most ambitious management initiative ever undertaken at GE began. The results have been nothing short of impressive over the course of

Sigma	Defects per million opportunities
1.5	500,000
2	308,537
3	66,807
4	6,210
5	233
6	3.4

FIGURE 7.3 Sigma level defects per million. (From Jean Cherry & Sashadri Sridhar, "Six Sigma: Using Statistics to Reduce Process Variability and Costs in Radiology," in *Radiology Management*, Nov/Dec 2000, p. 1.)

five years: over $3 billion in savings and annual productivity increases consistently in the double digits. The impact of Six Sigma improvement on bottom-line costs, return on investment (ROI), and profitability caught the attention of every industry, from merchandising to hospitality services. This interest also prompted a company like GE to begin taking the Six Sigma methodology to its customers, including those in health care. The impact on early adapters in the medical industry has been impressive and has continued to grow.

Six Sigma Health Care Pioneers

Example 1. One of these early health care adapters is the Mount Carmel Health System of Columbus, Ohio. The organization was barely breaking even in the summer of 2000 when competition from surrounding providers made things worse. Employee layoffs added fuel to an already all-time low employee morale.

Chief Executive Officer Joe Calvaruso was determined to stem the bleeding, break the cycle of poor financial performance, and return the hospital system to profitability. He sought the potential of Six Sigma and began a full initiation of its methodology. The plan was an audacious one, as the organization ensured that no one would be terminated as a result of a Six Sigma project's eliminating his or her previous duties. These employees would be offered an alternative position in a different department. Moreover, top personnel were asked to leave their current positions to be trained and work full time as Six Sigma expert practitioners overseeing project deployment while their positions were backfilled.

The Six Sigma deployment was the right decision. More than 50 projects were initiated with appreciable success. An example of one of these early Mount Carmel success stories was the dramatic improvement of their Medicare+Choice product reimbursements, previously written off as uncollectible accounts. These accounts were often denied by Health Care Financing Administration (HCFA) due to coding specifically around those patients classified as "working aged." Since the treatment process status often changed in these patients, HCFA often rejected claims or lessened reimbursement amounts, effectively making coding a difficult and elusive problem. The employment of Six Sigma process improvement tools fixed the problem, resulting in a realized gain of $857,000 in previously uncollected funds. The spillover to other coding parameters also has dramatically boosted revenue collection.

Example 2. With the help of GE, Commonwealth Health Corporation of Bowling Green, Kentucky, within 18 months of its Six Sigma launch realized nearly $1 million in annualized billing improvement savings and reduced radiology expenses. The cost savings came from recognizing specific opportunity areas in which productivity could be improved so that patient throughput could be increased by 25%. The changes resulted in a reduction in cost per procedure by 21.5%, although fewer resources were expended. Its CEO, John Desmarais, became a passionate believer of the impact Six Sigma has had on his company, and he says, "It's the single most important thing we have done in the history of our organization."

Example 3. Scottsdale Health care in Arizona used consultants from Creative Health care USA on a project, rather than doing a full deployment of Six Sigma in its organization to analyze its problem of emergency department (ED) "diversions." Diversions happen when emergency departments are too full in capacity to handle acute emergencies and a decision is made to close its doors to patients and ambulances are diverted elsewhere. The issue of closed and diverted emergency rooms is a growing nationwide phenomenon because of fewer EDs and a growing aged and uninsured population. The consultants, using Six Sigma principles, mapped the ED process and found multiple bottlenecks that have a direct effect on the probability of evoking a "diversionary" status in the emergency room.

One bottleneck process deemed to be "out of control," in Six Sigma jargon, was the issue of bed control. A process is considered "in control" when operating within acceptable specification limits. It was found that the average transfer time for a patient admitted to a hospital bed from the emergency department was 80 minutes. Half of this time a bed is available and waiting. The process was a significant waste of time and, moreover, it was complicated by an administrative nurse "inspector" locating beds on different floors. Two tenets of Six Sigma level of quality were violated: one, having an inspection is a correction for an inefficient process, and two, the more steps involved the less is the potential yield of a process. Through this revelation, the hospital eliminated the administrative nurse, reduced cycle time by 10% in bed control, and improved ED throughput, resulting in greater turnover, and, thereby, improving revenue by nearly $600,000.

The addition of a nurse inspector and waiting patients in a busy ED is an example of Little's Law, sometimes referred to as the first fundamental law of system behavior. When more and more inputs are put into a system, such as more ED patients and an additional nurse employee, and when there is variation in their arrival time (no control over patient arrivals) or process variation (different people doing the same things differently), there becomes an exponential rise in cycle time. Productivity of the system begins to fall, and inefficiency and variation creeps in, as seen in Figure 7.4.

And an examination of the project types to which health care provider organizations have utilized Six Sigma methodology reveals that almost any hospital process is a candidate.

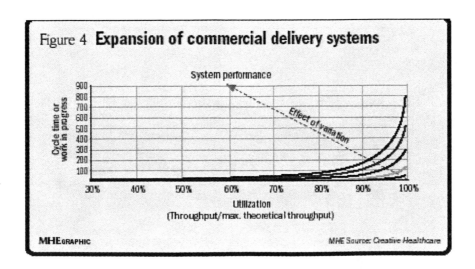

FIGURE 7.4 Expansion of commercial delivery systems. (From Keith Butler, MD, & Ian Lazarus, FACHE, "The Promise of Six Sigma," in *Managed Healthcare Executives*, October 2001, p. 4)

Example 4. The Charleston Area Medical Center (CAMC) in Charleston, West Virginia, chose to start implementing Six Sigma techniques in its supply chain management. The initial savings from a just-in-time inventory management system may have been merely $163,410, but projected long term savings is expected to be over $800,000. The Six Sigma staff of CAMC moved on to other projects and produced remarkable results, as exemplified in Figure 7.5.

Continuing Six Sigma Results for CAMC were as follows:

Medical Error Reduction

- Reducing patient falls
- Reducing medication errors
- Improving pharmacy turnaround times

Business Operations

- Improving the revenue cycle
- Improving human resource recruiting and retention
- Improving operating room scheduling and throughput

Patient Case Management

- Decreasing length of stay in long-term patients
- Decreasing length of stay for cardiac-patient types
- Reducing emergency department diversions
- Improving radiology scheduling, operational flow, resource maximization, and patient satisfaction

Figure 5 **Six Sigma project potential**
One hospital's experience

Project	Validated savings ($)	Long term savings ($)
Supply chain management	163,410	841,540
"Captain of the ship"	519,000	790,000
Denials	232,637	425,000
Results reporting	367,621	341,000
Medication safety	31,774	242,777
ED wait time	100,000	202,428
HR recruitment	32,000	124,430
Physician satisfaction	39,780	66,000

MHEGRAPHIC   MHE Source: Creative Healthcare USA

FIGURE 7.5 Six Sigma project potential. (From Bea Stamps, MD, MBA, & Ian Lazarus, FACHE, "The Promise of Six Sigma. Part II," in *Managed Health care Executives,* **January 2002, p. 6.)**

The Roadmap to Success

Six Sigma is a rigorous systematic discipline that demands the use of various problem-solving tools and a particular methodology to drive process improvement. While the approach is best known for its basis on quantitative metrics of quality, it is the approach to improving quality and reducing variation that separates Six Sigma from other quality campaign methods. In fact, many organizations use the measurable feedback data provided by Six Sigma to augment other ongoing quality initiatives, like total quality management (TQM) or the Balanced Scorecard. By validating the impact of defects and improvements as well as the use of small scale experiments, reaching the optimal solution to a problem makes implementing a change more believable to the organization. One chief of staff of a major metropolitan hospital has stated that the medical staff respects the statistical rigor of the methodology. Data and evidence gathered by stakeholders gets their attention. Root causes to variation suddenly emerge as a result of the problem-solving discipline. Many times, according to practitioners, the real problem is not what you thought after you look at the data. It becomes a real education to project stakeholders on an "out of the box thinking" approach to not only finding solutions to improving a process but, also, finding a solution that sustains itself in the long term.

At the heart of the Six Sigma management philosophy is the scientific approach known by the acronym **DMAIC (DefineMeasureAnalyzeImproveControl).**

(D) Define. This is the first phase of the Six Sigma practitioner's process. The team in charge of the project must clearly define the problem and the factors critical to quality (CTQ) that are important to the customer. An examination of the business process through mapping techniques correlates those CTQ factors with gaps in which the process falls short. An example of the delivery of patient test kits to a hospital by a laboratory highlights a basic definition problem.

On the surface, CTQ factors are found in the steps in the kit preparation process. One step—the assembly of patient test kits, for example—may involve a multitude of component activities, all of which may introduce variables of error into the process, leading to a cycle of error management. In further defining the process, these hidden factors add to the cost of quality, such as mistakes or defects in kit components, handling, or delivery.

Once a process is mapped out, the Six Sigma practitioner then begins isolating all the variables that enter into the fulfillment and delivery of patient care kits. Sometimes, the "low hanging fruit" of simple error correction is revealed by the basic process map.

The "hidden hospital," therefore, becomes all the redundant factors that do not add true value to the patient-care delivery system.

The diagram shows all the "hidden" or non-value added sidesteps a process may incur along its main path. Examples are redundant paperwork, a technician having to find supplies not readily available, or a physician having to redictate a lost case history.

It is said that Six Sigma turns a physical problem into a mathematical problem. The statistical nature of Six Sigma customer focus, for example, can best be expressed as a mathematical equation of $Y = f(X)$, where Y is the variables of output in a process. This output can mean patient satisfaction, accuracy of lab results, cycle time, or quality of a process. The X variables are the inputs that go into delivering or producing Y (Y is a function of X), such as essential strategy or critical processes. The exercise of defining the variables can often be quite revealing in what the customer really wants and, in turn, actually gets.

$Y = f(X)$, where Y = Outputs, X = Inputs or variables that determine output

(M) Measure. After a defined problem is established, the next step is to determine what the metrics are for this process. How do you determine if you are successful? One way is an establishment of base-level benchmarks of what the ideal process should be so that it can be compared to measures of defects. What is the process capability? What is the process "entitled" to be and what are the measurements? Are these measurements reliable and valid? These are the critical questions asked of "out of control" conditions. It is the measurement phase in which basic probability training and statistical analysis comes into play as part of the Six Sigma practitioner's armamentarium.

(A) Analyze. This is the phase in which underlying root causes for a problem are explored. Statistical analysis is used to examine potential variables that may contribute to the underlying defect. The multiple tools used in this phase include multivariate analysis, ANalysis Of VAriance (ANOVA), regression analysis, normality tests, and correlation. The questions to be asked at this point are whether the process can be improved, what can be done to improve it, what resources are needed to accomplish it, and what will undermine improvement efforts.

(I) Improve. The definitive answer to $Y = f(X)$ is answered. What is the effect of implementing this particular solution and is it the optimal one. A plan of action is measuring the outcome of several potential solutions to find the answer. Training in experimental design and multiple linear regression refines the decision making process and helps leave nothing to assumption or intuition.

(C) Control. Once a possible solution is found, critical ongoing measures are put in place to ensure consistency and quality in the changes made. The use of control charting techniques ensure costs, schedules, and so on are maintained and strategic goals are aligned with the organization.

The control phase concept is what separates the use of Six Sigma from other quality initiatives that may unravel over time or have no discipline for long-term payoffs in quality and revenue.

The Six Sigma Tool Box

A list of the tools in the Six Sigma box that practitioner's can call upon to arrive at a solution. Each phase has multiple tools in which the practitioner can use to approach the problem.

HOW IS SIX SIGMA EMPLOYED?

When an organization chooses to employ Six Sigma techniques in solving a problem, it has the choice of hiring a consultant practitioner to either help find a solution or jumping in and having the consultant incorporate the capability in-house through training and deployment of its own employees. Outside consultants work with staff to introduce them to the concepts and help them realize the potential effect on operations. Either way, the projects are supported by Green-Belt practitioners, who are supervised by Black Belts or, even more experienced, Master Black Belts. Black Belts have had the most intensive training in the tools and problem solving techniques employed through Six Sigma methods. Green Belts are often the process owner or "champion" of the process change.

The first step for an organization, before it decides to employ Six Sigma, is to define its strategic objectives and set forth its goals. The organization must have a clear vision of where it wants to go, what kind of organization it wants to be (preferably world class), and whether satisfying the customer as well as the stakeholders involved in the process is the key to long term success. The continuous pursuit of excellence is the ever-present hallmark of Six Sigma companies.

The incorporation of Six Sigma into an organization is not about a one-time effort to right the ship; it is about a strategic decision to be always customer focused, vigilant, and agile in order to stay on top of the marketplace. In essence, Six Sigma becomes a cultural change in philosophy and mind-set. It is a vigilant focus on what the customer wants. The traditional philosophy of ensuring that operations stay within lower and upper specification limits or "goalpost mentality" is replaced with customer-driven measures to achieve specific target goals. Any deviation from the target becomes a loss to the organization and, ultimately, a loss to society.

The Japanese engineer Genicihi Taguchi suggested a paradigm shift function to describe the loss to society of not having reached a more exact specification target.

Consider the financial and social implications in pharmaceutical errors incurred by institutions alone. This is one issue of quality in which vigilant focus on minimal variation is truly warranted.

In order to accomplish this cultural change, the business must give Six Sigma Projects the momentum and support it need through the proper alignment of organizations. Without the proper environment for cultivating change, initiatives never develop the momentum needed to reach critical mass. A supportive critical mass or a guiding powerful coalition is necessary for organization to gain wide acceptance and belief. Leadership must be the biggest supporter of Six Sigma Projects through a top down quality agenda. They must create the vision, communicate it and encourage a sense of urgency to "get it done." Management must reward those employees who are diverted from their usual duties to become Six Sigma trained. These employees will bring a skill set needed to reinforce Six Sigma at the process level and to drive and sustain quality improvement.

Six Sigma Projects must support also the strategic goals of the organization, and quantitative metrics must reflect the achievement of those goals. In health care, Six Sigma aligns patient goals with strategic goals, as illustrated in Figure 7.6.

A project such as ED throughput makes sense because patient satisfaction, and the perception of quality as well, is known to be directly related to patient waiting time as seen in many patient surveys. Improving ED throughput, not only decreases patient waiting time, but increases satisfaction, improves ED revenue generation, and minimizes diversion time.

Keys to Making Six Sigma Work

To summarize the key elements necessary for successful implementation of Six Sigma performance improvement methodologies, Jerome Blakeslee, Jr. (1999), names several key principles for organizations to reap the most benefits:

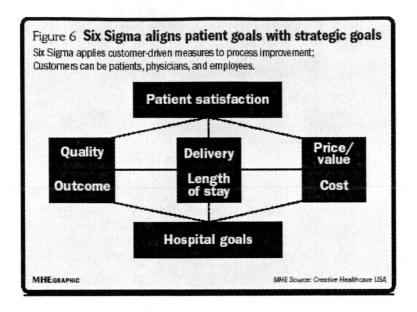

FIGURE 7.6   Six Sigma aligns patient goals with strategic goals. (From Bea Stamps, MD, MBA; and Ian Lazarus, FACHE, "The Promise of Six Sigma: Part II," in *Managed Health care Executives,* **January 2003, p. 4.)**

1. Six Sigma must be driven by committed leaders. To paraphrase the points made by Blakeslee, leaders must be willing to go against the grain in recommending unpopular or nonconventional management ideas. Their hands-on leadership and personal responsibility for driving Six Sigma efforts would leave little room for delegation to others.
2. Six Sigma efforts must be integrated with current quality, management, and strategic initiatives. This is good news to those who thought Six Sigma would have to replace the investment in existing management techniques. On the contrary, the quantitative metrics of Six Sigma enhances TQI, continuous quality improvement (CQI), or, more recently, Balanced Scorecard measures with feedback data that extend beyond assumptions.
3. Process thinking is the supporting framework for success with Six Sigma efforts. The organization must be rigorous in mapping existing business processes to see where it falls short of meeting customer expectations and market demand.
4. The organization must be vigorous in intelligence gathering on what the market and the customer wants. This means figuring out what hard-data measurements reflect customer satisfaction or loyalty on a continual consistent basis. A good closed feedback loop ensures the maximization of company output to match customer requirements.
5. The Six Sigma Projects must be designed to produce real savings and return on investment. Short-term payoff projects are designed to engage Six Sigma principles quickly, engender belief in the system, and establish a foundation for long-term Six Sigma success. Projects initially are designed to have short (less than six months) completion deadlines with significant payback. Long-

term payoffs are often the result of incremental short-term benefits, as well as long-term design.

SIX SIGMA AND PREVIOUS INITIATIVES SUCH AS TQM

Many organizations have quality initiatives in place and are possibly seeking to improve or replace current organizational improvement methods. To better understand where Six Sigma might fit in, a summary comparison of several key differences in the quality initiatives of TQM versus Six Sigma helps us to improve our understanding of where TQM measures have fallen short and where Six Sigma initiatives may succeed in picking up where TQM left off.

I. Customer Focus

TQM

- The early mantra of TQM policies and mission statements was to "meet or exceed customer requirements."
- If customers were happy before, let's keep it that way.
- Unfortunately, customers have dynamic and ever changing requirements that often were measured on a one-time, or sporadic, if not ongoing, basis.
- No one took the time to truly understand the customer needs and to adjust the process to constantly fit those needs.
- Lack of control mechanisms to sustain change.
- Quality also meant that as long as the customer was happy, the process was fine. There was with little regards as to the possibility of making it more efficient and less costly.

Six Sigma

- The customer focus is top priority.
- The goal is to truly understand the customer
- Before defining the problem, the customers of the process and their requirements must be fully understood. This is important, particularly in designing a controllable and sustained improvement with the appropriate metrics that allow the organization to stay on top of customer developments and unmet needs.
- The solutions are dynamic and ever changing in order to achieve Six Sigma level qualities.
- Control mechanisms of a process are designed to be sustaining but constant monitoring signals need for modification and change.

II. Goals

TQM

- The achievement of quality was a fuzzy concept with a specific quality department focused on quality control or quality assurance.

- The emphasis was on stabilization rather than on improvement of existing processes.
- The answers to improvement were, at times, based on assumptions and hypotheses, not hard data.
- Not having the tools to understand customer needs meant the possibility of an "open-loop" system.
- The quality initiatives were often separated from management objectives and strategic goals.

Six Sigma

- Solutions are data driven and fact driven with evidence based improvement. For the first time, questions are being asked as to what measurements are needed to gauge the performance of business processes.
- The difference is now managers are asking what is essential information is needed and how can this information be used to optimize results?
- The integration of Six Sigma, employing its tools and practices, require a proactive management philosophy.
- In order to cultivate support for improvement changes, process owners must build buy-in at all levels, from top down and across departments.
- Management is constantly aware of improvements and therefore, process ownership and accountability.
- In a culture of continual adaptation to a changing environment, management must stay on top of its business practices in order to achieve its ambitious goals.
- The "closed-loop" of a Six Sigma system allows organizations to track customer needs and adjust accordingly.

III. Organization

TQM

- There is inconsistent integration of quality policies, reforms, and decisions across the organization.
- Managers are sometimes left out of the circle while "quality councils" made changes.
- There is leadership apathy, possibly as a result of the above.
- Little attention is paid to process ownership, acceptance, and accountability.
- There are incremental changes
- Training is ineffective.

Six Sigma

- Clear, consistent, and focused emphasis on customer requirements, process improvement, and management are key.
- Implementation of Six Sigma methodology begins at the top leadership, where the vision to drive cultural change is derived. The passion for constant reinvention of the business is essential for survival.

- Training is in-depth and ongoing. Mentoring and coaching nurtures the infrastructure for sustainable change.
- Incremental exponential change is the rule.

CONCLUSION

Critics of Six Sigma have called it "TQM on steroids" or just a passing fancy as if it were the flavor of the month management program. The reason for this misunderstanding is that the differences of the methodologies are not well understood. Moreover, while success stories of TQM/CQI abound and these initiatives provided the fertile impetus for Six Sigma genesis, previous failures of half-hearted TQM implementation have left some with a bad taste for quality programs. These opinions have left many to be skeptical of Six Sigma's quality focus and methods. The misconceptions of TQM/CQI, and possibly failings, have had more to do with the introduction and management of these ideals than an actual failure of the system itself. These errors in implementation could also be repeated by organizations wanting to try Six Sigma as well. That is why an organization must take the time and make the commitment to truly educate itself on the successful ways of implementing Six Sigma into its culture. It is not for everyone, and there have been success stories for those who decide to take a quantum leap forward in competitive edge thinking.

Whichever initiative is chosen, be it TQM/CQI or any other improvement style, Six Sigma, or a combination of both, a successful implementation requires a hands on leadership approach that should be intimately involved in making sure there is a supportive environment for cultural change. In the spirit of Six Sigma's mathematical emphasis, the formula for putting it altogether is seen in Figure 7.7.

The key to driving any initiative is the urgency on the part of leadership to find a solution to today's marketplace forces. As stated before, the vision must be carried forth from the top down, and encouragement from management starts from the bottom up.

There is strong support for health care professionals to use Six Sigma methods for improvement of quality and reduce costs. Health care is a complex process with a lot of variability, diversity in specialty arenas, different patient needs, and professional skills. Managing this variability and improving efficiency while reducing costs is the greatest challenge for providers today.

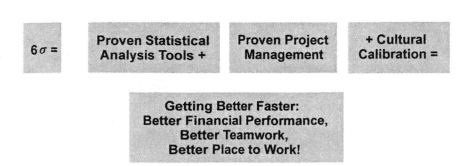

FIGURE 7.7

The ever-changing environmental challenges of lowered reimbursements, increased competition, and increased demands to improve and maintain safe patient care delivery make walking the tightrope of quality versus fiscal solvency a critical choice of management decisions. Physicians and health care executives are in a better position to make decisions when presented with credible, measurable, and controllable results. Buy-in for improvement changes within Six Sigma organizations is higher because of the collaboration required from multiple stakeholders in different departments. The process improvements become more robust and decisive rather than relying on intuition and on second-guessing. Six Sigma improvement methodologies are the competitive edge an organization needs to sustain long-term results.

REFERENCES

Arnold, Jennifer: "Six Sigma reveals astounding results." P. 4 of reprint from *www. GEMedicalSystems.com/education.*

Blakeslee, Jerome. Jr. Implementing the Six Sigma solution. *Quality Progress,* July 1999.

Ettinger, W. Six Sigma: Adopting GE's lesson to health care. *Trustee,* September 2001, 4.

Pande, P., Neuman, R., & Cavanagh, R. *The Six Sigma way: How GE, Motorola, and other top companies are honing their performance.* New York, NY. McGraw-Hill Publishing, 2000. 11–13.

Scalese, D. Six Sigma: The quest for quality. *Hospital and Health Networks,* December 2001.

Venable, S., & Silverman, P. "Six Sigma Methodology. Applying a corporate model to Radiology enabled MDACC to boost CT capacity." *Journal of Imaging and Technology Management,* Nov/Dec 2000, *(13)*7.

CHAPTER 8

Process Improvement Reporting for Physicians and Health Plans

Brent A. Metfessel

> Continuous improvement means augmenting quality and reducing costs by enhancing efficiency of the medical care delivery processes. These processes involve several departments and have substantial impact on how a hospital operates. Examples that continuous improvement teams address include the efficient distribution of supplies, the transfer of patients from the emergency department to patient rooms, changes in the chemotherapy admission process, and the verification of insurance data for the purpose of expediting and ensuring reimbursement.
>
> —Ohio State University Medical Center, Columbus, Ohio

Physicians and health plans use practice pattern information for a number of initiatives, including network optimization; incentive pool, bonus or withhold distribution; and provider education. No matter what the purpose of the profiles, it is imperative that the relationship between providers and managed care organizations (MCOs) move toward a spirit of partnership. Other stakeholders are also interested in physician cost effectiveness and quality profiles, including consumers, accrediting bodies, and referring practitioners.

USING INFORMATION FOR DECISIONS THAT AFFECT PROVIDERS

Health plans, consumers, and employer groups desire to use information from practice pattern profile reports for decision making concerning providers, including their status in the health plan. There exist several areas where such decisions affect providers.

Network Management

Some MCOs use practice profiles to determine which providers should be brought into the network or maintained as a network member. With such MCOs, providers with high cost variances or performance ratios, as well as those with significantly lower than average quality performance indices, may be relegated to out-of-network status. Although this provides an incentive for providers to perform optimally in the provision of cost-effective and high quality care, such action on the part of the MCO may be viewed as threatening and impair the relationship between the provider and the MCO. Generally, if a provider already has a relationship to the MCO in question, some type of provider education should be attempted prior to taking the action of moving the provider to out-of-network status. If possible, the health plan should allow up to two to three years for such education to reflect itself in improved practice patterns.

There also needs to be trending over time of cost-effectiveness and quality indices to make sure that the provider is not excluded from the network due to a single "bad" reporting period. A typical reporting period is one to two years long and is based on rolling quarters. It is important that an MCO does not make a decision based on a single snapshot profile in time but looks at trends from a number of reporting periods.

Bonuses and Incentive Pools

Some MCOs use provider profiles to allocate funds to the top-performing providers. The MCO may give additional bonuses or preferential allocation of incentive pool funds to providers that perform well on particular cost-effectiveness and quality indices. Incentive pools are often built based on a certain percentage or "withhold" of dollars that are taken from the providers' usual reimbursement and placed in a pool. Top performers would be allocated the greatest percentage. One mid-sized health plan in the Southeast paid a 20% bonus to providers with a case-mix adjusted performance ratio (actual/expected cost) of less than 1.3. Once again, although such allocation schemes might give providers the incentive to practice efficiently and with high quality, the MCO should attempt provider education as to the most appropriate practice patterns for the first one to two years after new profiles are introduced. This education should occur prior to introducing monetary incentives, since otherwise the relationship between providers and MCOs may ultimately become strained. Money can become a major point of contention between providers and between providers and the health plan.

Provider Education in a Spirit of Partnership

The basic idea would be to develop a continuous quality improvement program that would aid providers in improving practice patterns in accord with advances in medical care. This method is clearly best for the relationship between providers and the health plan, but it is also the most resource-intensive to implement on both the provider and MCO end.

WORKING IN PARTNERSHIP WITH HEALTH PLANS

The provider-health plan relationship necessitates a partnership rather than a relationship in which the MCO plays a strictly regulatory and payer role. Certain practice regulatory procedures, such as prospective utilization review, still have a place in modifying practice patterns for the better as long as the methods used are based on scientific evidence as to what treatments are most efficacious for specific clinical conditions. Evidence-based clinical guidelines provide a critical source for scientific grounding in utilization review. Some MCOs, however, have dropped the requirement for preauthorization of procedures. This was done in order to streamline health care administration. In such a case, providers are given more freedom to provide treatments of their choosing without necessitating health plan involvement, although the providers will still likely be profiled retrospectively. MCOs need not use either utilization review or provider profiling in a threatening or antagonistic manner; rather, more and more MCOs are adapting a partnership approach. The components of the health plan-provider partnership relationship include provider education on reporting and case-mix methodologies, clinical guideline dissemination, and provider education on best practices and care improvement.

Provider Education on Reporting and Case-Mix Methods

A partnership relationship means that the health plan, as much as possible, opens the "black box" in terms of its case-mix and reporting algorithms and methods. As for case-mix and risk-adjustment methods, providers should obtain answers to the following questions:

1. *Is it a major methodology?* Companies exist that are completely dedicated to developing case-mix methods. Some examples of widely used commercial case-mix algorithms are discussed in the previous chapter. Less well-known proprietary case-mix adjustment products also exist on the market as well. In addition, some MCOs have an informatics department that develops a custom case-mix methodology. Such algorithms are not necessarily inferior to the more widely used methods. In fact, custom methodologies developed by smaller vendors or by the health plan itself may show more flexibility in meeting local needs, such as tertiary care practices or urban versus rural practices. In contrast, the more well-known algorithms have the advantage of being on the market for usually 10 or more years and thus are more tried and true.

2. *Is it adequately tested?* A case-mix package should be tested against a number of scenarios and types of patients, including patients of different age groups, severities, and number and types of comorbidities. The health plan should be able to provide at least a high-level analysis of the test results such as explanatory power (R-squared). Some case-mix adjustment algorithms actually have different models depending on patient demographics, such as a Medicare model or a Medicaid model, that assigns a different risk profile to more elderly patients and to patients on public assistance, respectively.

3. *Does the case-mix adjuster make clinical sense?* A sound risk-adjustment model would have been developed with an abundance of clinician input into the process. Most of the well-known adjusters mentioned in the previous chapter do have extensive clinical experience built into the packages. Often the companies that create and maintain the models have multispecialty physician panels

that meet periodically and evaluate the algorithm development and enhancement process. As an example, Episode Treatment Groups™ (ETGs) deal with the process of care, and many of the episode classes correlate well with the way a provider sees the disease condition (see Table 8.1). Consequently, ETGs can be used for both primary care and specialist profiling, but they have particular strength with specialist profiling, since specialists deal mainly with specific illnesses rather than with patient-population management. Adjusted clinical groups (see Table 8.2) are more morbidity based, and at the end of the algorithmic process, these groups classify patients according to the type of behavior the disease condition exhibits rather than into classes that correspond directly to names of diagnoses. ACGs are particularly strong on classifying patient populations with multiple comorbidities. As a result, ACGs are well-suited for primary care profiling since these physicians usually manage patient populations, especially in "gatekeeper" model health plans where a member usually needs to obtain an evaluation by a primary care physician in the specialties of family practice, internal medicine, pediatrics, or sometimes OB/GYN prior to visiting a specialist. Other adjusters, such as distributed common ground systems(DCGS), use risk scores based on a profile of clinical conditions that the member shows during a reporting period. All of these adjusters are based on clinical conditions or clusters of diagnoses at some point in the process.

4. *Does the case-mix adjuster have adequate explanatory power?* Some MCOs still use a form of age-gender risk adjustment methodology similar to that used in

TABLE 8.1 Examples of Episode Treatment Groups™ (ETGs)

ETG	ETG Description
Gastroenterology	
436	Ulcer, complicated, with surgery
437	Ulcer, complicated, w/o surgery
447	Appendicitis, w/o rupture
Cardiology	
260	Coronary disease, w/o AMI, with coronary artery bypass graft
261	Coronary disease, w/o AMI, with angioplasty
263	Coronary disease, w/o AMI, with arrhythmia, with pacemaker implant
267	Congestive heart failure, with comorbidity

TABLE 8.2 Examples of Adjusted Clinical Groups (ACGs)

ACG	ACG Description
0200	Acute minor, age 2–5
0600	Likely to recur, with allergies
2800	Acute major and likely to recur
4430	4–5 ADG combinations, age > 44, 2 + major ADGs

some actuarial models. Age-gender adjustments tend to have low explanatory powers, explaining only about 3–7% of the variation in resource utilization among patients, as shown by the statistic called the *R*-squared. Well-known commercial case-mix packages explain about 25%–50% of the variation in health care resource utilization when used retrospectively (with data from past experience). An explanatory power in that range is a reasonable expectation. No case-mix algorithm that is based on claims data will ever obtain an explanatory power close to 100%, since there exist many random factors that affect resource utilization that adjusters cannot pick up using claims databases. Further explanatory power improvements may occur when clinical data is added to the claims, such as lab results.

5. *Is the algorithm a black box or an open methodology?* Most of the well-known case-mix packages have publications in peer-reviewed journals that describe the basic algorithm used in the adjuster. A health plan's analytic or informatics department should be able to provide practitioners with publications or at least publication references. For more locally-developed or proprietary case-mix approaches, the developers or provider relations personnel should have the ability to describe the model on request, or preferentially put out descriptive white papers, mailings, or literature that practitioners can access through the Internet.

6. *How are the provider reports developed, and what are the processes behind them?* More specific questions to ask yourself in this area include the following:

   • How are the expected values calculated? Do they consist of weighted averages based on a norm for each case-mix category? That is, are the norms weighted according to my specific patient experience?
   • With what norm am I being compared? Am I being compared to a plan average for each case-mix category or to another benchmark?
   • Am I being compared to all providers or just to those within my specialty? Comparison by specialty, where possible, allows more precise comparisons to peers. For example, if congestive heart failure (CHF) is one of the case-mix classes, the fact that cardiologists likely see more severe cases of CHF than internists needs to be taken into account.

7. *Is there drill-down capability?* A sound reporting system allows drill-down into more detailed data. Merely an overall performance ratio (e.g. actual/expected cost) is not adequate for the understanding of how to improve practice patterns. The drill pathways, as much as possible, need to allow the provider to see precise areas of variation that are systematically different than his/her peers or the norm. The cost variance (actual–expected cost) should be significant. Since the cost variance is approximately normally distributed, simple *z*-scores based on standard deviations can be utilized to select providers needing further practice pattern investigation. A good rule of thumb is to drill down on providers that differ from the norm by two standard deviations or more. Note that this includes "underutilizers" as well, since there may exist access difficulties. Such access difficulties may later result in increased emergency room or hospital utilization due to patient illness conditions that worsen due to under-treatment, not to mention the effect on the patients' quality of life. A scatterplot depicting both likely overutilizers and underutulizers is displayed

in Figure 8.1. Furthermore, trending of measures such as cost variance over time is also important to determine if the high variance maintains itself, thus adding evidence that the practice pattern variations are systematic rather than random.

In a partnership relationship, once the reasons for a provider's variation are noted, an education process needs to take place. One part of this education process is the dissemination of information that details more appropriate practice patterns for a wide range of specific common conditions.

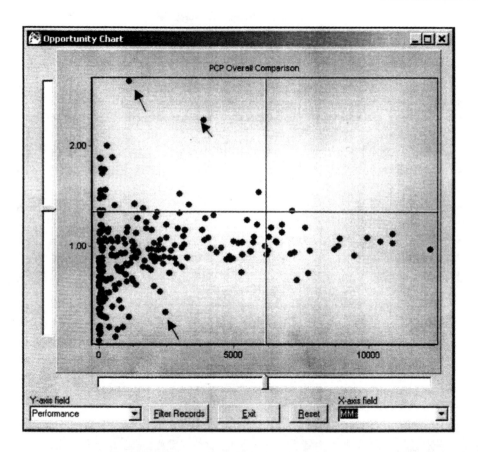

FIGURE 8.1 **Scatterplot of primary care providers (PCPs) showing performance ratio (actual/expected cost) plotted against total member months in the provider's patient population. The greater the number of member months, the more significant a high- or low-performance ratio becomes. Note that variation tends to increase as member-months decreases. This is likely due to random factors from a small patient population, and, consequently, such a plot normally has a "reverse megaphone" appearance. The arrows point to providers that appear to be significant outliers and in need of drill-down analysis. Note that this includes an underutilizer as well. For this analysis, members with greater than $25,000 in cost for the reporting year are excluded.**

Clinical Guideline Dissemination

Few clinicians can keep up with the full wealth of medical literature in their respective fields. Evidence-based clinical guidelines that summarize medical literature for specific medical conditions can be enormously helpful by making the information much more digestible. Individual guidelines are generally structured around single disease classes such as asthma diagnosis and treatment, or around major medical procedures such as the appropriate use of knee arthroscopy. Most of the over 600 MCOs in the United States utilize some type of guidelines—either evidence-based or an expert opinion consensus—to help analyze and improve practice patterns. This is particularly true of the larger MCOs.

The strongest type of clinical guideline is the evidence-based guideline, which synthesizes the most appropriate clinical studies into a white paper and/or a decision tree diagram. Evidence-based guideline developers generally have staff dedicated to reviewing medical studies. These staff members usually consist of registered nurses and personnel with advanced public health education. The evidence is graded based on reliability and strength of study design. For such grading analyses, double-blind studies would rate high on the rating scale; case-control studies might rate slightly lower, then review papers, then consensus expert opinion, and last, case studies, which would rate the lowest. The evidence is then combined and synthesized into a clinical guideline that discusses the most appropriate diagnostic tests and treatments for a disease condition, and under what circumstances the relevant procedures should be performed.

Disseminating guidelines so that they impact clinician practice is not a trivial task. There needs to exist a clear plan for distributing the guidelines to providers and holding them accountable for their implementation into clinical practice. One suggested method is to disseminate the guidelines initially to physician leaders. Such physicians would have a strong relationship with both the health plan and local providers, practice cost-effective and high quality medicine, and have a clear understanding of the practice pattern profiling and reporting process. Physician leaders can take the guidelines and apply them to the needs of local clinicians. In addition, such leaders can significantly help remove some of the provider educational burden from the health plan. Physician leaders can educate providers through didactic lectures, discussion groups, and one-on-one meetings.

The Institute for Clinical Systems Integration (ICSI) is a strong proponent of the value of evidence-based clinical guidelines, and cite the following objections that make their implementation and acceptance more difficult:

- **Guidelines are a legal hazard:** The fear is that if a guideline contains a major error, increased litigation may result from following such a guideline. Good guidelines, however, are evidence-based and not opinion-based drivers of care. Furthermore, once a review of the literature takes place and is synthesized into a preliminary guideline, multispecialty physician focus groups review the guidelines prior to finalization. This provides additional checks and balances to guideline development.
- **Guidelines are cookbook medicine:** Guidelines are just that—guidelines. Each patient is allowed treatment according to his or her individual needs. Evidence

based clinical guidelines are based on extensive reviews of the literature and are applicable to the vast majority of cases for a particular clinical condition. In the case of practice pattern evaluation or profiling, comparisons of such patterns to medical guidelines can help identify overall *systematic* variations from the norm rather than variations due to particular patients with special needs.

- **Guidelines do not work:** When used as the sole basis for practice improvement, this statement contains some truth. However, when incorporated into a systematic continuous quality improvement approach, they have been shown to improve practice patterns and reduce variation.

- **Physicians will not use guidelines:** Once providers know that the guidelines are based on a sound review of the medical literature, practitioner buy-in greatly increases. In addition, clinicians need to realize that clinical guidelines are only one part of the total treatment picture, since a team approach to patient care is becoming the norm.

- **Guidelines need validation through actual outcomes data:** This is correct when based on a continuous quality improvement approach, but is incorrect if outcomes are based on individual events. Local implementation of guidelines can be compared to outcomes data one or two years after implementation. Depending on the actual level of practice pattern improvement, minor alterations can be made to the guidelines to reflect local needs.

It is important to note that national guidelines may need adaptation to local patient needs and concerns. Accordingly, providers should be allowed to give feedback to the MCO or health plan on the usability of the guidelines to their specific practices. For example, a practice in a major metropolitan area where specialty care is readily available differs in major ways from a rural practice which is based more on primary care. Practices where many patients are poor or on public assistance also differs from practices in affluent areas. All of these aspects are local needs that guideline implementation plans must take into account; thus, one needs to avoid the *rigid* application of guidelines to clinical practices. However, when used as basic guides to appropriate practice, clinical guidelines can significantly decrease practice variation.

The development of accountability programs that track how providers follow basic guideline standards is critical to continuous quality improvement programs. The program needs an approach that enables providers to positively view the accountability process rather than consider it a threat or an attempt to take away clinical discretion from the providers. Health plans can develop such accountability programs after the guideline set has become widely accepted by providers, possibly with some additional local modifications. Information systems exist that measure compliance to simple guidelines, such as providing beta-blockers after an acute myocardial infarction (MI), prescribing angiotensin converting enzyme (ACE) inhibitors for congestive heart failure (CHF), and the presence in the claims record of a follow-up visit 30 days after a psychiatric hospitalization. Creating more sophisticated measures that reflect the true richness of clinical guidelines is also of great importance. Many of these measures can be obtained using commonly available claims and administrative data. Categories of measures for guideline compliance include the following:

- A procedure or treatment is commonly indicated for a clinical condition and should generally be performed. Many of these measures have already been developed, such as the measurement of hemoglobin A1c testing frequency for diabetic members. It is important that measurement of guideline compliance would not end up as an "all or nothing" algorithm. For example, the ideal measurement frequency for hemoglobin A1c in order to properly assess long-term control would be about three times a year. If a member receives the test just once per year, any "guideline compliance score" would be "partial credit," that is, the score would not be as great as if three tests were given but more than if the member had no tests in a given year. This "approximate reasoning" would also apply to the other suggested guideline compliance measure categories that follow.

- A procedure is indicated, but only after a certain time interval from the illness onset. A new episode of low back pain is usually treated conservatively for about 30 days. If the pain persists after the time period has elapsed, an MRI should be performed. However, multiple MRI scans for the same episode of care for back pain would be discouraged.
- A procedure is indicated, but only after another procedure is performed first, such as the need in certain conditions to perform a screening lab test prior to a more extensive diagnostic workup.
- Issues concerning inpatient utilization and setting of care: This includes hospital admissions to perform surgeries generally done on an outpatient basis, consistently long lengths of stay for various illnesses (exposing patients to risks such as nosocomial infection), and unnecessary use of assistant surgeons.
- Pharmaceutical practice patterns: These measures range from simple metrics such as the use of beta-blockers after acute MI to the appropriate use of first- and second-line hypertension medications prior to third-line medications in patients with new onset hypertension.

Provider Education

Physician leaders can once again have high influence on physician practice patterns as long as they are trusted colleagues of local physicians. Such physician leaders should have strong relationships with medical directors of dominant health plans in the geographic area. The medical directors can then educate physician leaders on plan-wide problems and issues, who can then educate local providers. These leaders can also have one-on-one sessions with providers having significant practice variation in an area, showing them peer-based comparisons and allowing feedback from the providers. This discussion can then lead to the dissemination of guidelines and best practices to aid the providers in improving their practice patterns. Other methods of education include discussion groups, written material and didactic lectures and conferences. These latter methods work best when educating multiple providers on overall plan-wide practice pattern issues. Physicians and other clinicians are busy people; therefore, education must be conducted efficiently. Furthermore, providers should be encouraged to discuss significant profile reports with other providers who receive similar reports. These discussions will help institute what is called the *Hawthorne Effect,* which, for care providers, means that merely having the knowledge of practice-pattern variation will enable providers on their own to seek ways to decrease their variation from peer practices. Clinical care providers do not like to be told by health plans how to practice medicine. However, it is ingrained in their culture to care about how they compare to their peers. This desire can be healthy and result in enhanced practices.

Goals of Performance Improvement

The major goals of performance improvement are twofold: First, for a particular practice pattern measure, the desire is to narrow the practice variation around the present health care mean. For instance, the spread of the distribution of a cost variance measure should decrease with process improvement. Second, clinical guideline-based best practices can be utilized to move the entire provider population mean toward better cost efficiency and quality. Although best practices may be guideline based, they should be adapted to local considerations and evaluated periodically through actual outcome analysis. Such outcome measures may include the following:

- Cost-efficiency improvement, showing a decrease in resource utilization.
- An increase in the performance of preventive measures, such as childhood immunizations, and various screening tests, such as breast and cervical cancer screening. This may increase costs initially but will more than pay for itself through a decreased illness burden and cost in the future.
- A decrease in episode length, usually implying a quicker resolution of symptoms.
- A decrease in emergency room visits and unplanned hospital admissions.
- A decrease in the rate of "sentinel events," such as status asthmaticus, hemorrhage during pregnancy, diabetic ketoacidosis, and ruptured appendix.

Many of these measures can be obtained using commonly available claims and administrative databases, although supplementation with clinical and functional status data will only increase the reliability and scope of outcomes analysis.

In order to see significant performance improvement in response to quality improvement initiatives, one must be patient. Two to three years may be needed to see this improvement. Trending of measures helps analysts to determine whether such improvement is occurring. Trending of data, however, can be quite resource–intensive, since there must be an adequate data set—usually requiring storage of data for several years of experience.

CONCLUSION

Health plans use physician practice pattern information for many reasons. Regardless, it is imperative that the relationships between providers and MCOs not be adversarial. Understanding the processes described in this chapter will assist in establishing a cordial relationship among all stakeholders, including patients, hospitals, health plans, accrediting bodies, and other providers for the development of their referral base.

ACKNOWLEDGMENTS

The author of this chapter for the first edition was Hope Rachel Hetico, RN, MHA.

REFERENCES

Frankel, H. L., Fitzpatrick, M. K., Gaskell, S., & Hoff, W. S. (1999). Strategies to improve compliance with evidence-based clinical management guidelines. *Journal of the American College of Surgeons, 189*(6), 533–538.

Bergman, D. A. (1999). Evidence-based guidelines and critical pathways for quality improvement. *Pediatrics, 103*(1 Suppl E), 225–232.

Onion, C. W., & Bartzokas, C. A. (1998). Changing attitudes to infection management in primary care: A controlled trial of active versus passive guideline implementation strategies. *Family Practice, 15*(2), 99–104.

Metfessel, B. (2001). An automated tool for an analysis of compliance to evidence-based clinical guidelines. *MEDINFO 2001*, V. Patel et al. (Eds.), © 2001 (International Medical Informatics Association).

Web Sites

www.symmetry-health.com

www.acg.jhsph.edu: J. P. Weiner, "Learn the ACG case-mix system, module 1", © 2003, Johns Hopkins University School of Hygiene and Public Health.

CHAPTER 9

Using Information Technology (IT) Systems to Track Medical Care

Brent A. Metfessel

> The most significant change in healthcare information technology (IT) would be the adoption of outsourcing. In the past couple of years, we have seen outsourcing move from a concept that didn't have much support to one where it is a normal consideration of the CEO. Recently, the Yankee Group issued a report describing how their propensity index indicated that healthcare providers would be turning to IT outsourcing.
>
> —Richard D. Helppie, CEO, Superior Consultant Company, Inc.

Computerized information systems are increasingly being used to analyze the cost-effectiveness and quality of care given by providers. A number of third parties show interest in such information, including health plans, federal and state governments, and consumer groups. Providers need clear awareness of the methods used to track their practice patterns, whether the tracking includes the cost of the practice, quality of care (such as frequency of preventive services that a practice provides), and/or outcomes monitoring. Using information systems for such purposes is part of the growing field of medical informatics, which can be defined as the applied science at the junction of the disciplines of medicine, business, and IT, which supports the healthcare delivery process and promotes measurable improvements in both quality of care and cost-effectiveness (source: Medical College of Wisconsin). Although a number of definitions of medical informatics exist, this definition is the one most relevant to the application of informatics to the tracking of care processes and provider profiling.

CATEGORIES OF DATA USED TO PROFILE CARE PROCESSES

Having the correct data to support the measures used in practice profiling is key to accurate reporting. The data must be "clean" and as free from errors as possible.

Errors in the data may occur due to a number of factors, such as poor diagnosis or procedure coding as well as the miskeying of data fields such as cost values. In addition, the category of data used needs to match the desired measures that one hopes to obtain. For example, if a health plan wants to look at the effect of a congestive heart-failure treatment regimen on exercise tolerance, claims data would not be the appropriate source. Functional status data would need to be collected as well. The following five data categories are of greatest interest in care profiling.

Claims, Encounter, and Other Administrative Data

This data category is the most readily available and abundant. Basically, all health plans have access to such data, which includes cost fields, member demographic information such as age and gender, International Classification of Diseases (ICD-9) codes for diagnoses, Current Procedural Terminology (CPT) codes for procedures, provider information including medical specialty, nine-digit National Drug Codes (NDC) to identify drugs, and other information. Claims databases can become quite large, and for major health plans, they often include millions of records. Economic and cost-effectiveness profiling are usually done using claims and administrative data. Some quality measures can also be obtained, but in a more limited fashion. These quality measures include frequency of preventive and disease monitoring services (such as the frequency of hemoglobin A1c tests to monitor diabetes), certain complications of care, and proxies for outcomes such as whether a treatment for a chronic condition leads to a decrease in emergency room visits and hospital admissions.

Functional Status Data

This category includes subjective data gathered from the patient in terms of his/ her view of the illness and the impact of the illness on activities of living, such as whether or not a congestive heart failure patient has the ability to walk up a flight of stairs without significant shortness of breath. The effect of a treatment regimen on such parameters can be performed to determine whether there is improvement in the patient's view, and whether side effects or complications are creating new difficulties for the patient. The SF-36 (QualityMetric, Inc.), a functional status survey with 36 query items, includes a scale that assesses eight health concepts:

- limitations in physical activities because of health problems
- limitations in social activities because of physical or emotional problems
- limitations in usual role activities because of physical health problems
- bodily pain
- general mental health (psychological distress and well-being)
- limitations in usual role activities because of emotional problems
- vitality (energy and fatigue)
- general health perceptions

Functional status data can be an excellent way to measure specific health outcomes in the patient's view, but the limiting factor is that data collection and analysis can be resource-intensive and expensive.

Patient Satisfaction Data

This is a subjective measure of what the patient perceives in terms of the level of service quality and care provided by the clinician. Many MCOs consider patient satisfaction an important measure of provider quality. Although not a direct measure of clinical quality, researchers often link patient satisfaction to clinical outcomes. This data, however, is also resource-intensive to collect and thus is not as abundant as certain other data sources, such as claims data.

Clinical and Medical Record Data

This category includes lab and radiology results along with other aspects of the medical record. Numerous companies exist that develop software for automated medical records, and the competition is intense. Nevertheless, some MCOs and vendors that do information reporting for MCOs do collect (or intend to collect in the near future) data such as lab results. Although, to repeat, this is very resource-intensive to collect and analyze, the proper use of such data can provide a much clearer picture of outcomes and treatment progress. Using diabetes as an example, claims data can provide information, such as the frequency of performance of hemoglobin A1c tests, but a separate lab result data feed can give the actual value of hemoglobin A1c, and thus the level of control of the diabetes over the past three to four months can be assessed as an outcome measure.

Health Risk Assessment (HRA) Data

Although HRA data are not generally used to profile care processes per se, such measures help to determine which members are at highest risk for chronic illness in the future, such as heart disease. Patients usually fill out such surveys directly, and many Internet sites have sprung up which include free HRAs and calculation of risk scores. Included in HRA surveys are smoking history, dietary habits, general health questions, level of energy, emotional health, driving habits, and other parameters. Providers can use such results as guides to ascertain which members need the most intensive intervention and thus help prevent poor future outcomes.

THE PROCESS OF CONVERTING INFORMATION TO VALUE FOR ORGANIZATIONS AND PROVIDERS

Data streams such as claims inputs are difficult to use in their raw form. Such streams may contain 50 or more fields (data items) per record and thus need processing in order to be useful in reporting and evaluating provider practice patterns. The following depict the six major steps in converting raw data to usable information that leads to action that benefits organizations (such as MCOs) and providers (see Fig. 9.1).

Data Collection

This involves inputting the data into the computer, which may range from a large mainframe to a personal workstation depending on the size of the database. Often

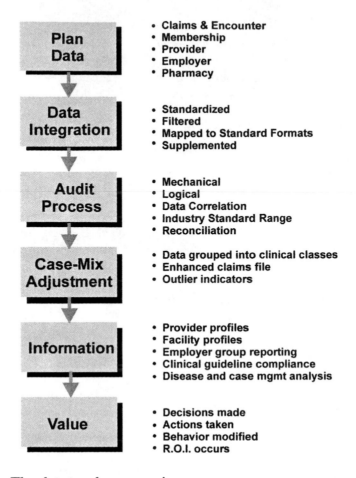

FIGURE 9.1   The data-to-value conversion process.

the data comes in the form of a tape and has to be input onto the disk. In this scenario, claims data is the data source, along with membership data (containing member demographics and eligibility information); provider identifying information; and pharmacy claims that contain NDC codes, fill dates, fill amount, cost data, and other fields.

Data Integration and Mapping

In the managed care industry, many different claims systems exist. National managed care organizations and third-party vendors of reporting software generally have to integrate the disparate systems together into a common format. This involves standardizing the data fields so that the same data items appear in the same location in the record and have a specified width. Thus, numeric fields such as cost will have the same number of digits no matter what claims system the values originally came from, and text fields such as provider specialty will have "mappings" so that the different specialty codes from the various systems that refer to the same specialty will be mapped to a single code in the final database. Such data standardization and mapping is critical to the accurate reporting on provider practice patterns, since the input into the reporting programs need to enter the system in a single standard format.

Processing of Data Audits

Also known as "data cleaning," the items in the database records are audited to check that they meet basic criteria. Usually the health plan either develops its own software to conduct the checks or purchases the software from a third party. Some examples of basic audits include the following:

- gender-diagnosis or gender-procedure mismatch, such as OB/GYN procedures in males
- age-procedure mismatch, such as pediatric procedures performed on adults
- notation of missing data or fields
- invalid values, such as an invalid provider specialty
- ICD-CPT mismatch, an example being a bunion procedure where the only diagnosis code is asthma
- data with out of range values; for instance, a claims record with a cost field value of $1,000,000

In many cases, the records with errors or audit flags are output as exception reports. In those cases, the health plan would decide whether to keep the record, modify it, or throw it out prior to input into the reporting system. In practice pattern profiling, it is critical that the data be as clean as possible. Incorrect data can seriously affect profiles, possibly to the point of mislabeling a very competent provider as having less than adequate cost-efficiency or quality of care.

Data Grouping for Case-Mix Adjustment

Proper risk adjustment or case-mix adjustment of the data is a necessary component of practice pattern profiles. Such algorithms help to level the playing field among providers or facilities (such as hospitals) that are being compared. Without such adjustment, a provider that receives a complaint from a health plan that his or her practice is too costly can easily come back with the argument that "my patients are sicker," which may very well be true. To adjust data for case mix, it needs to be fed into a grouper that clusters the data into clinical classes or risk groups. The class in which a data record belongs can then be added to the claims record as an additional field(s). These fields are then input into the reporting system along with the rest of the record and used to calculate "expected" values for providers or other comparative groups. The cost of practice is a commonly used value that is adjusted by case mix, but other metrics can undergo adjustment as well, such as visit rates and procedure utilization.

Information Reporting

In this step, the case-mix adjusted data is run through the reporting software systems to generate graphical or tabular reports that provide information on practice pattern performance. Such reports may be displayed either in Microsoft Excel or another third-party reporting platform. Furthermore, some health plans have developed their own reporting platforms for tables and displays. Commonly reported items include total cost of practice, cost by service category (such as lab costs, specialist professional costs, and facility costs), visit rates, preventive services rates (such as mammography screening), complication rates, and case-mix adjusted performance ratios (actual/expected cost) or cost variance (actual/expected cost). Many of the numeric measures on a report can undergo case-mix adjustment and the provider can be given a performance ratio. A performance ratio of 1.0 means the provider is practicing at the norm for the comparison group, and practice variation can be investigated further through other reports if the performance ratio deviates significantly from that number. Typically, reports are distributed quarterly to providers and generally cover one year of experience.

The Value of Information

Both providers and health plans can benefit from information reporting. Unless a provider with high variance from the norm is unwilling to change or is not open to education on more appropriate practice patterns, a provider profile from a health plan should not be viewed as a threat. Rather, it can open up discussion with peers and result in the wider dissemination of best practices. The consequence of decreased practice variation as a result of case-mix adjusted reporting improves both the quality and cost-effectiveness of care, since high quality of care usually leads to lower cost (e.g., savings in emergency-room usage, unplanned hospitalizations, and decreased resource use from complications). Thus, both the provider and the health plan can benefit.

CASE-MIX ADJUSTMENT: THE CENTERPIECE OF PRACTICE PATTERN PROFILES

It is difficult to construct an adequate practice pattern profile without case-mix or risk adjustment. There needs to be an algorithm that adjusts for the severity of patient mix. A tertiary care center in New York City cannot be compared using unadjusted data with a community hospital outside the city. The tertiary care center will use more resources, and thus cost more, than the community hospital no matter how exemplary the tertiary care center. A cardiologist cannot be compared to a family practitioner, since in general the cardiologist will see patients of greater severity. Providers have the right to ask that reports dealing with health care resource utilization have proper case-mix or severity of illness adjustment, and that resources are available at the health plan or MCO to answer questions concerning the adjustment algorithm and to offer a complete explanation of the case-mix methodology used. Many MCOs now provide literature to providers that discusses the reporting and case-mix methods when the profile reports are distributed.

Algorithms for Case-Mix Adjustment

A wide variety of methodologies exist that are useful for case-mix, risk, and severity of illness adjustment. A number of third-party vendors exist that sell software groupers for case-mix categorization. Since each methodology has different strengths, some MCOs have purchased more than one software package. There is no such thing as a "perfect" adjuster. Five examples of commonly used algorithms follow:

- *Diagnosis Related Groups (DRGs) and related adjusters:* Originally put into use in the early 1980s, DRGs were intended for use mainly as a methodology for Medicare to determine reimbursement for hospital stays. Nevertheless, DRGs and their more recent derivatives (revised DRGs [RDRGs], and All Patient Refined DRGs or APR-DRGs, both of which subclassify each DRG category into three to five severity strata using various algorithms) are useful for inpatient case-mix adjustment. An example of a DRG category is DRG 89, "simple pneumonia & pleurisy, age > 17, with CC (complications).

- *Episode Treatment Groups*™ or ETGs (Symmetry Health Data Systems, Inc.): This data grouper classifies the claims records into episodes of care that track the progress of an acute illness from onset to resolution, and it includes related diagnoses and treatments. For more chronic illness episodes, where there is really no defined "onset" or "resolution," one usually profiles providers on a predefined time window, such as a year-long episode. To capture enough episodes for analysis, ETGs generally require a two-year reporting period. Since this case-mix adjuster depicts the longitudinal aspects of care, ETGs are a process-based adjuster, meaning that they emphasize the process of care and the treatment the patient receives over a time course. A member can, and often does, have more than one ETG during a reporting period. An example of an ETG is "Obesity, morbid, with surgery." There exist over 600 ETG categories, which are granular enough to detect nuances in illness classes and severity but not so large as to lead to significant small cell size problems. ETGs also group pharmacy claims and attach them to the most relevant episode based on priority tables. Over 400 health plans have purchased the grouper as of May 2003. In addition, Episode Risk Groups™, a derivative of ETGs, can be used prospectively for predictive modeling of cost as well.

- *Adjusted Clinical Groups or ACGs* (Johns Hopkins University): ACGs group illnesses into morbidity clusters rather than specific diseases as do ETGs. An example of an ACG is "Acute major and likely to recur." Since ACGs are based on morbidity clusters, patients with multiple complex illness conditions can be readily identified. Since each patient has only one ACG for an entire reporting period, such an adjuster is called *population-based.* The process of care over time is not as important with such algorithms. In fact, ACGs do not require procedure or CPT codes at all—just ICD diagnoses, age, gender, and member and provider identification fields, which gives the methodology the advantage of input simplicity. There exist over 100 ACGs at present, and they are in use at nearly 200 organizations worldwide. In general, there are fewer categories in population-based adjusters than in process-based adjusters, since process-based algorithms need to account for specific diseases.

- *Diagnosis Cost Groups*™ *or DCGs* (DxCG, Inc.): DCGs are also a population-based grouper. Although the grouper begins with 184 condition categories (e.g., "Benign neoplasm of skin"). These Condition Categories are also sorted into hierarchies and aggregated into broader categories. The combinations of condition categories that a member has can then be used to predict health care resource utilization based on an overall risk score for each member. This prediction can either be for the current year or for the subsequent year, depending on the model used. Over 100 organizations now use DCGs, and, like ACGs, they do not require procedure codes. One important feature of DCGs are their ability to be used in predictive modeling of prospective resource use, using a different model than that used for retrospective analysis

- *Age-gender:* In these models, various age and gender strata are used to account for risk. Generally there are about 9 to 20 strata for age gender, depending on the needs of the health plan. Basically, resource use is moderate in the early years up until about age 5, then decreases through adolescence and the 20s, then slowly rises again in a nonlinear fashion until it becomes quite high in the senior years. Females also tend to use more resources during their reproductive years. Of all the models described, age-gender has the least explanatory power for the prediction of resource utilization either retrospectively or prospectively. The ability of a case-mix adjuster to explain variation in resource utilization is determined by the "R-squared" (the square of the correlation coefficient), with the case-mix categories or risk score as the independent variables and a measure of resource use (such as cost) as the dependent variable. Age-gender models have an explanatory power of about 3%–7%, while publications on proprietary adjusters have generally shown that they explain about 30%–50% of the variation for retrospective analysis. Prospective explanatory power is somewhat less, usually around 15%–25%.

Calculation of Expected Values

The purpose of a case-mix adjustment algorithm is in the calculation of the expected value of a measure for a provider or facility. The expected value is what a provider "should" obtain based on normative values for the individual case-mix or risk groups. To calculate the value, a weighted average is performed where the normative cost, such as a plan average, for each case-mix unit or group is weighted according to the provider's individual experience. Thus, for a provider who saw 50 cases of an expensive disease and 20 cases of an inexpensive disease, the expected value will be much more weighted toward the more resource-intensive illness, since more cases were seen (see Table 9.1).

Case-Mix Indices

Once an expected value is calculated for a provider or facility, comparison of the provider's actual practice patterns to the expected value can take place. In reporting, there exist three basic measures that utilize expected values:

- *Ratio of actual to expected (actual/expected).* This measure is in terms of a "performance ratio" or an "efficiency ratio." A value of about 1.0 would mean that

TABLE 9.1 **Example calculation of expected cost for a provider using medical and pharmacy claims. An episode of care case-mix adjuster is used in this case.**

Episode Type	Number of Episodes	Normative Cost per Episode	Total Expected Cost
Depression, Minor	45	$725	$32,625
Hyperlipidemia	60	$900	$54,000
Coronary Artery Disease, w/o MI	18	$2,490	$44,820
Totals	123		$131,445

Final Expected Cost per Episode: $1,069.00

practice patterns are close to the expected target or plan average. For cost comparisons, a value of slightly below 1.0 might even be more ideal, as long as the provision of high-quality care is maintained.

- *The difference between actual and expected values (actual/expected).* This measure is termed the "cost variance" and is very useful for looking at the cost impact of practice variation. An additional advantage of this measure is its approximately normally distribution, unlike performance ratios that are skewed toward the high end. This means that relatively simple statistics can be used to isolate providers or facilities with high positive cost variances for further analysis. Often, a z-score (number of standard deviations from the mean) of +2 or more is used as the approximate criteria for overly high utilization. It needs to be noted that a highly negative cost variance can point to care problems as well, in particular, problems with patient access to care or underutilization of services, so the reasons for very low cost variances also need to be discovered.
- *The ratio of the expected value to the unadjusted plan average (expected/average).* This measure is the "illness burden" of the provider and becomes a measure of the level of illness in the provider's patient panel. A high illness burden means that the provider or facility treats patients that are more ill than the average provider or facility. A provider with a high illness burden and yet a reasonable performance ratio is likely to be highly competent with complex patients, and the health plan should give special attention to such providers to keep them as active as possible in the network.

Other Considerations in Analyzing Case-Mix Methodologies

When an MCO analyzes provider practice patterns, it is imperative that the organization educates providers on the methodology and validation of the adjuster, since provider buy-in to the adjuster cannot be obtained otherwise. Such education may consist of readings provided with the distributed performance reports that explain the algorithm as well as evidence for the algorithm's validity. The MCO needs to be open to questions from providers and show willingness to open the "black box" as much as possible. There are further considerations and questions that are relevant to providers when dealing with case-mix adjusted reports:

1. *Are the reported performance measures adjusted by specialty?* The rationale for the additional adjustment comes from the fact that even though a number of specialties may treat congestive heart failure, for example, an internist or family practitioner generally treats less severe cases than would a cardiologist.

    Thus, even if a report is case-mix adjusted by illness class, the adjuster may not fully account for the differences in patient acuity within the illness class. Adjusting by specialty will enable a more "apples to apples" comparison and achieve greater provider buy-in to the process. However, for less common illnesses, the additional specialty adjustment may cause the cell sizes to become too small, causing the adjustment to lose meaning since there would not be enough patients in some cells for meaningful comparisons. Overall, whether or not specialty should be added as an additional adjustment is an individual decision made by the health plan. The larger the health plan, the less chance that cell sizes may become too small and the greater the advantage of the additional specialty adjustment.

2. *What are the exclusion criteria?* After the case-mix adjustment is performed, it is important that prior to reporting there exists an outlier exclusion criteria. Without such criteria, there is a much greater chance that a good provider may perform poorly on a performance report, since a few high-cost outliers, which may occur due to no fault of the provider, can strongly skew the case-mix indices and lead to artificially high cost variances and performance ratios. Some methodologies exclude general catastrophic cases, such as members with costs above $25,000, or there may be a truncation calculation in which catastrophic members are included in the reporting information but are truncated to the criteria amount. Thus, if a patient has costs of $50,000, the costs will be truncated to $25,000 prior to reporting. This has the advantage of including all patients but the disadvantage of not knowing the actual cost of the patient panel.

Another way to exclude outliers involves excluding them at the case-mix class level. This means that illnesses that generally use less resources will have different criteria—in this case a lower high outlier exclusion boundary—than would an illness class that typically has high resource use. If cost is used as the measure of interest, the distribution curve of cost for a particular illness is skewed to the high side and thus does not look like the bell-shaped normal distribution. This makes developing proper exclusion criteria more complex. For greater accuracy, a "nonparametric" or "distribution-free" test is useful. One such test was developed in 1993 by Sprent and consists of the following equation:

$$(|X_i - M| / MAD) > Max \qquad \text{(Equation 1)}$$

Where X_i represents any value being evaluated for outlier status, M represents the median (the value for which 50% of sample values are above, 50% below) of the sample (such as all cases in a disease class) and *MAD* is the median absolute deviation. To calculate the *MAD* value, first obtain the absolute value of the difference between each value and the sample median. Then, sort the difference scores in ascending order. The median of the difference scores is the *MAD* value. Max is then the criteria point for excluding outliers. A reasonable value of *MAD* would be five. Both low and high outliers would be excluded, based on this equation.

Outliers still may have useful information in themselves. Consequently, after excluding them from the comparative analysis, it still is wise to report on them separately, since such patients, particularly high outliers, may in some cases be steered to case-management protocols.

THE CONTENT OF PRACTICE PATTERN PROFILES AND REPORTS

This section deals with the kind of measures and information that a provider may see in a performance report as well as information in reports internal to the health plan. Providers need a strong knowledge base about commonly used metrics in reporting so that the provider can intelligently discuss the report content with his or her peers when needed as well as with the health plan that delivered the reports.

Economic Profiling

This type of practice pattern profiling emphasizes the economic impact of practice variation. Usually, a cost data field is used as the measure of interest, and variation from the norm is often determined through such case-mix indices as discussed previously. Costs may also be broken down into service categories, such as lab, surgical, radiology, other professional, facility, drug, and other cost categories. Each of these service categories should also be case-mix adjusted so that a performance index and/or cost variance can be provided for each one.

Areas that can be profiled in economic and resource utilization profiling include the following:

- Consulting, specialty, and subspecialty referral practices.
- Prescription habits, including sample dispensation and using generic equivalents, especially for chronic conditions such as hypertension and Type II diabetes.
- Use of invasive and interventional tests, such as angiograms, IVPs, bone scans, and certain biopsies.
- Use of noninvasive procedures and tests such as CT and MRI scans, cardiovascular stress tests, chest x rays, and ultrasounds.
- Average length of hospital stay (ALOS), surgical operating times, use of assistant surgeons, and other utilization parameters.

If a provider receives a report that points to significant practice variation, the question comes up as to what factor(s) caused the variation. This is where the capability of "drill-down" analysis becomes important. In this method, an area of variation is pinpointed and reports are brought up in greater detail specifically concerning that area of variation. For example, if a physician shows a high cost variance for migraine headache, a drill-down analysis into the disease state may show that the provider uses CT and MRI scans of the head significantly more frequently than his or her peers. The provider can then be educated about the need for fewer scans, reserving them only for cases having a high index of suspicion for a tumor.

The importance of balancing economic or cost-based profiling with quality of care profiling must be stressed. Managed care has been purported in many areas of the media to be concerned primarily with profits and costs of care to the detriment of quality. Such instances include reports of overly short maternity lengths of stay, difficulty obtaining access to care, and rushed physician visits. Health plans increasingly extent are including various quality measures in their practice pattern profile reports in an effort to show the community that they desire to maintain quality while keeping costs down. Hopefully this trend will continue.

Quality Profiling

Such metrics attempt to look beyond cost. Typically, good quality care leads to improved costs since stable patients have fewer unplanned visits, less emergency room usage, and a reduced frequency of hospital admissions, all of which save money.

The *Health Plan Employer Data and Information Set* (HEDIS®) contains measures obtainable from claims, survey, provider, membership, and medical record data. HEDIS® was developed in conjunction with the National Center for Quality Assurance (NCQA) and is a widely accepted specification for quality measures. Consumers, managed care organizations, and accrediting bodies have a high level of interest in the HEDIS® 2004 metrics. These measures are divided up into a number of categories:

- *Preventive services.* Includes childhood and adolescent immunization status, breast and cervical cancer screening rates, chlamydia screening in women, assistance with smoking cessation, and well-child visits.
- *Access to care:* Includes access to preventive, primary care, and prenatal and postnatal care services.
- *Utilization.* Contains measures of frequency of selected procedures, inpatient utilization such as average lengths of stay for maternity and mental health patients, C-section and VBAC rates, and other measures of inpatient and outpatient utilization.
- *Acute and chronic illness care.* Examples are rates of beta-blocker use post–myocardial infarction (MI), comprehensive diabetes care (such as annual retinal exams), control of high blood pressure, appropriate medications for asthma patients, and follow-up within 30 days after hospitalization for mental illness.
- *Provider data and statistics.* Includes residency completion information, board certification, and provider turnover.
- *Membership statistics.* These measures deal with member demographics and total membership in the health plan.
- *Survey data.* Includes member satisfaction survey results.

The NCQA is continually revising its measures in the HEDIS® product and provides new versions annually. Although HEDIS® contains many measures of quality of care, it provides few measures of actual clinical outcomes.

Outcomes measures are an important component of quality reporting. There exists a number of ways to use data to measure outcomes:

Outcomes Obtained from Claims Data

Claims data has clear limitations for outcomes analysis. It only deals with the process of care and does not have information directly pertaining to outcomes except where specified in the ICD-9 codes. Thus, one must rely in many cases on *proxy* measures for outcomes. Proxy measures are process of care metrics that can imply certain outcomes, such as length of an illness episode. The following are some ways to ascertain outcomes of care using claims data:

- *Complications of care.* The ICD-9 codes directly contain language for denoting outcomes. There exist codes for wound infection and dehiscence, miscarriage in pregnancy, and general surgical complications. The coding of a major infection in a cancer patient on chemotherapy is another example of complications-based outcomes obtainable through claims data.
- *Procedure reperformances.* Two coronary artery stent procedures within a six month to a year period may imply failure of the first stent. However, a medical record check may ultimately be needed, since the second procedure could also be a stent placed in a new vessel. Returns to the operating room within a few days of a surgical operation or an outpatient procedure that turns into an inpatient stay within a few days also implies poor outcomes.
- *Readmission rates.* Two or more hospitalizations for the same episode of care within 30 to 60 days also implies poor outcomes.
- *Episode length analysis:* The length that an episode of care lasts can be compared between providers. Shorter episodes for acute illnesses imply better outcomes unless it is due to the expiration of a patient or poor access to care.
- *Medication prescribing patterns.* In some conditions the drugs prescribed may imply certain outcomes. A rheumatoid arthritis patient that needs Remicade® probably has a more severe form of the illness. Frequent antibiotic switching for an infectious disease such as pneumonia either implies a resistant organism or difficulties in quality of care.
- *Emergency room and hospital utilization.* Frequent ER use or hospitalizations for chronic conditions such as asthma or congestive heart failure imply a poor outcome from outpatient treatment.

Outcomes Obtained from Non-Claims Data

- Patient satisfaction data may be an indicator of outcomes, since patient satisfaction with care often relates directly to how well a patient has progressed with respect to his or her illness.
- Functional status survey data provides a direct subjective account of the severity of illness and/or outcome of treatment, depending on when the survey was given. A congestive heart patient that reports in a survey that he/she cannot walk up a flight of stairs may show nonresponsiveness to treatment that needs addressing.
- Clinical data analysis is becoming important as more and more organizations are adding clinical data to the claims, such as lab values. Hemoglobin A1c

values, for example, hold the key to how well controlled a diabetic is over the long term.

The difficulty with nonclaims data is that collection of such data can be resource-intensive and costly, depending on the sophistication of the information systems available.

Drill-down Analysis

If a provider or facility is found to have a significant variance from the norm on a measure, such as cost, drill-down analysis is important to find the reason behind the variance. Episodes of care case-mix adjustment is naturally suited to this kind of analysis, but other population-based groupers such as DCGs also allow drill-down if the clinical categories that are precursors to the assignment of a risk score are used. The idea behind drill-down is to obtain greater and greater detail on an area of interest. Thus, if a provider is found to have a high overall cost variance or performance ratio, a user can select the provider and drill-down into emergency room usage, hospitalization frequency, types of illnesses seen, or procedures performed. Case-mix is useful even for the more detailed reports since if, for example, emergency room (ER) use or the utilization of specified procedures is not adjusted for illness burden the "my patients are sicker" argument can easily hold. However, if the procedures are related to illness classes, providers can be compared to their peers on procedure use for that illness class.

Scenario. Dr. Jones is a family practitioner who had a high patient load from a single large health plan. These patients under his care had a total of 450 episodes over a two-year period. His case-mix adjusted performance ratio was 2.28, and cost variance was $157,400. Dr. Jones requested a drill-down analysis to determine why his practice patterns showed such a high variance from the norm. One area that the health plan data analysts found had high variance were patients he saw with tendonitis of the lower extremity. He saw 30 episodes of care for this condition, having a total performance ratio for the illness class of 6.0 and a cost variance of $25,300. On further drill-down, the analyst found that the major cost center included the frequency of MRI scans of the lower extremity for the tendonitis patients. His scan rate was 0.4, which means an average of 4 out of 10 episodes received scans, making a total of 12 scans in all. His peers of the same specialty showed 0.1 scans per episode of tendonitis of the lower extremity. Dr. Jones showed a performance ratio of 3.0 and a cost variance of $10,800. On learning this information, Dr. Jones decided to alter his referral patterns so that his scan rate was brought closer to the norm.

Trend Analysis

One report that shows high variance does not necessarily mean that the provider is outside the norm in that area as a matter of course. There may be, for example, a number of high-cost cases during the reporting period that were not excluded as outliers but had a higher severity during that time period that the case-mix adjuster did not take into account. There tends to be a "regression on the mean" phenomenon wherein a provider or facility with high variance during one period does not show the same high variance on the next reporting period due to the fact that possible random or severity factors have become more normalized. There exist methods to analyze in a formal way the time course of practice pattern measures and what it means for the provider's method of practice as a whole. A well-known method is process control charting, in which the measure's value is plotted against the progress of time. At least eight data points are needed to make an adequate process control chart, although preferably there exists a greater number of points for analysis.

The purpose of the chart is to let one know whether the practice variable is "out of control" in a systematic way. To determine this, the upper control and lower control limit lines are drawn on the chart, which are also called the "three sigma" lines. These lines are criteria for determining if a process is out of control in a statistically significant manner. The mean of the variable is noted as a line in between the three sigma lines, equidistant from both the upper control limit and the lower control limit. If a single point is above or below the upper control limit or the lower control limit, respectively, the process during that time was out of control and needs to be analyzed. If there exist only one or two points in time that are out of control for a provider variable, such as actual/expected performance ratio on cost, the overall performance ratio may be high on the report due to reasons beyond the provider's control, such as temporary patient factors not accounted for in the case-mix methodology. Health plans and providers would need to take this into account when evaluating provider or facility performance.

Also important is the direction of the trend. If there are eight or more points above or below the mean, it indicates that the overall process has changed significantly. Thus, for a control chart of 24 points (such as a monthly analysis of two years of data), if there are eight points above the mean in performance ratio, it likely means that during those eight months either practice patterns have changed toward less cost efficiency or more severe patients were brought into the provider's panel and that this was not taken into account by the case-mix methodology. Drill-down analysis will help distinguish between those two possibilities. In addition, seven points in a row that show a steady trend of increasing or decreasing values is also significant. For example, if a high performance ratio shows a decreasing trend for seven months in a row, this may mean that the provider is responding to quality initiatives or has realized through another way that his or her practice patterns were not as cost-efficient as the provider's peers and thus decided to bring practice patterns more in line with the norm over time (see Fig. 9.2).

Control charting is becoming increasingly important in profiling applications as the desire grows for more accurate information on providers and facilities.

CONCLUSIONS

Health plans, consumers, employer groups, government groups, and accrediting bodies are increasingly asking for more detailed information on provider and facility practice patterns. For the information to accurately portray practice patterns, the case-mix tool must be reliably account for the illness burden of the population that a provider or facility sees. This methodology must be open to those being profiled in order to obtain the much needed provider buy-in. Important report content

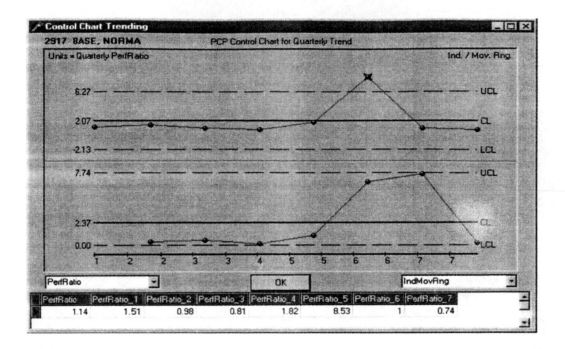

FIGURE 9.2 Two control charts for primary care providers, plotting performance ratio against time for quarterly data. The first one depicts a single "out of control" point (shown by the *X*). The second depicts a brief trend toward a lower performance ratio. This may be in response to practice improvement measures, but one actually needs at least seven points trending in the same direction to be assured of statistical significance.

issues include the need to balance cost indicators with quality metrics, drill-down methodologies to help determine the reason for practice pattern variation, and trending capability to look at practice pattern changes over time. Where possible, commonly available claims information should be supplemented with member satisfaction data, functional status surveys, and clinical values, such as lab results, in order to obtain better information on quality and outcomes of practice patterns.

ACKNOWLEDGMENTS

The author of this chapter for the first edition was Hope Rachel Hetico, RN, MHA.

REFERENCES

Goldfield, N., & Boland, P.(1996). *Physician profiling and risk adjustment.* New York: Aspen Publishers.

Kelley, D. L. (1999). *How to use control charts for healthcare.* American Society for Quality.

Sheshkin, D. J. (2000). *Handbook of parametric and nonparametric statistical procedure,* Boca Raton, FL: Chapman & Hall/CRC, 2000.

Metfessel, B. (Fall 1998). Specialist profiling using claims and administrative databases. *American Journal of Integrated Healthcare, 1*(4), 168–174.

Web Sites

www.dxcg.com
www.symmetry-health.com
www.acg.jasph.edu

Quantitative Aspects of Medical Practice

CHAPTER 10

Capitation Econometrics Revised

Angela Herron and Allan Gordon

> **Q:** Is a physician's prospect for being reasonably remunerated for treating Medicare and Medicaid patients diminishing hopelessly?
>
> **A:** Hopeless is in the eye of the beholder. But, yes, it's certainly diminishing. The government has fewer resources. The demographics are getting worse. Managed care offers the possibility of improving the financial standing of providers in Medicare. You know, fee-for-service can only ratchet fees down, because it has no controls on volume, only on price. Managed care can have an influence on volume as well, and when you do that, there is less pressure on price.
>
> —Dr. Peter R. Kongstvedt, FACP
> Partner-Health and Managed Care Consulting Division
> Cap Gemini Ernst & Young, LLC

This chapter identifies the key questions that physicians should ask about capitated contracts and provides a methodology for evaluating the potential impact of the contracts on practice economics. The model demonstrates the impact on a solo family practice physician's office. However, the method is applicable to any specialty and to small or medium group practices.

MARKET DYNAMICS

Continuing changes in the healthcare marketplace make evaluating capitated contracts both more difficult and critical to the success of a physicians practice. Market dynamics have been shifting to a less restrictive form of managed care arrangements. This shift has resulted in the prevalence of more preferred provider organization (PPO) products than the more restrictive HMO coverage. Since 1988, the percentage of workers with choice in a PPO program has quadrupled from 18% to 76% per Kaiser Health Foundations 2002–2003 Employer Health Survey. This shift in insurance coverage may initially appear to favor the physician's ability to remain in fee-for-service-based contractual arrangements, however, it also makes any remaining capitated contracts (if any) more critical to evaluate. The fewer patient members under capitated arrangements the more financial risk the physician may incur.

CAPITATED CONTRACTS

For physicians in solo practice or in small group practices, the common path to capitated contracting comes through membership in an independent practice association (IPA) or similar affiliation that has the legal authority to secure health plan contracts on behalf of its members. Even though the individual members of the IPA may not be involved in negotiations with the health plans, it is important for any physician to understand the terms of each contract. The key areas of concern are the following:

- patient mix
- capitation rate and contract terms
- service responsibility
- stop loss

Patient Mix

Health plan contracts are marketed to specific population groups, and the demographic characteristics of the patient populations will vary accordingly. Typically, the target population is identified in terms of the health plan's "product"—commercial plan, Medicare plan, or Medicaid plan. It is important for the physician to know about the population that is covered by the contract in anticipation of the types of services that those patients will require. Physicians should inquire about the age/sex/health status characteristics of the population the health plan expects to enroll and compare those to the current profile of the practice.

Capitation Rate and Contract Terms

The most important considerations are the actual capitation rate and the factors that can affect that rate, either up or down. It is also important to have a sense of market comparison on the capitation rate provided under the contract. Here is a list of specific questions physicians should ask:

- Which Health Plans can access this contractual arrangement? Is the Health Plan limited to just the one negotiating the contract or are there silent or affiliated plans that can access the agreement? This will impact the number of lives covered under this agreement.
- What is the monthly capitation rate paid to the physician? How much is the IPA taking from the health plan's payments to cover the cost of their services?
- Is the capitation rate a fixed amount per member per month, or will it be age/sex adjusted based on the actual blend of patients who are assigned to the physician?

- What day of the month will the capitation payment be paid? Does the contract stipulate that the IPA must pay interest charges for late payments?
- Are there any "low enrollment guarantees" built into the contract to provide for minimum payment amounts in the early stages of contract enrollments? Some contracts provide for fee-for-service payments until enrollments reach an effective level for capitation, such as 500 members.
- Are there provisions for retroactive changes in the enrollment assigned to the practice, and are there specific time limits on those provisions, such as 30 or 60 days? Failure to include time limits on retroactive enrollment adjustments may result in disruptions to cash flow and increased administrative paperwork.
- How are bonuses, if any, earned and paid? What are the specific measures if bonuses are based on performance?
- What penalties and deductions from the capitation payment can be imposed for actions such as "inappropriate referrals" or for referrals to noncontracted providers?
- How often can the capitation rates be renegotiated?
- What are the physician's financial obligations upon termination of the contract? Does the contract convert to a fee-for-service agreement or is continuing care for the patient covered under the existing capitation rate? If so, what is the contract time limit for providing continuing care?

Service Responsibilities

Physicians should ask for a copy of the list of the services that are included in the capitation payment. All rendered services should be defined by current procedural codes (CPTs) or similar billing code. Physicians who take primary care contracts and who also practice in specialty fields, such as allergy, cardiology, gastroenterology, or pulmonology, should have a clear understanding of how these services are managed under the contract—whether they are included or excluded in the capitation payment; whether these services can be billed separately. Other key questions about services include the following:

- What are the restrictions or limitations on billing patients for services that are not covered by the responsibility matrix? If it is permissible to bill for these services, are there restrictions on the billing rates?
- How is the physician reimbursed for nonphysician services, such as supplies, lab tests, and injections? This is particularly important if the practice has a high number of pediatric patients or provides allergy shots.
- What are the financial responsibilities of the practice for call coverage? Does the contract require that the physician pay for call coverage out of the capitation payment? If so, how is this payment handled—physician to physician, or as a deduction from the capitation payment?

Stop Loss

Another critical factor is reinsurance for high cost cases. This is called stop-loss coverage. Physicians should know if the contract has stop-loss provisions and what the costs are for coverage and the effect on the capitation rate once the stop-loss level has been reached. In some cases, the contract may convert to a new capitation rate. In others, payment may be on a predetermined fee-for-service arrangement. It is also important to know who is responsible for identifying cases when they reach the stop-loss limit and whether there is a time limitation when filing a stop-loss case.

In addition to these key points in capitation contracts, physicians should also anticipate that there will be "administrative burdens" related to new contracts. In most situations, the IPA or other physician organization will take responsibility for credentialing for the provider network, for utilization management and quality management programs required by the health plans, and for claims administration. Each physician, however, will be required to submit encounter data and respond to various queries and requests for information. In some cases, health plans or IPAs may stipulate financial penalties for failure to comply, for poor timeliness, or for administrative errors.

EVALUATING THE ECONOMICS OF SHIFTING TO AND FROM CAPITATION

Shifts in payor mix can cause dramatic impacts to the financial performance of a medical practice. While it is important to try to evaluate the impact before taking on capitated business, similar principles apply as physician practices shift back to fee for service business from capitation.

Before taking capitated contracts, physicians should answer three questions:

1. How much capitation should I accept as a percent of my total business?
2. How will the shift to capitation affect my practice financially?
3. How much will I need to reduce operating expenses in order to break even or profit from capitation?

As physicians' practices shift back to fee for service from capitation, two additional considerations must be addressed:

1. How much capitation is too little?
2. How will another shift in payer mix impact my practice cost structure?

Whether shifting to or from capitation, it is important to understand the factors that contribute to overall practice economics. The following examples can help a physician answer these questions by demonstrating the effect of changes in payor mix on a solo primary care physician practice. The methods described can also apply to other specialties or group practices.

THE SHIFT TO CAPITATION

To determine the impact that a capitated contract might have on a practice, it is necessary to analyze the economics of that practice. In traditional fee-for-service practices, there are three key financial measures:

1. Net revenue and net revenue per patient visit.
2. Office expenses, including fixed expenses such as rent, and those that vary with patient volume, such as medical supplies.
3. Net income, the amount remaining to be paid as physician compensation or reinvested in the medical practice.

By adding capitation to the practice, a physician must consider two additional factors:

- The capitation rate per member per month.
- The estimated number of visits for each capitated patient.

It is often difficult to isolate the financial performance related to one specific payor contract because the same resources are used to care for all the practice's patients. One way to evaluate the impact of a new contract is to determine what the practice's breakeven volume level is before and after the shift to capitation. Breakeven can be described as the level of patient volume required to cover all practice expenses. It is an important measure because once a practice achieves breakeven volume, each additional visit contributes to practice net income. Two variables that impact breakeven are revenue per visit and variable cost per visit. Breakeven volume equals—

$$\frac{\text{Total Fixed Expenses}}{(\text{Net Revenue per Visit} - \text{Variable Expenses per Visit})}$$

In some cases, the impact of a shift in payer mix on breakeven volume can be dramatic. This is illustrated in the following examples.

BASELINE

The baseline example is an internal medicine physician in solo practice. Currently, payment for services is from traditional fee for service sources including indemnity insurance, some discounted rate plans, self-pay patients, and Medicare. To analyze the potential financial impact of a shift in payor mix to or from capitation, it is necessary to establish a few key statistics from the practice's most recent 12-month period. Total net patient revenue and total operating expenses can be easily identified. Next, it is necessary to identify fixed operating expenses, which are those costs that generally do not change with volume within a defined range of capacity, such as space, most staffing needs, and utilities. Subtracting fixed expenses from total operating expenses provides total variable expenses, or those costs that are directly related to patient volume, such as medical supplies. Average variable expense per visit is calculated by dividing total variable expenses by the number of patient visits. The baseline practice profile is shown in Table 10.1.

In the baseline example, the practice needs 2,028 annual visits to break even. Any additional visits contribute $81.38, or the difference between net revenue and variable expenses, to net income.

TABLE 10.1   Baseline Practice Profile

	Total Annual	Average per Visit
Patient visits fee-for-service (FFS)	4,800	
Total net revenue	$480,000	$100.00
Fixed expenses	$165,000	$34.38
Variable expenses	$89,400	$18.62
Total practice expenses	$254,400	$53.00
Net income	$225,600	$47.00
Breakeven visits	2,028	
Contribution to net income after breakeven		$81.38

PAYOR-MIX SCENARIOS

We can now develop scenarios to help evaluate the impact of changes in payor mix. In each scenario, we assume that the practice is at capacity with 4,800 visits, so new capitated patients represent a shift from fee for service business and are not incremental business to the practice.

Scenario 1

Let's assume that 333 of the practice's patients shift to a capitated plan, and that on average, a capitated patient has three visits per year, which equals a total of 1,000 visits to the practice. The physician receives a capitation payment of $12 per member per month. The average revenue per visit under the capitated agreement is $48 ($12 per month times 12 months, divided by three visits), a substantial reduction from the fee for service average of $100. Therefore, the breakeven number of visits for the practice increases to 2,339, as the overall average net revenue per visit decreases to $89.17. In order to maintain the fee for service breakeven level of 2,028, the practice would need to reduce total costs significantly. However, even modest reductions in operating expenses can help to compensate for the downward pressure of capitated contract rates on net revenue. In Scenario 1, total expenses are reduced by 10% through a combination of fixed and variable cost reductions. Scenario 1 is shown in Table 10.2.

As a medical practice shifts back from capitation to better paying fee for service business, it is important to remember two things:

1. Increasing revenue per visit does not mean costs should increase.
2. Maintain enough capitated business to average out the effect of a few high utilizers, or get out of capitation entirely.

MAINTAIN PRACTICE COST SAVINGS

Let's assume that the practice was able to decrease operating expenses by 10%. With the shift to capitated business, the practice's net income is $199,060. What happens

TABLE 10.2   Payer-Mix Scenario 1: Shift to Capitation

	Total Annual w/ No Expense Reductions	Avg per Visit w/ No Expense Reductions	Total Annual w/ Expense Reductions	Avg per Visit w/ Expense Reductions
Patient visits—FFS	3,800		3,800	
Patient visits—capitation	1,000		1,000	
Total net revenue	$428,000	$89.17	$428,000	$89.17
Fixed expenses	$165,000	$34.38	$148,500	$30.94
Variable expenses	$89,400	$18.62	$80,440	$16.76
Total practice expenses	$254,400	$53.00	$228,940	$47.70
Net income	$173,600	$36.17	$199,060	$41.47
Breakeven visits	2,339		2,051	
Contribution to net income after breakeven		$70.55		$72.41

if the practice's business shifts back to fee for service? If the costs revert back to the levels before cost savings were implemented, the practice's net income and breakeven volume are the same as they were originally under the Baseline Scenario. But if the practice is able to maintain the cost savings it experienced, net income increases by $25,460, breakeven volume decreases by 244 visits, and each visit above breakeven contributes $83.24 to the bottom line. This is shown in Table 10.3.

MANAGE THE LEVEL OF CAPITATED BUSINESS

Physicians are paid a fixed amount per member per month to care for capitated patients. Capitation rates paid to the practice are determined actuarially based on demographics of the patient population covered, including their anticipated utilization of resources. When a practice has a significant number of capitated patients, the effects of a few high utilizers are usually offset by the utilization patterns of the rest of the population.

TABLE 10.3   Shift from Capitation to Fee for Service

	With Old Cost Structure	With New Cost Structure
Total visits	4,800	4,800
Net revenue	$480,000	$480,000
Total expenses	$254,400	$228,940
Net income	$225,600	$251,060
Breakeven visits	2,028	1,784
Contribution to net income after breakeven	$81.38	$83.24

TABLE 10.4   Shift from Capitation to Fee for Service

	333 Capitated Patients	50 Capitated Patients	15 Capitated Patients
Capitated patient visits	1,000	220	115
Average visits per capitated patient	3.00	4.40	7.67
Annual capitation revenue	$48,000	$7,200	$2,160
Capitation revenue per visit	$48.00	$32.73	$18.78
Variable expense per visit	$16.76	$16.76	$16.76
Contribution to net income after breakeven	$31.24	$15.97	$2.02

For example, if the average number of visits per year for a capitated patient is three, it is likely that a few patients will have more visits, but that most patients will visit the physician less frequently. In a practice, with a large capitated population, those patients offset the additional use of resources (cost) required to care for the higher utilizers.

Assume the practice's capitated enrollment shifts mostly back to fee for service, so that only 50 capitated patients remain. Ten of those 50 are high utilizers, requiring 10 visits per year. The contribution to net income drops by nearly half, from $31.24 to $15.97. As an extreme example, assume that only 15 capitated patients remain and that 10 of them are high utilizers. The contribution drops to only $2.02 per visit, barely enough to cover variable costs. The impact of this is shown in Table 10.4.

CONCLUSION

Changes in payor mix, to and from capitation, have significant impacts on practice economics. It is important that physicians understand the financial, service responsibility, and administrative terms of payor contracts. It is also important to test the potential financial impact of a shift in payor mix. By applying basic economics described in this chapter, a physician can anticipate and prepare for the changes that are likely to occur.

CHAPTER 11

Cash Flow Analysis and Management

David Edward Marcinko

> Cost reductions have been the focus of many health care providers for years. But in order to successfully fulfill core missions, such as providing effective patient treatment and curing diseases, it is essential that emphasis be placed on cash flow analysis and management.
>
> —Altary, Inc.

T he statement of cash flows (SCF) is the lifeblood of any medical practice. It summarizes the effects of cash on office operating activities during an accounting interval. In periods of rapid growth, as can occur with the acceptance of some managed care contracts, increased revenue actually equates to less cash and potential trouble in terms of practice survival. Therefore, accurate cash flow analysis (CFA) will allow the physician executive to determine the effects of past strategic business decisions in quantitative form. The accurate and proactive nature of this analysis may spell economic success or failure in the competitive health care environment.

PURPOSE OF CASH FLOW ANALYSIS

The primary purpose of CFA is to answer important questions such as how much cash was generated by the practice? How can the office's cash account be overdrawn when the CPA said we were profitable? How much was spent for new equipment and supplies and how was the cash for the expenditures acquired? Most important, the cash-flow statement is then used to review past fiscal decisions and make a predictive leap into the economic future concerning the acceptance of contemporary managed-care contract arrangements. The business tool of CFA will allow the doctor to evaluate revenues and more effortlessly make the translation to fixed reimbursement contractual remuneration and corporate health care.

FINANCIAL ACCOUNTING STATEMENTS

Financial statements report practice activity for a specific accounting period through horizontal or linear analysis. Showing changes in this fashion forms a perspective for variances that have taken place. The three traditional statements are (1) net income statement (NIS), also known as the profit & loss statement, (2) balance sheet (BS), and (3) SCFs. In order to fully understand the significance of cash flow, it is vital to briefly review these two statements in relation to the SCFs.

Net Income Statement

The net income statement (NIS) and the profit and loss (P&L) statement, reflect patient revenues and those medical expenses considered general overhead. The NIS may report physician compensation and benefits as an expense category, during a specified interval or period of time. Smaller practices report income and expenses on a "cash accounting" basis, reflecting income actually received and expenses actually paid. The accrual method of accounting records expenses when they are incurred and income when earned, not when paid or received as in the cash method. The cash method is easier, but the accrual method is more accurate, and most surgical practices use this method. Accrual accounting will increase because of the nature of discounted contracts, capitated contracts, or other fixed reimbursement arrangements. Moreover, for medical groups wanting to switch from the cash method to the accrual method, it is best to make the change after a fiscal calendar quarter. However, accountants may be leery of the shift because they are filing taxes on a cash basis.

Balance Sheet (Statement of Financial Position)

The balance sheet (BS) reports the practice's financial position in terms of its assets, liabilities, and owner's equity in the practice at a specified point in time. Fixed assets are furniture, equipment, and property. Current assets include those that can be converted into cash within a short period of time, such as accounts receivable (AR), checking accounts, and money funds. Intangibles include goodwill. Accounts payable (AP) and current liabilities are short-term debts and notes, while long-term liabilities are loans repaid over many years. The last category reflects ownership in the form of retained earnings or equity and represents the difference between the total assets and total liabilities of the unit.

Statement of Cash Flows

The cash-flow statement is the lifeblood of a medical office because it summarizes the affects of cash on three activities.

- *Operating* activities include cash inflows (receipts, interest, and dividends) and outflows (inventory, supplies, and loans.
- *Investing* activities include the disposal or acquisition of noncurrent assets, such as equipment, loans, or marketable securities.
- *Financial* activities generally include the cash inflow or outflow effects of transactions and other events, such as issuing capital stock or notes involving creditors and physician/owners.

TABLE 11.1   Cash Flow Adjustments

For changes in these current assets and current liabilities:	Make these adjustments to convert accrual basis net income to cash basis net income:	
	ADD	DEDUCT
Accounts Receivable	Decrease	Increase
DME Inventory	Decrease	Increase
PrePaid Expenses	Decrease	Increase
Accounts Payable	Increase	Decrease
Accrued Liabilities	Increase	Decrease

Prior to 1988, the formal SCFs were known as a statement of changes in financial position; they projected estimated cash flows by month, quarter, and year, along with the anticipated timing of cash receipts and disbursements.

A practice's bills and obligations are paid out of cash flow, not net income. Therefore, the direct method of cash flow evaluation deducts from cash revenues only those overhead operating expenses that consume cash. Under this method, each item on the NIS is directly converted to a cash basis. For example, assume that office revenues are stated at $100,000 on an accrual accounting basis. If ARs increased by $5,000, cash collections from patients and third-party insurance companies would be $95,000. All remaining items on the income statement are also converted to a cash basis.

As a general rule, an increase in a current asset (other than cash) decreases cash inflow or increases cash outflow. Thus, when ARs increase, professional service revenues on cash basis decrease. When cast materials, splints, or other DME inventories increase, the cost of goods sold on a cash basis increases (increasing cash outflow). When a prepaid expense, such as malpractice liability insurance, increases, the related operating expense on a cash basis increases. The effect on cash flows is just the opposite for decreases in these other current assets.

Similarly, an increase in a current liability increases cash inflow or decreases cash outflow. Thus, when APs increase, the cost of goods sold on a cash basis decrease. When an accrued liability such as salaries payable increases, the related operating expense on a cash basis decreases. Decreases in current liabilities have just the opposite effect.

Alternately, the *indirect* (add-back) method starts with accrual net income and indirectly adjusts it for items that affect reported net income (accrual) but do not involve cash. For instance, net income is adjusted (rather than adjusting individual items in the income statement) for (1) changes in currents assets (other than cash) and current liabilities, and, (2) items that were included in net income but did not affect cash. The most common example of an expense that does not affect cash is *depreciation*.

The following table can be used to make the adjustments to net income for the changes in current assets and current liabilities.

Notice in the above table that all changes in current assets are handled in a similar manner. Also, all changes in current liabilities are handled the same way, but in the opposite manner from that of current asset changes. In applying the rules, a decrease in a current asset is added to net income and an increase in a current asset is deducted from net income. For current liabilities, increases are added to net income, and decreases are subtracted from net income.

The financial accounting standards board (FASB) encourages the use of the direct method but permits use of the indirect method. Regardless of the method used, the SCF reflects the internal generation of funds available to owners, investors, and creditors to assess the following:

- The practice's ability to generate positive future net cash flows.
- The practice's ability to met its financial obligations.
- The practice's ability to generate profits and dividends.
- The practice's need for external financing.
- Reasons for differences between net income and cash receipts/payments.
- Effects on financial position for both investing and financing transactions.

CASH FLOW IN A MANAGED-CARE EXAMPLE

Given:

Suppose that a medical practice was awarded a managed care contract that increased revenues by $100,000 for the next fiscal year. The practice had a gross margin of 35% that was not expected to change because of the new business. However, $10,000 was added to medical overhead expenses for another assistant and all ARs are paid at the *end* of the year, upon completion of the contract.

Costs of Medical Services Provided

The costs of medical services provided (COMSP) for the managed care organization (MCO) business contract represents the amount of money needed to service the patients provided by the contract. Since gross margin is 35% of revenues, the COMSP is 65%, or $65,000. Adding the extra overhead results in $75,000 of new spending money (cash flow) needed to treat the patients. Therefore, divide the $75,000 total by the number of days the contract extends (one year) and realize the new contract requires about $205.50 per day of free cash flows.

Assumptions

Financial cash flow forecasting from operating activities allows a reasonable projection of future cash needs and enables the doctor to err on the side of fiscal prudence. It is an inexact science, by definition, and entails the following assumptions:

- All income tax, salaries, and APs are paid at once.
- Durable medical equipment inventory and prepaid advertising remain constant.
- Gains/losses on sale of equipment and depreciation expenses remain stable.

- Gross margins remain constant.
- The office is not efficient, so major new marginal costs will not be incurred.

Physician Reactions

Since many physicians are still not entirely comfortable with fixed-price medical payment contracts, practices are loath to turn away business. Physician/executives must then determine other methods to generate the additional cash, which include the following general suggestions:

1. **Extend Accounts Payable**
   Discuss your cash flow difficulties with vendors and emphasize their short-term nature. A doctor and her or his practice still has considerable cachet value, especially in local communities, and many vendors are willing to work with them to retain their business.
2. **Reduce Accounts Receivable**
   According to most cost surveys, about 30% of multispecialty group's ARs are unpaid at 120 days. In addition, multispecialty groups are able to collect on only about 69% of charges. The rest was written off as bad debt expenses or as a result of discounted payments from Medicare and other managed care companies. In a study by Wisconsin-based Zimmerman and Associates, the percentages of ARs unpaid at more than 90 days is now at an all time high of more than 40%. Therefore, multispecialty groups should aim to keep the percentage of ARs unpaid for more than 120 days, down to less than 20% of the total practice. The safest place to be for a single specialty physician is in the 30%–35% range; anything over that is just not affordable.

   The slowest paid specialties (ARs greater than 120 days) are multispecialty group practices, family practices, cardiology groups, anesthesiology groups, and gastroenterologists, respectively. So, work hard to get your money faster.
3. **Borrow with short-term bridge loans**
   Obtain a line of credit from your local bank, credit union, or other private sources. Beware the time value of money, personal loan guarantees, and usurious rates.
4. *Do not* **stop paying withholding taxes in favor of cash flow because it is illegal.**

Hyper-Growth Model

Now, let us again suppose that the practice has attracted nine more similar medical contracts. If we multiply the above example tenfold, the serious nature of potential cash-flow problem becomes apparent.

In other words, the practice has increased revenues to one million dollars, with the same 35% margin, 65% COMSP, and $100,000 increase in operating overhead expenses.

Using identical mathematical calculations, we determine that $750,000 divided by 365 days equals $2,055.00 per day of needed new free cash flows! Hence, indiscriminate growth without careful contract evaluation and cash flow analysis is a prescription for potential financial disaster.

OPERATIONAL METHODS TO INCREASE CASH FLOW

There are other specific strategies to increase medical office cash flow. A few are listed below:

- Post your office collection policy for copays and deductibles so that your patients know that you will require their payment at the time services are rendered. It is also a good idea to have your collection policies on the patient statement so that they have a written copy of your policies with every bill. If your policy states that payment is expected before the visit, be sure that you collect that payment so that your patients know you are serious about reconciling their account.

- Coordinate benefits, since some patients don't immediately pay unless you collect the copay up front. These patients are waiting to see how much their insurance company will pay. While they wait, they are getting billed statements from their health care providers detailing recent submissions. If they do not receive paperwork on a recent visit, many will assume you have not submitted the claim to their insurance carrier and will not pay. A clear, easy-to-use billing statement, providing information that can be compared with insurance payments is a huge first step toward meeting the patient's needs and expectations. Be sure that your account reconciliation for the patient reflects what the insurance company reflects for payment.

- Maintain credentialing files, since a patient may be covered by numerous insurance plans. Because they have seen you many times, changes in their insurance may not prompt them to notify you that their insurance has changed. But what if you are not a member of their new insurance plan or your provider status has expired? How will you know? By maintaining credentials and provider status, you will be aware of an expiring or need for renewal status. In addition, if your client base continues to add insurance carriers, even for secondary payment, you will have contact information for contracting with new insurance carriers to provide services to an even wider range of patients, meaning greater opportunity to expand your practice.

- Create separate accounts, especially in pediatric cases, since typical divorce judgments include provisions that hold both parents equally responsible for the health care bills of their children. Try to gain an understanding of payments from both parents so that the bills for each child are sent to the correct parent and insurance carrier. If your practice continues sending bills to only one of the parents or the wrong insurance carrier, the parent who gets the bill can quickly find an account that is difficult to decipher and quickly becomes past due. The other parent, meanwhile, gets only information that is filtered through their ex-spouse, which can already be past due before an opportunity to reconcile is available.

- Do not wait for patients to be released to the insurer. Invoice all hospital patients daily, or as soon as a procedure is performed within the global surgical period. Realize that payers are constantly shrinking the claim submission time window or filing limits, now often between 31 days and 24 months. And, know your state insurance laws and review all new managed-care contracts to eliminate wording and phrases that give payers more time to hold onto your compensation.

- Reconcile patient visits with claim submissions every day. You may have actually treated 30 patients in your office, but only billed for 29. Audit charts and missing claims. This internal audit control is also a good method to identify and reduce mere accidents, or purposeful fraud. Following a random and individual patient's path of care is another good method to ensure that all charges have been filed.

- Update International Classification of Diseases (ICD-9) codes and use either a certified medical coder, or have the doctor or medical care provider directly provide the procedural code to your insurance staff. Know Medicare policy, rules, and regulations and make sure you have a copy of the most current *Medicare Provider Manual* (www.HCFA.gov). Read the monthly *Medicare News* and understand the *CMS Correct Coding Initiative*. And, review all claims denials, Explanation of Benefits (EOBs), vouchers, and unpaid professional invoices at least biannually to determine aberrant patterns and trends, and then fix them. A practice may lose up to 25% of revenues through improper coding. And, copy both sides of drivers' licenses and insurance cards for coverage verification and personal identification. Update patient contact information, in accordance with the Health Insurance Portability and Accountability Act of 1996 (HIPAA) guidelines, regularly.

- Use electronic claims (e-claims), despite the HIPAA *deminimus* exemptions. Payments are faster, and rejections are noted sooner. Private carriers will require it eventually, and major insurance carriers such as Blue Cross or Blue Shield, and Medicare encourage e-claims submission, since costs are 18% to 63% less than paper claims. The American Medical and Dental Associations report the cost of paper claims processing ranges from $6 to $12 per claim in labor and overhead. This equates to over $300 million per year in potential savings for the health care industry, according to the following segmentation from AmeriScan, Inc.

  - 90% of all corporate memory exists on paper.
  - Of the pages that get handled each day in the average medical office, 90% are merely shuffled.
  - The average document gets copied 19 times.
  - A practice may spend 5% of total filing cost on equipment, 20% on space, and 70% on labor.
  - A four-drawer file cabinet holds 17,000 pages, and it costs $25,000 to fill and $2,000 per year to maintain.
  - Costs to store information:

    - Paper $4.55/mg
    - Computer green-bar paper $2.73/mg
    - Floppy disk $1.25/mg
    - Microfilm $0.76/mg
    - Digital Disk $0.06/mg

  - Companies spend $20 in labor to file a document, $120 in labor to find a misfiled document, and $220 in labor to reproduce a lost document. And, 7.5% of all documents get lost completely.

- As added encouragement for e-claims submission, many insurance carriers have mandated that e-claims be reimbursed as a first priority. As an example, it traditionally takes Medicare about 27 days to review paper claims. Then it takes an additional 14 days to cut a reimbursement check. This totals an excess of 40 days to receive reimbursement for the services that were rendered, assuming the claim was filed correctly, since the AMA also reports an average of 33% of those paper claims submitted contain errors. If there are any problems with the claim, regardless of how minor, the claim is returned to the doctor after the initial review period, and the process begins again. Claims that are submitted electronically to Medicare do not have to go through this 27-day review period. Therefore, reimbursement checks can be cut within 7 to 14 days. If there happened to be a problem with the claim, that claim is returned electronically for correction. Once the claim is corrected, it can be resubmitted with almost no delay. Furthermore, 15% of denied claims are never resubmitted, reducing revenue. By filing claims electronically, expenses can be decreased and cash flow can be accelerated and improved by 20–30 days. But, do not send procedural reports or other attachments unless requested.

ASSESSMENT

The statement of cash flows has been reviewed in order to understand its importance and the potential pitfalls of practice growth in a managed care environment. Known as cash-flow analysis, it is determined using two different methods (direct and indirect). It is an important technique that allows the physician to make proactive business decisions regarding the direction and growth of a practice by reviewing changes in past operating, investing, or financial activities.

If the medical executive becomes skillful at performing this analysis, much can be ascertained about the operational efficiencies of the medical practice.

CONCLUSION

Cash-flow analysis is the comparative norm for all business organizations, and a medical practice is no exception. Having access to the analytic tools needed to derive such information is vital to practice survival. Furthermore, CFA and related economic research will only add value to the services rendered by the modern physician, much to the benefit of patient, doctor, and payer alike.

CHAPTER 12

Medical Office Expense Modeling

David Edward Marcinko

> As managed care, capitation, and cost-based forms of reimbursement continue to develop as the predominant methodologies in health care, the identification, control, and reduction of health care costs (resource consumption) will become increasingly important for all health care entities. The consumer will become a more discerning purchaser of services, the physician must treat the patient in a cost-effective manner while maintaining quality of care, and the hospital must manage the delivery of services to maximize efficiency while minimizing cost. The strategies and processes that are and will be available to accomplish the control and reduction of costs will be numerous, but the foundation for most will be the accuracy and validity of the fully allocated procedural cost data on which decision-support reporting will be based.
>
> —Health care Concepts, Inc.

In today's competitive marketplace, managerial cost accounting is often used to set short- and long-term medical office business policy. The information is used to increase profitability by either decreasing costs, increasing revenues, or decreasing operating assets. More than ever, cost accounting can mean the difference between a successful medical practice or a mediocre one. It consists of five goals:

- Providing vital costing information for internal office use.
- Developing proactive future office strategic plans information.
- Accentuating the relevancy and flexibility of financial data.
- Reviewing real-time service segments rather than just total office operations.
- Acquiring nonfinancial business data.

Cost accounting is not governed by the Financial Accounting Standards Board (FASB) as is a CPA. Rather, a costing expert may be a certified cost accountant (CCA) or certified managerial accountant (CMA), designated by the Cost Accounting Standards Board (CASB), an independent board within the office of management and budget's (OMB) Office of Federal Procurement policy. As such, practitioners are obligated to comply with the cost accounting standards (CAS) promulgated by its federal agencies:

- CAS #501 requires consistency in estimating, accumulating and reporting costs.
- CAS #502 requires consistency in allocating costs incurred for the same purpose.
- CAS #505 requires proper treatment of unallowable costs.
- CAS #506 requires consistency in the periods used for cost accounting.

Again, this is much different from traditional financial accounting that is concerned with providing static historical information to creditors, shareholders, and those outside the private medical practice.

OFFICE COST STRUCTURE AND BEHAVIOR

Cost behavior is the study of how medical office costs change in relation to variations in activity or use. *Kaizen* costing is the continual pursuit of reducing those costs. Medical office costs may be divided into several categories (fixed, variable, mixed, marginal, direct, indirect, and differential, etc.) through a relevant range* as described in the following paragraphs.

Fixed Costs

Fixed costs can be viewed in the aggregate or on a per unit basis, but they always remain constant, period. That is why they are called *fixed*. For example, your office rent doesn't increase if you expand office hours into Saturday or Sunday (see Fig. 12.1).

Total fixed costs are not usually affected by changes in activity (e.g., office rent, taxes, insurance, depreciation, salaries of key personnel). Your rent is still due even if you spend two weeks diving in Aruba and see no patients. A fixed cost remains constant, over the relevant range, even if the activity changes (e.g., a busy summer or a winter slowdown). On the other hand, fixed costs decrease per unit as the activity level rises and increase per unit as the activity level falls. Generally, fixed costs are not altered by decisions or changes in the short term. They remain constant in total amount throughout a wide range of medical office activity, and they vary inversely with activity if expressed on a per-unit, or per-patient, basis.

Example

Assume that a physical-therapy practice dispenses custom-made orthotic devices for various biomechanical conditions. The office rent is fixed over the course of its lease at $9,000 per month. Therefore, the total and per unit rent costs at various levels of orthotic activity would be depicted as follows:

---

*The relevant range is an economic principle that can be defined as the range of office activity within which certain assumptions are neither too high nor too low. These assumptions relate to variable and fixed cost behavior with statistical validity.

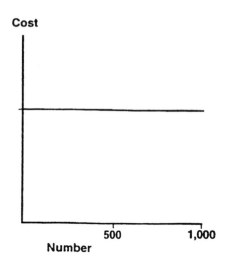

FIGURE 12.1 **A fixed cost remains constant in total amount throughout a wide range of medical office activity.**

TABLE 12.1 **Fixed Rent**

Cost per Month	Number of Devices	Rent Cost Per Device
$9,000	-0-	Fixed
9,000	1	$9,000
9,000	10	900
9,000	100	90
9,000	200	45

The table shows the affects of volume (cost per month and number of devices) on the cost of rent per item. If office hours are begun on Saturday, the cost of the rent is less per device because there are more items to disperse it across. However, the cost per item does increase with the vacation trip.

Variable Costs

Total variable cost increases and decreases in proportion to activity, while per unit variable costs remain constant per unit. In other words, a variable cost changes in total in direct proportion to changes in the level of activity but it is constant on a per-unit basis. Practice costs that are normally variable with respect to volume include durable medical equipment (DME), indirect labor, and indirect materials such as utilities, air conditioning, clerical costs, and other medical supplies. Generally, variable costs change as a direct result of making a decision or altering a course of action (see Fig. 12.2).

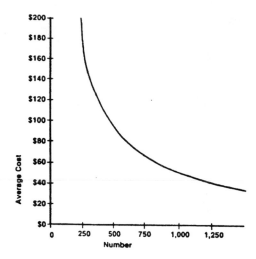

FIGURE 12.2   A fixed cost varies inversely with activity if expressed on a per-unit basis.

TABLE 12.2

Cost Per Splint	Number Splints Dispensed	Total Variable Cost per Splint
$30	1	$30
30	10	300
30	100	3,000
30	200	6,000

Example

The same large physical-therapy practice dispenses a custom-made latex elbow splint for $30 per device. The per unit and total costs of the splints at various levels of activity would be depicted as follows:

Generally, the manufacturing community has embraced the trend toward fixed business costs. Conversely, the medical community is trending toward more variable costs because (1) medicine is a personal-service industry, and (2) movement is toward *locum tenens* and hired physician employment (i.e., nonowner physicians).

Simple Cost Calculations

From the above, we intuitively realize that: Total Costs (TC) = Total Fixed Costs (TFC) plus Total Variable Costs (TVC), or: TC = TFC + TVC.

Furthermore, Total variable costs for a physician group practice can be further equated to TVC = (TVC per visit) × (number of visits). So that: TC = TFC plus {(VC/visit) × (number of visits)}.

And, if given Total Profit = Revenue (Price [P] × Volume [V]) − Costs then Total Profit = (P × V) − (Fixed Costs [FC] plus Variable Costs [VC])

Mixed Costs

A mixed (semivariable) cost is one that contains both fixed and variable elements. Although the definition may change from office to office, consistency is important for cost behavioral purposes. For example, an x-ray unit is leased for $2,500 per year, plus five dollars per sheet of film. In this case, the yearly lease is the fixed element, while the per unit film charge varies depending on use (see Fig. 12.3).

Direct and Indirect Costs

A *direct* cost can be obviously traced from its destination and can specifically be traced to the performance of a procedure. The more procedures done, the higher the direct costs. In a medical office, radiographs, surgical supplies, blood panels, durable medical equipment, and other procedures can be traced to a specific patient, while labor is traced to the office staff. An *indirect* cost must be allocated to general office overhead rather than specifically assigned to the *cost driver* in question. Such expenses as the rent, the mortgage, or the office manager's salary are constant. They have no relationship to frequency of use. Of course, some expenses are *mixed costs* and combine both indirect and direct costs. For example, in analyzing your billing department's costs, the purchase expense of the system would be considered the indirect element, while the cost of electronic medical claims filing would be considered the direct element, as the more claims filed, the greater the expense.

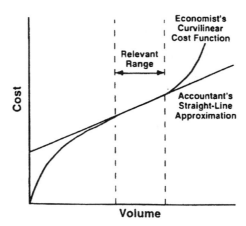

FIGURE 12.3 **The relevant range is an economic principal that can be defined as the range of office activity within which certain assumptions relative to variable and fixed costs behavior are valid.**

Differential Costs

Any cost that is present under one alternative but is absent in whole or part under another alternative is known as a differential cost.

Example

Dr. Lindsay is a chiropractor with a solo office but has been offered a job in a rural medical center. The differential revenue and costs between the two jobs is depicted in Table 12.3.

Controllable Costs

A controllable medical cost occurs at a particular level of the office if the owner physician has the power to authorize the expenses. There is a risk/benefit and time dimension to controllable costs. For example, costs that are controllable over the long run may not be controllable over the short time. In the very long term, however, all costs are variable and controllable.

Opportunity Costs

An opportunity cost is the potential advantage or benefit that is either sacrificed or lost when selecting one course of action over another. It is also known as an *either-or* decision. For example, if Dr. Jones was invited to speak at a local Lion's Club meeting, will the publicity garnered help his reputation enough to compensate for the actual time, and revenue, lost from the office? Some intangible opportunity costs cannot be mathematically calculated.

Interest Rate Costs

Recently, several major banking institutions have addressed the problem of escalating debt upon graduating physicians, midlife practitioners, and even seasoned health

TABLE 12.3

	Office	Medical Center	Differential Cost
Weekly Salary	$900	$1,200	$300
Weekly Expenses:			
Commuting	30	90	60
Lab Coat Rental	-0-	50	50
Food	10	-0-	(10)
Total Weekly Expenses	40	140	100
Net Weekly Income	**$860**	**1,060**	**200**

care providers; despite historically low rates for prime customers. Unfortunately, one may still wonder how many clinicians truly appreciate the risks associated with usurious interest rates for medical equipment and other consumer items. The following review is offered to reduce this peril.

Simple Interest

Simple interest is merely the pro-rata interest on a loan or deposit and represents the most basic interest rate type. For example, for every $100 Dr. Smith borrows at 12% annual interest, he pays 12 dollars per year. The interest is calculated by multiplying the principal, or original amount, by the interest rate in decimal form ($100 \times .12$). The interest remains the same, year after year, until the arrangement is terminated. Unfortunately, simple interest rarely applies to real life since it is usually compounded.

Add-on-Interest

Add-on-interest immediately attaches the annual interest amount to the principal amount at the beginning of the payment period. Payments are then made according to the number of years required. The following formula is useful:

$$\text{Add-on-interest minus payment} = \frac{\text{Total interest on balance}}{\text{Number of payments}}$$

For example, if Dr. Smith borrows $10,000 at 8% add on interest, he will repay $10,000 plus $800 ($10,000 \times 8%$) or $10,800, divided by 12 months, for a total of $900 per month, since $900/month \times 12$ months equals $10,800. This is an expense way to borrow money, but not as expensive as the discounted method discussed below.

Discounted Interest

When using the discounted interest method, the interest amount is deducted from the principal right up front. Notice that this the opposite of add-on-interest, which is applied up front. For example, if Dr. Smith borrows the same $10,000 at a discounted interest rate of 8%, he will only receive a $9,200 loan, since $10,000 − $800 is $9,200. Obviously, the discount method is the most expense way to borrow money and the most profitable way to lend money. Always avoid borrowing money according to this method, if possible.

Annual Percentage Rate

Most financial institutions advertise an annual percentage rates (APR) for loans, deposits, and investments. The APR is the periodic interest rate multiplied by the number of periods a year. If the APR is 12%, and interest is compounded monthly, you receive (or pay) 1% of your balance each month, and the balance shifts with each compounding. If Dr. Smith deposits $100 dollars at 12% APR compounded monthly, he receives $1 interest the first month (1% of $100), $1.10 the second month (1% of $101), and so forth. If compounding is daily, the interest accumulates at the rate of 1/365 of the APR each day. Unless interest is compounded annually, the APR will be lower than the effective annual interest rate, which is discussed in the following section.

Effective Interest Rate

It is important to differentiate between the effective interest rate and the APR, which is often the most prominent figure in advertisements for business equipment, consumer goods, and financial services (loans, annuities, IRAs, CDs, investment analysis, college funding, or retirement planning). Although the APR is the periodic interest rate multiplied by the number of periods per year, the effective annual interest rate is the periodic rate, compounded.

In our case, if the APR is 12% compounded monthly, the monthly interest rate is 1% and the effective annual rate is the monthly rate compounded for 12 periods. Therefore, if your calculation is for a single year, you can treat the effective rate as simple interest. If you deposit (or borrow) $1,000 at 12% APR, the effective rate is 12.68%, and interest for the first year is about $126.80 (12.68% of $1,000). For longer periods, you can use the effective interest rate as the periodic interest rate, compounded annually.

"Rule of 72" (Double Your Money)

The number of periods required to double a lump sum of money can be quickly estimated by using what is known as the Rule of 72. To get the number of periods (usually years), just divide 72 by the periodic interest rate, expressed as a whole number (not a decimal).

For example, if the annual interest rate is 10%, it will take about 7.2 years (72/10) to double any lump cache of money. Conversely, you can also calculate the interest rate required to double your money in a given period by dividing 72 by the term. Thus, to double your money in 10 years, you need to earn about 7.2% annual interest (72/10) = 7.2%). This "quick and dirty" method is mentally performed and is very useful when your stockbroker, bank officer, or spouse calls for a loan or sale. It allows you to determine approximately how much the call will cost.

"Rule of 78"

According to this method, interest is front-end loaded, like a home mortgage, to discourage prepayment of a loan and consequently preserve the lender's profit.

In other words, it is a method of calculating installment-loan interest rebates. The number 78 comes from the 1954 Congress approved method of accelerated tax depreciation, known as the *Sum of the Years Digits* (SOYD) method (i.e., 12 + 11 +

10 + 9 . . . = 78). This fact is important because, throughout the period of a loan, even though the payments are all the same, the portions that are interest and principal are very different. The calculations are very difficult, and lenders use standardized charts or sophisticated computer software to determine rebates.

Using such methods, for example, a one-year loan shows that, in the first payment, 15.38% of the interest due is paid off, and by the sixth month, 73.08% of the interest is paid off. This means that if a doctor make a one-year equipment loan with a total interest charge of $100 and pays the loan off in full with the sixth payment, he or she will not get an interest rebate of $50 but only a rebate of $26.92, since $73.08 of the interest has already been prepaid. Most ethical lenders use simple interest rates for loan rebates, and the Rule of 78 is considered unfair by many authorities. Therefore, it is important to check any loan agreements before you sign if there is a chance you will prepay, in order to avoid this penalty.

"Rule of 116"

A derivative of the Rule of 72 is the Rule of 116. This determines the number of years it takes for a principal amount to be tripled and is calculated by dividing the annual interest rate into 116. The Rules of 72 and 78 are very handy for figuring the amount of interest payments made or growth of funds invested. They can also be used in reverse to calculate at what rate of interest money must be invested to double or triple in a certain number of years.

The "Magic" of Compound Interest

Common to most lending institutions today is compound interest. In this case, the fee for borrowing money includes not only interest on principal, but also interest on interest. The interest is compounded, or added-up, at regular intervals. The actual dollar amount of interest grows more rapidly as the number of compounding periods increases. Obviously, interest charges accrue due much faster using this method. It is the cause of much consumer debt and financial misery in this country. Of course, compound interest is beneficial if you receive the interest, rather than pay it. In fact, Albert Einstein called this almost magical growth of interest, the Eighth Wonder of the World.

Example Scenario

Dr. Jones is about to purchase some short-lived medical office equipment, and the sales representative tells him that the most important financial consideration is the monthly payment (i.e., "keep it as low as possible"). However, Dr. Miller, a friend, suggests the annual percentage rate is a better measurement. Who is correct and what is the cheapest way to borrow the money?

Solution

The salesman wants to close the deal and minimize cash outflow at the expense of increasing and prolonging the debt burden. This is no bargain! Fortunately, Dr.

Jones was given better information by his colleague about the APR, which allows consumers to compare apples to apples when considering interest rate expenses; all else being equal. The annual percentage rate is a federally mandated method of determining the true cost of a loan and is calculated based on time value of money principles. The APR must be disclosed to the consumer under the Consumer Credit Protection Act of 1968. This requirement is also known as the Truth in Lending legislation.

The method is advantageous because, except for simple interest that is almost never used in business, the APR is one of the least expensive ways to borrow money. For example, when we compare the above interest rate methods on a $10,000 loan, compounded monthly at 8%, for one year, we note the following comparisons:

	SIMPLE	ADD-ON	DISCOUNT	RULE 78
APR:	8%	14.77%	16.05%	8%

For more practice, use the above examples to crunch the numbers and satisfy yourself of these figures. Of course, a favorable APR is no bargain if the purchase price is exorbitant. Therefore, shop around for price and quality and don't forget that used but functional office equipment may be the best transaction of all. Remember, it is usually always wise to decrease your operating assets.

Sunk Costs

A sunk cost is an expense that has already been incurred and cannot be changed by any decision, either now or in the future. It is committed and irreversible. For example, the fancy new treatment chair purchased by Dr. Haley, for cash, is a sunk cost. Nothing can be changed since she owns the chair outright.

Relevant Costs

A relevant medical office cost is avoidable as a result of choosing one alternative over another. All costs are considered avoidable, except sunk costs and future costs that do not differ between the alternatives at hand. The physician owner should follow the steps below to identify the costs (and revenues) that are relevant in any costing decision:

- Assemble all of the costs and revenues associated with the alternative.
- Eliminate sunk costs.
- Eliminate those costs and revenues that do not differ between alternatives.
- Make a decision based on the remaining costs and revenues. These are the costs and revenues that are differential or avoidable, and, therefore, they are relevant to the medical-business decision to be made.

Example

Dr. Hartwell, an orthopedic surgeon, is considering replacing an old x-ray processing machine with a new, more efficient and automatic one. Data on the machine is listed below:

New Machine:

List price new $9,000
Annual variable expenses 8,000
Expected life ....5 years

Old machine:

Original cost $7,200
Remaining book value 6,000
Disposal value now 1,500
Annual variable expenses 10,000
Remaining life ....5 years

Dr. Hartwell's office revenues are $200,000 per year, and fixed expenses (other than depreciation) are $70,000 per year. Should the new processing machine be purchased?

Erroneous Solution

Some physicians would not purchase the new machine since disposal of the old machine would apparently result in a loss:

Remaining book value $6,000
Disposal value now 1,500
Loss from disposal 4,500

Correct Solution

The remaining book value of the old machine is a sunk cost that cannot be avoided by Dr. Hartwell. This can be demonstrated by looking at comparative cost and revenue data for the next five years.

FIVE YEARS TOGETHER

	KEEP	PURCHASE	DIFFERENTIAL
Sales	$100,000	$100,000	-0-
Less variable expenses	50,000 (5 × 10k)	40,000 (5 × 8k)	10,000
Less other fixed expenses	35,000	35,000	-0-
Depreciation (new)	-0-	(9,000)	(9,000)
Depreciation (old)/ book value	(6,000)	(6,000)	-0-
Disposal value (old)	-0-	1,500	1,500
Total net income	**9,000**	**11,500**	**2,500**

Using only *relevant costs*, the correct solution would be—

Sales in variable expenses provided by new machine ($2,000 × 5 years) $10,000*
Cost new machine 9,000
Disposal value old machine 1,500

Net advantage new machine **2,500**

* **Note:** $10,000 − 8,000 = $2,000

Economic Order Quantity Costs

Economic order quantity cost (EOQC) is a standard accounting model for minimizing medical business inventory, such as DME costs. The EOQC makes three key assumptions: (1) revenues (inventory depletion) are constant, (2) costs per order are stable, and (3) just-in-time-delivery allows the placement of orders so that new orders arrive when inventory approaches zero.

The mathematical formula for EOQC is the square root of $2SO/C$, where: $S =$ annual sales in units; O is the cost per order; and C is the annual carrying cost per unit.

Example

Suppose that a large urban hospital performs a good deal of orthopedic Surgery and uses 10,000 special self-absorbing bone screws every year. The cost per screw is $200, and the annual inventory carrying cost per screw is $10. According to the formula, the EOQC is 632, the orders per year is 16, and the time between each order is about 3.3 weeks.

Carrying Costs

Represents the cost of maintaining inventory (DME) in your office or storage facility. This cost includes things like rent, utilities, insurance, taxes, employee costs, and also the opportunity cost of having your space or capital tied up in them.

Marginal Costs and Marginal Revenue

Marginal Cost (MC) is the expense incurred to treat one additional unit (patient), while Marginal Revenue (MR) is the revenue received for treating that patient (unit). These two concepts are among the most important in the entire business universe environment of medicine today.

In the office "clinical pathway" or "flow process," we are assuming that extra time remains on the doctor's schedule to see patients, and that an existing financial base exists to cover all fixed costs. This means a managed care contract might be considered if the MR received By treating the patient is greater than the MC (i.e., MR > MC) incurred to treat that patient. Profit (total) will continue to increase up to the point where MR = MC; and then it will decrease as additional costs (more office space, equipment, or assistants) are incurred to accommodate the increased volume.

In other words, maximum office efficiency (MOE) occurs where: MR = MC. Since marginal cost can be thought of as the change in total costs associated with any given change in output quantity(Q), MC can be calculated from the following formula(s):

TABLE 12.4 Example Marginal Cost*

Patient Vol. (A)	(Price) Marg. Rev. (B)	(A × B) Total Rev. (C)	Marginal Cost (D)	Total Cost (E)	(C – E) Total Profit (F)
0	20.1	00.00	NA	50	−50.00
1	20.1	20.10	15	65	−44.90
2	20.1	40.20	10	75	−34.80
3	20.1	60.30	8	83	−22.70
4	20.1	80.40	7	90	−9.60
5	20.1	100.50	6	96	4.45
6	20.1	120.60	4	100	20.60
7	20.1	140.70	4	104	36.70
8	20.1	160.80	6	110	50.80
9	20.1	180.90	10	120	60.90
10	20.1	201.00	12	132	69.00
11	20.1	221.10	16	142	73.10
12	20.1	241.20	20	168	73.20
13	20.1	261.30	22	190	71.30
14	20.1	281.40	25	215	66.40
15	20.1	301.50	30	245	56.50

*Note: Total Costs (column E) are cumulative, derived by adding the marginal cost (D) to the prior total cost figure. This keeps a running total, adding each additional marginal cost to the total cost number.

$$MC = \text{change total costs/change in output quantity, or,}$$
$$MC = \text{change TC/change Q, or,}$$
$$MC = CTC/CQ$$

Note that marginal costs depend only on changes in variable costs. Because fixed costs do not change as output quantity changes, fixed costs don't even influence marginal costs. MC is only influenced by VC.

The goal of such marginal cost and revenue analysis is to treat the appropriate (optimum) number (quantity) of patients, not necessarily the most (maximum) number of patients. This may be contrary to the norm established in the heretofore fee-for-service medical payment environment, but this mindset must be broken to be most efficient in the year 2004 and beyond.

Dr. Jon Hultman, MBA, gives the following examples of how, as a new medical office grows, marginal costs decline. Later, as volume and capacity related inefficiencies begin to occur, marginal costs again increase. Notice, that in the table, marginal costs almost always equal marginal revenue at a patient volume of 12 units, and total profit is the greatest at this point. When volume increases beyond 12 patients however, total revenue increases, but total profit declines.

If the practice were to add patients beyond 12 units, the price (fee) would have to be raised to make the addition of these patients profitable. This cost and volume relationship exists in any mature medical office, and it emphasizes the point that the goal of an efficient office should be profit *optimization*, rather than revenue or volume *maximization*.

Additionally, the point of MOE is where V, per patient fee (PP), and cost per patient (C) produces the most profit (P), not necessarily the most revenue (R). "It

TABLE 12.5   Breakeven Analysis

FC	VC/PP	REV/PP	Volume	Total Costs	Total Revenue	Profit
200-K	$22	$102	2,500	$255,000	$255,000	-0-
200-K	$22	102	3,000	266,000	306,000	40-K
200-K	$22	102	6,000	332,000	612,000	280-K
200-K	$22	102	9,000	398,000	918,000	520-K

is a unique equilibrium efficiency point for each medical practice and individual health care provider."

In terms of managed-care contracting, understanding the dynamics behind these numbers may provide an insight into making informed volume, fee, and profit decisions. Recall that fee pricing and profit are "made at the margins," *and that an office with 60% overhead, for example, does not produce a marginal profit of 40%. Rather, the total profit margin* is 40%, but the *marginal profit* might be only 10% or 15% for each *new* patient visit; and; expense reduction programs will be more effective in increasing profit than in increasing patient volume. Furthermore, consider that if marginal profit for new patient business is 10%, cutting marginal costs by one third (33%) will produce the same profit as would increasing patient volume by almost 300%!

BREAK-EVEN ANALYSIS AND PROFITS

To illustrate the concept of breakeven analysis relative to profit maximization and the costing concepts just discussed, let's use three more modified examples, again given by Dr. Hultman.

Example One

The three doctors of ABC practice own a clinic whose fixed operating costs are $200,000. The average variable cost per patient is $22. The breakeven point (BEP) is reached when revenue and total costs intersect at about 2,500 patients. The variable costs (VC) ($22 × 2,500 = $55,000), plus the fixed costs (FC) ($200,000), equal the total costs of $255,000, which, at the BEP, are equal to the total revenues, resulting in an economically neutral (breakeven) clinical operation, as seen in the spreadsheet following:

Furthermore, it can be appreciated that when volume increases, total profit increases at a faster rate than total costs. This is known as *high* or *positive clinic operating leverage.*

Example Two

Now, if the doctors of ABC clinic accept a discounted managed care contract where the average revenue per patient (REV/PP) declines from $102 to $75, the BEP in-

TABLE 12.6   Leveraged Breakeven Analysis

FC	VC/PP	REV/PP	Volume	Total Costs	Total Revenue	Profit
200k	$22	$75	2,500	$255,000	$187,500	−67,500
200k	$22	75	3,000	266,000	225,000	−41,000
200k	$22	75	3,774	283,000	283,050	22
200k	$22	75	6,000	332,000	450,000	118,000
200k	$22	75	9,000	398,000	675,000	277,000

TABLE 12.7   Nonleveraged Breakeven Analysis

FC	VC/PP	REV/PP	Volume	Total Costs	Total Revenue	Profit
250-K	$22	$75	2,500	$305,000	$187,000	−$67,500
250-K	$22	75	3,000	316,000	225,000	−41,000
250-K	$22	75	4,717	353,774	353,775	1
250-K	$22	75	6,000	382,000	450,000	68,000
250-K	$22	75	9,000	448,000	675,000	227,000

patient volume is now increased to 3,774 patients. At this volume, profit is at $22, and total revenue and total costs are about equal. At 6,000 patients, profit is $118k (77% decline) and at 9,000 patients, profit is at $277k (47% decline). To get an appreciation for the leveraging effect of this decline in price, recognize a price decrease of 26% (from $102 to $75), as seen in the spreadsheet following:

Example Three

The final example for ABC clinic is a very likely scenario under many managed care contracts today. That is to say, a decrease in fees (from $102 to $75), combined with an increase in fixed costs ($250,000) involved in servicing the contract.

At a patient volume of 9,000, profit declines by 56%, along with the salaries of each doctor. If volume dropped to 6,000 patients, profit would decline to 87%. In order to produce the original profit of $520k, volume would have to increase by 61% (14,528 patients), an unlikely scenario. ABC clinic profit, then, will be determined by it's cost position and efficiency in managing a larger volume of patients, along with clinic overhead expenses.

In other words, as long as the revenues received from a medical service is above the variable cost of providing that service, it is said to be making a contribution to fixed costs.

In addition any managed-care contract that is below a practice's variable costs, will lower its profit and should not be considered. Therefore, an aggressive cost reduction program (as described in other chapters), along with more modest patient-volume increases, might be a prudent strategy for the doctors of ABC clinic to pursue.

EQUIPMENT PAYBACK METHOD OF COST ANALYSIS

The payback method (PM) of cost analysis involves making capital budgeting decisions that do not involve discounting cash flows. The PP, expressed in years, is the length of time that it takes for the investment to recoup its initial cost out of the cash receipts its generates. The basic premise is that the quicker the cost of an investment can be recovered, the better the investment is. The PM is most often used when considering equipment whose useful life is short and unpredictable. When the same cash flow occurs every year, the formula is as follows:

Investment required ÷ net annual cash inflow = PP

Example

Dr. Feelgood, a chiropractor, wants to install a new large piece of equipment in place of several smaller modalities in his office. He will need to hire a therapist to administer the larger modality, and he estimates that incremental annual revenues and expenses associated with the equipment would be as follows:

Revenues	$10,000
Less Variable Expenses	3,000
Contribution Margin	7,000
Less Fixed Expenses	
Insurance	900
Salaries	2,600
Depreciation	1,500
	5,000
Net Income	**$2,000**

Parts for the equipment would cost $15,000 and would have a 10-year life. The old machines could now be sold for a $10,000 salvage value. Dr. Feelgood requires a payback of five years or less on all investments.

Net Income (above)	$2,000
Add: Noncash deduction Depreciation	1,500
New Annual Cash Flow	3,500
Investment in the New Equipment	15,000
Deduct: Salvage value old machines	1,000
Investment Required	14,000

Payback Period = $140,000 ÷ $35,000 = 4.0 Years

CONCLUSION

The cost and managerial accounting techniques presented in this chapter are drastically different than what your accountant may tell you, since he or she only reports total or average office cost data to you. While helpful, this general overhead costing information may produce the wrong data to use when making managed-care contracting decisions. And so, an informed practice management consultant might be a more helpful to work with in this case.

CHAPTER 13

Accounting for Mixed Practice Costs

David Edward Marcinko

> Mixed (medical) cost accounting is an activity that provides financial and nonfinancial information to business managers, (physician-executives) and other internal decision makers of an health care organization (e.g., a health care organization).
>
> —Skill-Soft Corporation

As we have seen, medical office business costs may generally be divided into fixed, variable, and mixed (micro) overhead costs. However, the concept of mixed (micro) costs has yet to be fully explored.

A mixed (semivariable) cost is one that contains both fixed and variable elements. For example, a photocopy machine may be leased for $1,500 per year plus 2 cents per copy. In this case, the yearly lease is the fixed element, while the per-unit element copy charge varies depending on use. Although the fixed element versus variable element distinction may become blurred and can change from institution to institution or office to office; definitional consistency is important for mixed-cost tracking purposes.

In another example, a CT scanner to evaluate orthopedic osteomyelitis can be leased for $150,000 per year plus $100 dollars per scan. In this case, the yearly lease is the fixed element, while the per-unit copy charge varies depending on use. To further illustrate, assume that during a particular year the CT scan is used 1,000 times. The cost of the lease will then be $250,000; made up of the $150,000 in fixed cost plus $100,000 (1,000 × $100) in variable costs. Even if the leased CT scan is not used a single time during the year, the hospital will still have to pay the minimum $150,000 charge; but for each time the machine is used, the total cost of leasing it will increase by only 100 dollars. Remember, this is a cost analysis and does not necessarily represent a revenue, charge, or profit analysis.

EVALUATION METHODS

There are two basic methods that can be used to further evaluate mixed office costs: the high-low method and the sum-of-the-squares method.

(1)   The high-low method (HLM) is a cost accounting technique concerned with determining the relative proportion of fixed, variable, and mixed costs associated with an expense. It uses a mathematical formula as a linear equation for determining mixed overhead business costs. The high-low method is particularly suited for certain disease states, such as severe orthopedic infections and significant lower extremity trauma, which require heroic treatment, costly interventions, multidisciplinary resource utilization, and prolonged hospital stays.

(2)   Similarly, the linear-regression analysis (LRA) method for analyzing mixed costs uses a mathematical formula to compute the regression line that minimizes the sum of the squared errors. This method is very precise, and practices are beginning to incorporate it into a cost accounting analysis in order to determine, evaluate, and reduce their own mixed costs. It is increasingly being used in the contemporary health care business setting.

Until recently, neither method has been regularly used in the medical arena. Now however, both are being applied to the in-patient and office settings because of the current insurance crisis. Going forward in time, the knowledge and use of these business management tool by hospitals, clinics, out-patient or ambulatory surgical centers, or the solo physician, will become more important as profit margins erode in the current competitive health care climate.

ANALYSIS OF MIXED COSTS

The concept of mixed (micro) costs is important, since it is common to a wide range of hospital or medical office types. Mixed costs include labor, production, electricity, carrying costs, material handling costs, heat and utilities, repairs, telephone, fax, computer, and many miscellaneous other costs. Of course, an important mixed cost, relative to orthopedic infection admissions, is the operating room (OR).

The fixed portion of a mixed OR cost represents the basic, minimum charge for just having the operating room service ready and available for use on an as needed basis. The variable portion represents the charge made for *actual consumption* or use of the OR room service. As expected, the variable element varies in proportion to the amount of the service that is consumed. Now, for economic planning purposes, the administrator or physician/executive must decide how to allocate mixed costs for the typical infected orthopedic admission.

The ideal approach would be to take each cost invoice as received and break it down into its fixed and variable elements. As a practical matter, even if it were possible to make this type of minute breakdown, the cost of doing so would probably be prohibitive since such tracking and allocation is a very time- and labor-intensive endeavor. Instead, analysis of mixed costs can be done on an aggregate basis, concentrating on the past behavior of a cost at various levels of activity.

HIGH-LOW METHODOLOGY

The HLM of analyzing mixed costs is based on costs observed at both the high and low levels of activity within the relevant range. The difference in costs observed at the two extremes is divided by the change in activity between the extremes in order to determine the amount of variable costs involved. Two examples are illustrated in the following section.

Example 1: High-Low Hospital Admissions

While performing due diligence in contemplation of a fixed price contract, the physician-executive of a large state hospital was required to develop a formula linking the costs involved in treating (medical and surgical) orthopedic infections to the number of patients admitted during a year.

For instance, the admitting department's costs and the number of patients admitted during the immediately preceding eight years are given in the following spreadsheet:

YEAR	NUMBER PATIENTS	HOSPITAL J COSTS
1998	1,800	$14,700
1999	1,900	15,200
2000	1,700	13,700
2001	1,600	14,000
2002	1,500	14,300
2003	1,400	13,100
2004	1,400	12,800
2005	1,100	14,600

CALCULATIONS

The first step in using the HLM is to identify from the above spreadsheet the periods of lowest and highest hospital admission activity. Those periods are the Year 2005 (1,100) and the year 1999 (1,900), respectively.

The second step is to compute the variable costs per unit (patient) using those two points.

YEAR	NUMBER	J COSTS
1999 high level	1,900	$15,200
2005 low level	1,100	12,800
Change observed	**800**	**2,400**

Variable cost = change in cost / change in activity
Variable cost = $2,400 ÷ 800 = $3 per patient admitted

The third step is to compute the fixed cost element (FCE) by deducting the variable cost element from the total cost at either the high or low activity. In the calculation below, the high point of activity is used.

$$\text{Fixed cost element} = \text{total cost} - \text{variable cost element}$$
$$= \$15,200 - (\$3 \times 1900 \text{ patients})$$
$$\text{FCE} = \$9,500$$

From the example given, we see that for every nonelective orthopedic service admission there were $9,500 of fixed costs per patient plus $3 of variable costs. This is noteworthy in that we now discerned this type of admission represents a high-fixed-cost–low-variable-cost service.

The fourth and final step is to combine the variable and fixed elements into a single cost formula, using the standard mathematical equation for a straight line $(Y = a + bX)$, over the relevant range of 1,100 to 1,900 patients.

High-Low Cost Formula Equation Per Orthopedic Admission:
$$Y = \$9{,}500/\text{patient} + \$3X$$

Example 2: High-Low Dental HMO Practice

Dr. Don and Dr. Bill have incurred certain medical office costs, as listed below, while providing dental care to a specific HMO population, during the past eight months.

MONTH	PATIENTS SEEN	J COSTS
January	600	$6,600
February	500	6,500
March	700	7,000
April	900	8,000
May	800	7,600
June	1,000	8,500
July	1,200	10,000
August	1,100	8,700

Analysis of their variable and fixed elements, by the high and low method of semivariable costing, reveals the following:

	PATIENTS SEEN	J COSTS ($)
High activity level	1,200	10,000
Low activity level	500	6,500
Changed observed	700	3,500

Variable rate: change cost ÷ change activity = 3,500 ÷ 700 = $5 ÷ Patient

$$
\begin{aligned}
\textbf{Fixed cost element} \;&=\; \text{Total cost} - \text{variable cost element}\\
&=\; \$10{,}000 - (1{,}200 \text{ patient} \times \$5/\text{patient})\\
&=\; \$4{,}000
\end{aligned}
$$

The cost formula for the HMO is a realistic:
$$
\begin{aligned}
Y &= a + bX\\
Y &= \$40{,}000 + \$5X
\end{aligned}
$$

where: a = fixed cost
b = variable cost rate
X = activity measurement (patients)
Y = total mixed costs

Unfortunately, the high-low method of mixed costing suffers from two major problems: (1) just two points are not enough to produce accurate results, and (2) the volume periods are often unusual. For a strictly controlled staff model HMO contract or for a deeply discounted medical provider with razor thin margins, it may just not be accurate enough for long-term use. Therefore, regression analysis may be used for more accuracy.

LINEAR REGRESSION ANALYSIS

Now, when considering a capitated or other fixed reimbursement medical contract, the practitioner, administrator, or physician executive must also decide how to allocate mixed costs for his or her facility. The ideal approach would again be to take each cost invoice as received and break it down into its fixed and variable elements. As a practical matter, even if it were possible to make this type of minute breakdown, the cost of doing so would, again, be prohibitive.

Instead, an analysis of mixed costs can be done on an aggregate basis, concentrating on the past behavior of a cost at various levels of activity. If this analysis is done carefully, good approximations of the fixed and variable elements can be obtained with little effort.

The result is known as a *linear regression analysis line,* and it merely represents a line of averages. If graphed visually, the average variable cost-per-unit of activity would be represented by the slope of the line, and the average total fixed costs would be represented by a point where the regression line intersects the cost axis. Considering the economic analysis of cost behavior, the least squares linear regression technique is useful for calculating the mixed cost portion of a fixed price (capitated) contract typically offered as reimbursement today

REGRESSION METHODOLOGY

The least squares method for estimating a linear relationship is based on the equation for a straight line: $Y = a + bX$.

The estimates of the vertical intercept (a) and slope (b), which minimizes the sum of the squared errors, are obtained by solving the following two simultaneous equations:

$$SUM\ XY = a\ SUM\ X + b\ SUM\ X^2$$
$$SUM\ Y = na + b\ SUM\ X$$

where:
X = independent variable (activity level)
Y = dependent variable (total mixed cost)
a = vertical line intercept (total fixed cost)
b = slope of Line (variable rate)
n = number of observations
SUM = sum across all n observations

The solution then involves four steps:

$$2$$

Step 1: Compute SUM X, SUM Y, SUM XY, SUM X, and n.
Step 2: Insert values of Step 1 into the simultaneous equations.
Step 3: Solve simultaneous equations for the variable cost rate (b).
Step 4: Solve one of the equations for the total fixed cost (a).

Example 1: Linear Regression

The executive of a large psychology group is interested in determining the relationship between material costs per patient and the number of patients treated. The goal is to keep material (variable) costs to a minimum, in this doctor (PhD) and time-intensive specialty. Located in an upscale neighborhood, the office has very high fixed costs; it is well appointed with antiques in a luxurious office complex.

The information is needed before the office can elect or reject its first all-risk managed care organization (MCO) contract.

To illustrate, assume material costs have been observed for the past seven years, as follows, within the relevant range of 5,000 to 8,000 patients per year.

Step one: Compute SUM X, SUM Y, SUM XY, SUM X squared, and n.

YEAR	(Cost Driver) PATIENTS (X)	J COSTS (Y)	(XY)	(X)
First	5,600	$7,900	$44,240,000	31,360,000
Second	7,100	8,500	60,350,000	50,410,000
Third	5,000	7,400	37,000,000	25,000,000
Fourth	6,500	8,200	53,300,000	42,250,000
Fifth	7,300	9,100	66,430,000	53,290,000
Sixth	8,000	9,800	78,400,000	64,000,000
Seventh	6,200	7,800	48,360,000	38,440,000
SUM Totals:	45,700	$58,700	$388,080,000	304,750,000

CALCULATIONS

From the above spreadsheet:

SUM X = 45,700
SUM Y = $58,700
SUM XY = $388,080,000
SUM X (squared) = 304,750,000

Step two: Insert the values computed in step one into the simultaneous equations. Substituting these amounts into the two equations given above yields the following:

(1)   SUM $XY = a$ SUM $X + b$ SUM X squared
(2)   SUM $Y = na + b$ SUM X

$388,080,000 = 45,700a + 304,750,000b$
$58,700 = 7\ a + 45,\ 700b$

Step three: Solve the simultaneous equations for the variable cost rate (b).

To solve the equations for (*a*) and (*b*), it is necessary to eliminate one of the terms. A term can be eliminated by: multiplying equation (1) times 7, multiplying equation (2) by 45,700, and then subtracting equation (2) from equation (1). The steps are—

Multiply equation (1) by 7:	$2,716,560,000 = 319,900a + 2,133,250,000b$
Multiply equation (2) by 45,700:	$2,682,590,000 = 319,900a + 2,088,490,000b$
Subtract (2) from (1):	$33,970,000 = 44,760,000b$
Divide by 44,760,000	**$0.759 = b**

Therefore, the variable material cost is 75.9 cents per patient.

Step four: Solve one of the equations for the total fixed cost (*a*).

The fixed cost can be computed by substituting the variable cost rate (*b*) just obtained into either equation (1) or (2). Then use equation (2) since the numbers are smaller and easier to calculate.

$58,700 = 7a + 45,700b$
$58,700 = 7a + 45,700 \times 0.759
$58,700 = 7a + $34,686$
$24,014 = 7a$
$3,431 = a$

Therefore, the fixed cost is $3,431 per year/patient and the formula for the material (variable) cost is

$$Y = a + bX$$
$$Y = $3,431 + $0.759X$$

Linear regression analysis material cost formula for office business unit:

$$Y = $3,431 \text{ per year} + 76 \text{ cents per patient}$$

Obviously, in this example, a fixed cost reduction program directed at reducing the recurring portion of practice overhead (large and fixed) might seem more prudent than the medical executive's original erroneous assumption of its material (minute and variable) costs!

Example 2: Linear Regression

In this real-life example, the Olympic Podiatry Group in Atlanta owns an outpatient surgical center. It is interested in the relationship between the center's surgical costs for a solitary hallux valgus bunion repair and the number of patients treated in its first MCO contract for the surgical center. Data is given below:

MONTH	SURGERIES (X)	COSTS $ (Y)	(XY)	(Y SQUARED)
JANUARY	4	$9,500	38,000	16
FEBRUARY	1	4,000	4,000	1
MARCH	3	8,000	24,000	9
APRIL	5	10,000	50,000	25
MAY	10	19,500	195,000	100
JUNE	7	14,000	98,000	49
Totals:	**30**	**$65,000**	**$409,000**	**200**

CALCULATIONS

(1) SUM $XY = a$ SUM $X + b$ SUM X squared $409,000 = 30a + 200b$

(2) SUM $Y = na + b$ SUM X $65,000 = 6a + 30b$

(1) $409,000 = 30a + 200b$

(2) Multiple by 5: $325,000 = 30a + 150b$

    Subtract (2) from (1): $84,000 = 50b$

    Divide by 50: $1,680 = b$

Therefore, the variable rate is $1,680 per bunion repair, or $1,680 per case.

Substitute in Equation (2): $\$65,000 = 6a + 30\,(1,680)$

    $65,000 = 6a + 50,400$

Subtract 50,400 $14,600 = 6a$

Divide by 6 $\mathbf{2,433} = a$ (rounded)

The linear regression cost formula is **Y = $2,433 per month + $1,680 per case.**

MIXED COST ASSESSMENT

The high-low method of mixed cost evaluation may not be as precise as linear regression analysis, but it is easy to perform and track. It may even be the method of choice for many medical offices; since the law of diminishing returns may preclude further cost element differentiation by using more sophisticated regression techniques.

On the other hand, for costlier and more time-consuming regression analysis to be meaningful, the relationship between the independent (X) and dependent (Y) variables must be linear. In many situations a series of data does not plot a straight line. If you graph either X or Y at an increase by 20% a year, for example, the plotted data points will be a curve, and the regression analysis will not be valid. You can, however, use data regression analysis with more than one independent variable. This is called *multiple regression analysis,* and spreadsheets are ideal for these calculations. In fact, with most computer programs, as many as 16 independent variables with as many as 8,192 data points can be used. However, the number must be the same for all, and, while with more than two variables you can't describe the results geometrically, the relationship between each independent and dependent variable must still be linear.

CASE MODEL: MIXED COSTING AT THE VETERAN'S ADMINISTRATION

Because the Veteran's Administration (VA) does not routinely prepare patient bills, VA researchers and analysts at the Health Economic Research Center (HERC) must rely on other sources to calculate the cost of patient encounters (*www.herc. research.med.va.gov*). Three cost accounting alternatives are available: mixed (micro) cost methods (MCM), average cost methods (ACM), and decision support systems (DSS).

Mixed (micro) cost methods. Mixed Cost Methods include three approaches: direct measurement, preparation of pseudo bills, and estimation of cost function.

- *Direct Measurement.* Direct measurement is used to determine the cost of new interventions and programs unique to the VA. Inputs such as staff time and supply costs are directly measured to develop a precise cost estimate. The time of each type of staff is estimated and its cost determined from accounting data. The analyst may directly observe staff time, have staff keep diaries of their activities, or survey managers. The cost of supplies, equipment, and other expenses must also be determined. Program volume is determined from administrative records, and average cost is estimated. When units of service are not homogenous, unit costs may be estimated by an accounting approach, by applying estimates of the relative cost of each service, or via an econometric approach.
- *Pseudo Bill.* The pseudo-bill method combines VA utilization data with unit costs from non-VA sources to estimate the cost of patient care. This is commonly referred to as the pseudo-bill method, because the itemized list of costs is analogous to a fee-for-service hospital bill. The unit cost of each item may be estimated by using Medicare reimbursement rates, the charge rates of an affiliated university medical center, or some other non-VA sector source.
- *Cost Function.* The cost function method requires detailed cost and utilization data for a specific, non-VA service to simulate the cost of a comparable VA service. If suitable non-VA data are available, a function can be estimated using cost-adjusted charges as the dependent variable and information about the encounter as the independent variable. VA costs are simulated using VA utilization data and the function's parameters. Its chief advantage is that it requires less data than is needed to prepare a pseudo bill, making it a more economical way of (micro) mixed costing.

Average cost methods. This method combines relative values derived from non-VA cost datasets, VA utilization data, and department costs obtained from the VA cost distribution report (CDR). Every encounter with the same characteristics is assumed to cost the same. Average cost estimates are needed because detailed mixed-costing is too time-consuming and laborious a method to apply it to all possible health care utilization. In many studies, and for some of the health care utilization in nearly every study, an "average cost method" can be used.

Decision support systems. Researchers are beginning to use the decision support system (DSS), a computerized cost-allocation system adopted by VA. DSS staff is undertaking the difficult task of allocating costs to VA health care products and patients' stays. If DSS is found to be accurate, it will be an extremely useful source of VA cost information. Validation is an important step in the use of DSS data. Work with DSS to date suggests that analysts should not rely exclusively on DSS cost estimates.

Which Costing Method Is Best?

The best cost accounting method to use depends on the level of accuracy required. Micro or mixed-costing methods are accurate but expensive to employ. Average cost methods are easier to undertake, but the cost estimate may not fully reflect how the intervention affects the resources used in providing care. In fact, it is often appropriate to use mixed methodologies in the same study. Usually, one uses a mixed-cost method to estimate the cost of care associated with an intervention or the issue under study and a simpler average cost method to find the cost of other unrelated care.

The physician/executive or analyst must consider whether the assumptions used to create average cost estimates are appropriate to all utilization within the study; for example, whether the intervention might affect the cost of hospital stays in a way that will not be captured by the diagnostic related group (DRG) or length of stay, or whether it will effect the cost of ambulatory visits in a way that will not be captured by the relative value units associated with current procedural terminology (CPT) codes.

Estimates of outpatient costs based on average cost methods do not reflect the cost of laboratory tests or prescriptions pharmaceuticals. An analyst who needs an estimate that reflects this type of utilization must turn to mixed-costing. Orders for laboratory tests must be extracted from the VA system, and information on filled prescriptions must be obtained from VA or the pharmacy benefits management system.

And so, as in most business expense modeling scenarios, the correct answer is: It all depends!

CONCLUSION

In today's competitive marketplace, the high-low methodology or linear-regression analysis may be used to set medical practice business policy regarding mixed overhead business costs. The information is then used to increase profitability by adjusting either the fixed or variable portion of each mixed costs. More than ever, these costing techniques can mean the difference between a successful medical practice, clinic, or hospital, and a nonexistent one.

READINGS

Marcinko, D. E. (2003). Adapted from *Business decision making in medical practice: Financial planning for physicians and healthcare professionals*. New York: Aspen Publishers.

CHAPTER 14

Medical-Activity–Based Cost Management

David Edward Marcinko

Activity Based Cost Management (ABCM) is a systematic, cause and effect method of assigning the cost of activities to products, (medical) services, customers (patients) or any cost object. ABCM is based on the principle that products or (medical) services consume activities. Traditional cost systems allocate costs based on direct labor, material cost, revenue or other simplistic methods. As a result, traditional systems tend to over-cost high volume products, (medical) services and customers (patients) and under-cost low volume.

—Tom Pryor
President, ICMS, Inc.

A stute physician/executives are becoming aware of the need to demonstrate the cost effectiveness of medical care since this can be an important competitive advantage over other providers. Whether this scenario occurs in the office, emergency, room or hospital setting, hard numerical business information is required. Such information may be obtained by using the managerial accounting tools known as: activity based cost management (ABCM) and the clinical (critical) path method (CPM). Here's how.

In the traditional financial accounting practice system, costs are assigned to different procedures or services based on average volume (quantity). So, if a general surgical service is doing a higher volume of surgical procedures than of primary care services more indirect overhead costs will be allocated to the surgical portion of the practice.

ABCM and CPM, on the other hand, determine the actual costs of resources that each service or procedure consumes. But, because primary care actually requires more service resources than surgery, ABCM will assign more costs to the medial (low volume) practice.

The idea is to get a handle on how much every task costs by factoring in the labor, technology, and office space to complete it. In this way, the next time a discounted managed-care contract is offered, or your medical office or hospital department is over budget, you will know how to accept or reject the contract or to solve the variance problem.

THE MEDICAL CRITICAL (CLINICAL) PATH METHOD

An activity is any event or service that is a cost driver. To "activity cost" any critical or clinical medical pathway, five steps are used:

1. Identify key transactions.
2. Identify the time and resources required for each step.
3. Define noneconomically valued activities.
4. Note office operational inefficiencies.
5. Determine the cost of each resource.

Examples of several specific medical office activities that are cost drivers include the following:

- Surgery set-ups
- Vital sign checks
- Cast changes
- x-ray processing
- Taking radiographs
- Blood test runs
- Records requests
- Insurance verifications
- Referral orders

ABCM improves managerial accounting systems and flow process reengineering in three ways:

1. It increases the number of cost pools (expenses) used to accumulate general overhead office costs. Rather than accumulate overhead costs in a single office wide pool, costs are accumulated by activity, service, or procedure.
2. It changes the base used to assign general overhead costs to services or patients. Rather than assigning costs on the basis of a measure of volume (employee or doctor hours), costs are assigned on the basis of medical services or activities that generated those costs.
3. It changes the nature of many overhead costs in that those formerly considered indirect are now traced to specific activities or services. The office service mix of procedures (Current Procedural Terminology codes) may then be adjusted accordingly, for additional profit.

In general, the most important end result of ABCM is the shift of general overhead costs from high volume services to low volume services.

ABCM/CPM IN THE EMERGENCY-ROOM SETTING

According to a CNN report of May 8, 2001, the "U.S. nursing shortage is going into crisis." But based on an ABCM analysis performed by the firm Integrated Cost Management Systems, Inc., of Arlington, Texas, there was no real shortage of nurses at a local St. Paul, Minnesota, hospital emergency room. Instead, there were too many nonmedical activities assigned to nurses. And managers experiencing a nursing shortage, with related P&L losses, turned to ABCM and the CPM for the solution.

Case Study: St. Paul Emergency Room

Upon CPM evaluation, it was discovered that about half of all activities performed at the St. Paul hospital emergency room by nurses and emergency room (ER) staff, were previously done by materials management, maintenance, admissions, or housekeeping employees. But, the work was not visible in traditional budget reports. On the other hand, ABCM analysis made both the work and the worker visible. ABCM helped the ER administrator eliminate non–value-added overhead activities, redeploy nonmedical activities from nurses to lower cost employees, improve nurse morale, improve processes, and much more (Figure 14.1).

Intuitively, it was obvious that increased overtime, or the importing of nurses from other countries, did not address the root cause of impending nurse shortages. ER managers benefited by using ABCM as a diagnostic tool to fully understand departmental concerns.

ABCM/CPM IN THE PRIVATE OFFICE SETTING

Dr. Smith works in a large medical group consisting of 25 healthcare practitioners. In the aggregate, they render 4,000 office visits to the patients from XYZ-MCO and 20,000 visits to patients from the UVW-MCO, each year. Each doctor averages 40 hours per week and dispenses various pieces of durable medical equipment (DME) to their elderly patient population. The office currently uses doctor hours (DH) to assign general overhead costs to medical services rendered. The predetermined (given) overhead rate follows:

$$\frac{\text{Office overhead costs}}{\text{Doctor labor hours}} = \frac{\$900,000 \text{ (given)}}{50,000*} = \$18/\text{DH}$$
$$*(25 \text{ docs} \times 40\text{hr/wk} \times 50 \text{ w/yr})$$

Traditional View		ABM View	
Emergency Room		**Emergency Room**	
Salary & Fringes	$1,460,000	Treat Patient	$1,250,000
Space	150,000	Resolve Problems	180,000
Depreciation	350,000	Do Paperwork	177,000
Supplies	330,000	Procure Supplies	348,000
Other	210,000	Expedite Supplies	177,000
		Do Housekeeping	368,000
	$2,500,000		$2,500,000

FIGURE 14.1 Traditional costing versus activity based costing methods.
Source: ICMS, Inc.

MCO-XYZ requires 2.5 DLH and MCO-UVW requires 2.0 DLH. According to a traditional general overhead cost system, the costs to treat one patient in each MCO is determined in Table 14.1.

Now, for simplicity, let's suppose that office overhead costs are actually composed of the five activities listed in Table 14.2.

Let us also assume that the below transactional data was collected by the medical office manager in Table 14.3.

These data can be used to develop general overhead rates for each of the five activities in Table 14.4.

The general office overhead rates can now be used to assign overhead costs to the respective services, in the following assigned overhead cost manner (Table 14.5A).

TABLE 14.1   Traditional Cost Method

	XYZ	UVW
Direct materials	$36.00	$30.00
Direct labor	17.50	14.00
General office overhead		
2.5 DLH × 18/DLH	45.00	
2.0 DLH × 18/DLH		36.00
Total Cost Per Patient	$98.50	$80.00

TABLE 14.2   Actual Activity Costs

CPM ACTIVITY	TRACEABLE COST ($)
Cast changes	$255,000
Radiographs	$160,000
Blood panels	$81,000
Dressings	$314,000
DME	$90,000
Total	$900,000

TABLE 14.3   Transactional Activity Costs Data

ACTIVITY	NUMBER OF EVENTS TOTAL	(XYZ)	(UVW)
Cast changes	5,000	3,000	2,000
Radiographs	8,000	5,000	3,000
Blood panels	600	200	400
Dressings	40,000	12,000	28,000
DME	750	150	600

TABLE 14.4   Overhead Rates

ACTIVITY	COSTS	TRANSACTIONS	RATE PER TRANSACTION
Cast changes	$255,000	5,000	$51 / change
Radiographs	160,000	8,000	20 / x-ray plate
Blood panels	81,000	600	135 / panel
Dressings	314,000	40,000	7.85 / bandage
DME	90,000	750	120 / DME

TABLE 14.5-A   Assigned Overhead Costs

XYZ-MCO ACTIVITY	RATE	TRANSACTIONS	AMOUNT
Cast changes	$51	3,000	153,000
Radiographs	20	5,000	100,000
Blood panels	135	200	27,000
Dressings	7.85	12,000	94,200
DME	120	150	18,000
Total overhead (*a*)			$392,200
Number units (*b*)			4,000
Overhead per unit (*a/b*)			$98.05

Medical service and product costs using the two different methods can now be contrasted, as follows in Table 14.5B.

Again, these spreadsheets demonstrate that the per-unit costs of the low-volume services increase and the per-unit costs of the high volume services decrease. These effects are not symmetrical, as there is a bigger dollar effect on the per-unit costs of the low-volume service (Table 14.6-A and Table 14.6-B).

TABLE 14.5-B   Assigned Overhead Costs

UVW-MCO ACTIVITY	RATE	TRANSACTIONS	AMOUNT
Cast changes	$51	2,000	102,000
Radiographs	20	3,000	60,000
Blood panels	135	400	54,000
Dressings	7.85	28,000	219,800
DME	120	600	72,000
Total overhead (a)			$507,800
Number units (b)			20,000
Overhead per unit (*a/b*)			$25.39

TABLE 14.6-A   Costs Using Activity Based Costing (ABC) Methodology

	XYZ-MCO	UVW-MCO
Durable Equipment	$36.00	30.00
Doctor Hours:	17.50	14.00
Office Overhead:	98.05	69.39
Total Cost per Unit:	151.55	69.39

TABLE 14.6-B   Costs Using Traditional Accounting Methodology

	XYZ-MCO	UVW-MCO
Durable Equipment:	$36.00	30.00
Doctor Hours:	17.50	14.00
Office Overhead:	45.00	36.00
Total Cost per Unit:	98.50	80.00

About ABCM and CPM

ABCM is not a new concept; it was born in the 1880s as manufacturers tried to get a handle on unit costs of production. For example, if a company built wagons, they could divide their total costs by the number of wagons to figure out how much it cost to build each one. But they couldn't use that formula if they built wagons of different size. So producers began to use direct labor, materials, and overhead to calculate ABC, as described earlier. By the 1970s, medicine was heavily skewed toward labor and technology costs making it more applicable to economic service sectors like medicine.

The CPM, on the other hand, is a concept that was originally developed by the DuPont Corp. as a system of project management in the late 1950s. Today, it is embraced by the health care system as a way to use deterministic time estimates to control the costs of medical care. In the CPM, medical activities can be *crashed* (expedited) at extra cost, deemed *critical* if unable to be delayed, or *slacked* if a moderate delay would not adversely affect patient care. Since, ABCM determines the actual costs of resources rendered for each medical activity, it is a defacto measure of profitability. To activity cost any medical office activity path,

- identify the key steps and individuals involved,
- interview staff and clinicians about the time or resources involved in each step,
- define nonclinical activities associated with patient care,
- define and assess possible efficiencies, and
- ask each caregiver to define the costs of each resource he or she applies to the pathways.

Then, *crunch the numbers* as presented above and be surprised at how low-volume medical costs increase and high-volume costs decrease. *In fact, medical practices still using traditional cost accounting systems will be clueless about the financial effectiveness of their care going forward.*

The Practice Expense Coalition

Recently, the Practice Expense Coalition (PEC) suggested to the Health Care Finance Association (HCFA), now Center for Medicare and Medicaid Services (CMS) that it produce a wide-ranging ABCM project to validate or disprove Medicare practice expense reimbursement fees. Specialties, such as gastroenterology, neurosurgery, thoracic surgery, and cardiac surgery, were especially interested. This occurred because physicians argued that HCFA uses inaccurate cost information to set practice-expense rates under Medicare guidelines. Surgeons and procedurally based practitioners were especially worried that greater emphasis on a resource based relative value system (RBRVS) would reduce their reimbursements. And, according to HCFA, some selected specialties will be affected by evolving resource based practice expense rules. Fortunately, a March 1, 2003, revision corrected a previously scheduled 4.4% negative update and implemented a positive 1.6% update, overall.

Meanwhile, organizations like the American Society of Cataract and Refractive Surgery (ASCRS), the American Academy of Orthopedic Surgeons (AAOS), and the American Podiatric Medical Association often use their own costing studies. DePaul University accounting professor Dr. Gary Siegel is a leader of this new movement.

"Risk Adjusters" in ABCM

Traditionally, physician payment risk adjusters focused on variables such as gender, age, and geography to predict an individual's health care cost variability at any given time. Such methods needed only to successfully explain 15–20% of all variation in order to adequately reflect selection; and/or predict 10% of healthcare claims variability on a prospective basis, and/or 33% variability on a retrospective basis, to be considered successful 4% of the time. Hence, accounting research has focused on ways to segment these variations in order to enhance the use of ABCM in medical practice and augment profitability. These newer methods use retrospective ICD-9 code utilization rates to indicate prospective healthcare needs for either an individual or cohort. Although methods differ as whether to a highest cost or multiple cost diagnosis should be used, as group size increases, costs trend toward the average regardless of the factors selected.

Thus, when considering diagnosis based "risk adjusters" with any capitated managed-care plan, the size of plan, its stop-loss arrangements, and sound medical management are the key to financial success, since higher cost patients typically require greater medical skills to manage successfully,

Medical Practice Cost Analysis with ABCM, CPM, RBRVs, and Relative Value Units (RVUs)

In actuality, using ABCM as described above is a difficult and cumbersome task at best. Still, you must know your office costs to treat patients and perform medical services and procedures.

An excellent way to do this is to perform a medical practice cost analysis (MPCA) for your practice and specialty, since it assigns the total costs of operating a practice to the various CPT codes and services you provide (Table 14.7). To measure such productivity, the Medicare resource based relative value scale system (RBRVS) sets benchmarks for the various procedures that may be used. In January 2000, this system originally served as a starting point for RVUs, which included the following:

- Physician's work component (PWC) for time, intensity and procedural effort (54%).
- Practice expense component (PEC) for equipment, rent, supplies, utilities, and general overhead (41%) with a geographic practice cost-index component (GPCIC).
- Malpractice liability insurance component (PLIC) for malpractice expenses (5%).

Each component was assigned a relative value unit, adjusted for local cost differences, and then multiplied by a conversion factor that translated them into dollars. The formula used to calculate payment rates is

$$(PW\ RVU + PE\ RVU + PLI\ RVU) \times \text{conversion factor}$$

Example

CPT code 27130 (total hip replacement arthroplasty) has a physician work relative value of 20.12, a practice expense relative value of 13.58, and a professional liability relative value of 2.82. The current conversion factor is $36.78. By including practice expenses in the mix, the incentive to perform equipment orientated procedures is reduced. Thus, the 2003 payment for a hip replacement was

$$(20.12 + 13.58 + 2.82) \times \$36.78 = \$1,343$$

TABLE 14.7   Aggregate Work RVUs per Physician Specialty per Year

SPECIALTY	Single Specialty Group Practices	Multi Specialty Group Practices
Allergy/immunology	—	3,677
Cardiology: Invasive	7,608	7,464
Cardiology: Noninvasive	5,475	6,530
Family practice (without OB)	4,091	3,749
Internal medicine	3,864	3,814
Obstetrics/gynecology	7,927	6,140
Pediatrics*	4,561	3,982
General surgery	9,497	6,042

Data source: Medical Group Management Association Physician Compensation and Production Survey: 2001 Report Based on 2000 Data © 2001
*"Pediatrics" excludes subspecialty pediatrics such as pulmonology, neurology, gastroenterology, and endocrinology.

Additionally, as the system evolves, pay and performance become even more closely linked, with about 10% of projected revenues at risk for so-called citizenship fees of administrative duties, cost efficiency, and quality measures. This allows the doctor to determine if the reimbursement for each service is enough to cover the cost of providing it. In other words, it will allow you to decide whether to participate in a certain discounted managed-care plan or if incurring the costs of more labor is justified.

To conduct a MPCA, the following information is needed.

Procedure code (CPT) frequency data, for your specialty or office for the prior 12–18 months. (Sample spreadsheet with projected utilization costs for 5,000 members).

CPT Code	Cost by Component	Projected Utilization	Projected Cost
Totals	Historical Data	Historical Data	$60,000.00

Per Member/Per Month Calculation

Total Costs divided by 5,000 members divided by 12 Months = $1.00 PMPM

1. Office Financial statements for the prior 12–18 months.
2. Medicare Fee Schedule for your medical specialty.
3. Computer spreadsheet, such as Microsoft Excel-TM.
4. Categorization all office expenses as *direct* or *indirect*.
5. Determine the best standard of measurement to assign costs to each work activity in the office (i.e., time, number of procedures or patients, or assigned Relative value units). The RVU system works best for most doctors. Data is available from the *U.S. Federal Registry.*
6. Separate the RVU of each CPT code into its component parts (physician labor component, practice expense component, and malpractice liability risk component).
7. List all CPT codes or the ones used most frequently, as demonstrated in the spreadsheet table below.

Now, according to ABCM methodology, divide total direct and indirect costs by the correct RVU component, as shown in the following chart, which will allow you to calculate the cost of one unit of the CPT activity.

Next, unit costs are multiplied by the appropriate work expense and liability component RVUs in order to arrive at a total unit cost per procedure, as seen in Table 14.8.

Finally, the results are added to the cost drivers, other than RVUs, such as the number of patient encounters, as seen in the table following.

The results are then benchmarked to determine reasonableness and compared with the HMO's fee schedule. The contract is then accepted, rejected, or renegotiated based on its fiscal merits. Alternatively, spreadsheet parameters can be changed and various *what if* scenarios can be manipulated in mere seconds.

TABLE 14.8 Sample Spreadsheet with Projected Utilization Costs for 5,000 Members

A	B	C	D (B×C)	E	F (B×E)	G	H (B×G)
CPT Code	Frequency (Number)	Work RVU[1]	Total Practice Work RVU	Practice Exp. Exp. RVU[1]	Total Practice Exp. RVU	Liability RVU[1]	Total Office Liability RVU
11111	115	0.91	105	0.40	46	0.04	5
22222	44	0.43	19	0.37	16	0.03	1
33333	59	0.32	19	0.32	19	0.03	2
44444	285	0.23	66	0.23	66	0.02	6
55555	528	1.13	597	0.45	238	0.04	21
66666	788	1.66	1,308	2.10	1,655	0.19	150
77777	445	4.39	1,954	4.11	1.829	0.37	165
88888	2,216	4.41	9,773	4.37	9.684	0.39	864
99999	1,103	6.24	6,883	7.05	7,776	0.74	816
12345	1,085	8.69	9,429	8.81	9,559	0.98	1,063
54321	2,764	0.51	1,410	0.30	829	0.03	83
73620	490	0.16	78	0.54	265	0.04	20
73630	373	0.17	63	0.59	220	0.04	15
99203	4,632	1.14	4,973	0.52	2,268	0.06	262
99212	3,753	0.38	1,426	0.28	1,051	0.02	75
99213	1,825	0.55	1,004	0.38	694	0.03	55
Others	2,006						
Totals	**32,241**		**39104**		**36,213**		**3,602**

CPT-4 codes denote common medical procedures. The figure presents the percentages of total office/outpatient visits, by CPT-4 codes, for MGMA groups in the first six months of 2001. The codes denote differences in the complexity of the case and in the time required to perform a procedure successfully. For instance, more than one tenth (10.9%) of all new-patient office and outpatient visits to noninvasive cardiologists were coded 99205 (high complexity).

Specific data available from current *U.S. Federal Registry.*

Another simple example would be the physician allocation of monthly payment using the cost per RVU methodology, as given the sample spreadsheet below:

Services Produced	Physician A	Physician B	Physician C	Physician D	Grand Totals
CPT Total	CPT Cost / CPT Revenue	CPT Revenue /	CPT Revenue /	CPT Revenue /	CPT Revenue / CPT Revenue

Thus, the financial power of ABCM for the physician, and, more specifically, MPCA, is demonstrated.

ABCM/CPM IN THE HOSPITAL SETTING

In order to be paid and maintain cash flow, hospitals set up levels of specialization. But, the result usually means more handoffs, delays, eroding financial positions, and a frustrated set of patients and physicians. Much seems out of control. And, when you factor in the maze of the new Health Insurance Portability and Accountability Act of 1996 (HIPAA) technologies, it becomes overwhelming.

At the hub of the patient hospital experience is access management, formerly know as admitting or registration. This department collects information for clinicians treating the patient; meets joint commission and other requirements, facilitates medical record documentation, patient flow, revenue capture, billing and collections; and ultimately begins to settle accounts. In other words, the access management area has numerous customers in addition to the doctor, patient, or family member sitting across from them.

Without the benefit of relevant information, managers attempt to staff access management departments based on past history—namely, if patient and physician complaints aren't too high, there is probably enough staff. However, staffing in access management has not kept up with the increased demands and complexity of the process, and other hospital areas often suffer. Clinicians and medical records personnel deal with incomplete or incorrect information. Even claims information is incomplete and left to a back office to sort through.

All of these deficits make for an unhappy set of customers (physicians and patients) as they continually live with the repercussions of inaccurate and incomplete information. This does not go unnoticed by patients and physicians, as these situations erode confidence in the hospital's ability to get things done correctly.

As Table 14.9 demonstrates, access management is the hospital's first chance to create an "emotional contract" with the customer. It is here that the tone is set for the patient on the issues with respect to their hospitalization. And, it is here that the provider has the chance to begin working on the patient's behalf so that clinical outcomes are appropriate. All of this must happen in an environment that minimizes

TABLE 14.9   Cost per CPT Procedure

A Expense	B Acct. Mgmt.	C MD Labor	D MPCA	E Staff Labor	F Misc.	G Insurance	H Other
MD Salary		1,362,300					
Staff Salary	257,635		111,378	42,600			55,000
Malpractice					58,100		
DME Lease				2,388			
Dues/Subs							13,850
File Fee	9,350						
Laboratory						1,428	
DME					201,366		
Other Exp.	30,000				22,000		368,850
Total Exp (2)	296,985	1,362,300	111,378	42,600	227,182	58,100	436,850
Total Units (1)	32,241	39,104	39,104	36,213	36,213	3,602	36,213
ABCM/Unit	**9.21**	**34.84**	**3.08**	**1.18**	**6.27**	**16.13**	**12.06**

(1) Total expenses for each column divided by total units
(2) = Total units from prior table, 14.8
Direct Costs = B, C, D, E, F
Indirect Costs = G, H

the likelihood of a favorable occurrence, and outside the realm of the complex legal requirements established by state and federal officials.

So why do we let unresolved issues out of the access management area? In a manufacturing environment, if there are problems on the front-end design, huge problems ripple downstream in terms of recalls, warranty related expenses, lawsuits, and customers that abandon the company's products. World-class manufacturers dealt with these issues with their ISO-9000, total quality management (TQM), and Six Sigma programs during the 80's and 90's. Hospitals, however, have allowed issues in their access management process to fester and create huge and costly problems in the downstream process beyond the near future.

The Physician's Role

So, every provider must take a proactive role in dealing with this trend. The next few years will be pivotal in adapting to the new age of empowered customers, Internet technologies, and more demanding payment plans. The first step in this journey is physician/executive assessment.

Rest assured, this assessment is not a management engineering set of time studies aimed at microcosting every second of work. The CPM information needed for this plan is reasonable and can be collected in a few days by talking to the people performing the work. Estimates are gathered based on workers' views about how they spend their time (Table 14.10). This information is combined with available workload measures and general ledger cost information, and then, activity based reports are produced.

Going forward, ABCM it is an exercise in planning. Activity-based information is used to look at areas where work can be restructured so that errors and rework can be eliminated. New technologies that target problematic activities are selected and implemented. Outside companies that can perform complex activities more economically can be used *(www.ICMS.net)*. So, change your mindset and plan to get started now (Table 14.11)!

ASSESSMENT

ABCM and the CPM hold great promise as a common-sense solution to the faults and frustrations of health care process budgeting, human resource management, access management (Figure 14.2), and aberrant cost allocation methods. Some reasons follow:

- Traditional budgets **don't identify waste.** ABCM/CPM **exposes nonvalue costs.**
- Traditional budgets **focus on office employees.** ABCM/CPM **focuses on workload.**
- Traditional budgets **focus on office costs.** ABCM/CPM **also focuses on process cost.**
- Traditional budgets **focus on fixed versus variable costs.** ABCM/CPM **focuses on used versus unused capacity.**
- Traditional budgets **measure "effect";** ABCM/CPM **measures "cause."**

TABLE 14.10   Patient Encounter Cost Drivers

A	B[1]	C[2]	D (BC)	E[1,3]	F[4]	G (EF)	H[1]	I[5]	J (HI)	K[1]	L[4]	M (KL)	N (D+G+ J+M)
CPT Code	Unit Cost	RVU	Unit Total	Unit Total	RVU	Unit Total	Unit Cost	RVU	Unit Total	Unit Cost	RVU	Unit Total	TOTAL
	Physician/MDs			RN Staff/Labor			Insurance/ Liability			Other Misc.			
11111	34.84	0.91	31.70	10.53	0.40	4.21	16.13	0.04	0.65	12.06	0.40	4.82	$41.39
22222	34.84	0.43	14.98	10.53	0.37	3.90	16.13	0.03	0.48	12.06	0.37	4.46	23.82
33333	34.84	0.32	11.15	10.53	0.32	3.37	16.13	0.03	0.48	12.06	0.32	3.86	18.86
44444	34.84	0.23	8.01	10.53	0.23	2.42	16.13	0.02	0.32	12.06	0.23	2.77	13.53
55555	34.84	1.13	39.37	10.53	0.45	4.74	16.13	0.04	0.65	12.06	0.45	5.43	50.18
66666	34.84	1.66	57.83	10.53	2.10	22.11	16.13	0.19	3.06	12.06	2.10	25.33	108.34
77777	34.84	4.39	152.95	10.53	4.11	43.28	16.13	0.37	5.97	12.06	4.11	49.57	251.76
88888	34.84	4.41	153.64	10.53	4.37	46.02	16.13	0.39	6.29	12.06	4.37	52.70	258.65
99999	34.84	6.24	217.40	10.53	7.05	74.24	16.13	0.74	11.94	12.06	7.05	85.02	388.60
12345	34.84	8.69	302.76	10.53	8.81	92.77	16.13	0.98	15.81	12.06	8.81	106.2	517.58
73620	34.84	0.16	5.57	10.53	0.54	5.69	16.13	0.04	0.65	12.06	0.54	6.51	18.42
73630	34.84	0.17	5.92	10.53	0.59	6.21	16.13	0.04	0.65	12.06	0.59	7.12	19.90
99203	34.84	1.14	39.72	10.53	0.52	5.48	16.13	0.06	0.97	12.06	0.52	6.27	52.43
99212	34.84	0.38	13.24	10.53	0.28	2.95	16.13	0.02	0.32	12.06	0.28	3.38	19.89
99213	34.84	0.55	19.16	10.53	0.38	4.00	16.13	0.03	0.48	12.06	0.38	4.58	28.23

Legend:
1 = Activity cost/unit from Table 14.9
2 = Same RVU from column C, Table 14.8
3 = Sum of activity cost/unit from columns D, E and F in second table
4 = Same RVU from column E in table 1
5 = Same RVU from column G in table 1
Direct Costs = Physicians/MDs, RN Staff/Labor
Indirect Costs = Liability Insurance, Other, miscellaneous

CONCLUSION

ABCM and the CPM will become the defacto managerial accounting method of choice for the modern medical office, clinic, or hospital. It will replace the traditional financial accounting methodology of average costs with the more specific methodology of tracing actual resources consumed. The idea is to appreciate how much every task costs by factoring in every resource used to complete it. Thus, by assigning overhead expense costs to low volume activities, a better idea of each activity's profit (or loss) can be ascertained and/or adjusted. In this way, when your next financial crisis occurs, you will know how to deal with the problem through ABCM/CPM, and this will allow you to return to profitability.

REFERENCES

Pryor, T. (1995). Using ABCM for continuous improvement. Arlington, Texas: ICMS.
Pryor, T. (2002). Activity based management: A healthcare industry primer, Chicago: American Hospital Association.

TABLE 14.11

A CPT	B[1] Account Mgmt.	C[2]D Patient Encounter	(B + C) Total Procedure Cost
11111	9.21	41.39	50.60
22222	9.21	23.82	33.03
33333	9.21	18.86	28.07
44444	9.21	13.53	22.74
55555	9.21	50.18	59.39
66666	9.21	108.34	117.55
77777	9.21	251.76	260.97
88888	9.21	258.65	267.86
99999	9.21	388.60	397.81
12345	9.21	517.58	526.79
54321	9.21	25.03	34.24
73620	9.21	18.42	27.63
73630	9.21	19.90	29.11
99203	9.21	52.43	61.64
99212	9.21	19.89	29.10
99213	9.21	28.23	37.44

(1) Activity cost/unit from Column B, Table 14.9

(2) From column N, Table 14.10

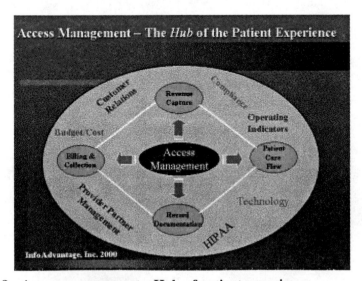

FIGURE 14.2   Access management—Hub of patient experience.

CHAPTER 15

Medical Practice Financial Benchmarking

Gary L. Bode

> I live in Alexandria Virginia. Near the Supreme Court Chambers is a toll bridge across the Potomac. When in a rush, I pay the dollar toll and get home early. However, I usually drive outside the downtown section of the city and cross the Potomac on a free bridge. This bridge was placed outside the downtown Washington, DC, area to serve a useful social service—getting drivers to drive the extra mile and to help alleviate congestion during the rush hour. If I went over the toll bridge and through the barrier without paying the toll, I would be committing tax evasion. If, however, I drive the extra mile and drive outside Washington to the free bridge, I am using a legitimate, logical, and suitable method of tax avoidance, and I am performing a useful social service by doing so. For my tax evasion, I should be punished. For my tax avoidance, I should be commended. The tragedy of life today is that so few people know that the free bridge even exists.
>
> —Justice Louis D. Brandeis

This chapter begins with the external point of view of your medical practice, as in the case of a banker considering your business loan. Financial statements are discussed, emphasizing their translation from financialease into English. Some useful financial benchmarking ratios are then explained, both at a specific point in time, and, as successive values over time for internal managerial purposes. The chapter makes a strong case for proactive practice management and illustrates some of the tools needed to do so.

YOUR MEDICAL PRACTICE AS AN ASSET

Your practice is a valuable asset in two respects. First, it provides the work environment that generates your personal income. Second, it has inherent sale value that can be part of an exit (retirement) or transfer strategy. Some of this inherent value lies in the current market value of medical equipment, minus any money owed. The other aspect of inherent value is goodwill, or the worth of the practice as an ongoing concern that allows you to sell it to another practitioner.

Despite the importance of the practice to the practitioner, some practices essentially run without a manager. This is like an orchestra without a conductor, in that the individual facets of talent have no common pathway to make music. Other practices evolve over time reactively and are not what the practitioner would have proactively defined as ideal.

FINANCIAL REWARDS OF A MANAGERIALLY EFFICIENT PRACTICE

Most medical practitioners are not well trained in business. However, your health care services are provided in an underlying business environment. Let's consider the financial rewards of a well-run practice, since they are the most tangible. Table 15.1 shows the financial benefit of improving practice performance 1% in three key parameters.

This example uses a practice with $500,000 per year of gross fees, a 20% contractual write off rate, 3% of bad debt, and 70% of overhead. The money available for pretax practitioner salary is $116,400.

The financial leverage inherent in a practice makes even small improvements in performance yield dramatic bottom–line, or "in pocket" results. Table 15.1 shows that cutting overhead 1% nets the practitioner an extra annual $3,880 of potential salary. Likewise, decreasing bad debt 1% yields $1200. A simultaneous 1% improvement in both parameters yields $5,120, *all for the same amount of patient care with no additional malpractice liability.*

Notice that increasing gross fees, the area most practitioners think of when discussing practice management, has the least financial impact of the three key parameters. While outside the scope of this chapter, good services marketing can improve any practice's gross fees, even in today's environment. The key to this is superb patient service, of which the clinical result is only a component. Making the patient's total perceptions exceed their prior expectations ensures a full appointment book.

COLLATERAL BENEFITS OF AN EFFICIENT PRACTICE

The rewards of a well-run practice transcend financial considerations. Other benefits include:

1. A better, more consistent clinical result.
2. Improved patient perception, which increases referrals and decreases liability.

TABLE   15.1   Managerial Benefits of an Efficient Practice

1. 80% (100% minus the 20% of contractual write off) of 500,000 in gross fees is $400,000.
2. 97% (100% minus the 3% of bad debt) of 400,000 is $388,000.
3. .30% (100% minus the 70% of overhead) of 388,000 is $116,400.

3. Less employee turnover.
4. Less stress.
5. More free time for the practitioner.

EXTERNAL EVALUATION OF FINANCIAL STATEMENTS

Financial Statements

Practice financial statements are usually provided by an independent accountant. External parties, like banks, often use these tools for evaluation of the practice, and financial ratios are the cornerstone of utilizing these statements. But, financial statements have potential problems, and are often suspect for several reasons:

1) First, they rely on unverified information from the practitioner. A practice's internal bookkeeping, even with the highest of intentions, is often sloppier than an accountant might hope. Professional liability with the IRS and time constraints keep the average accountant from doing anything but merely compiling figures given them. The standard disclaimer on their financial statements states this fact.

2) Most accountants are generalists in that they service other industries, like hog farms and flower shops, besides health care. Specialization developed in health care for a good reason: it became too complex for a single person to have a comprehensive grasp on all of it. The accounting industry has not followed suite. Thus, they often have little direct experience in the health care profession.

3) Accountants generally limit their scope of service to interfacing with the government for you on tax issues. Thus, their statements reflect tax position, which is only one component of the practice's total financial condition. While important, this is hardly all your accountant is capable of. See the sidebar on what your accountant can do for you when asked.

The common result of this is financial statements, though accurate for tax compliance, are less than optimal for managerial purposes. Unfortunately, many practitioners never even look at their financial statements or ever learn how to interpret them. The accounting expense is viewed as a necessary evil for tax compliance. This is a shame because such information, properly derived and presented, can be an important managerial tool. The following is a concise presentation of what each type of statement is, along with the common problems encountered in interpreting them.

Income Statement

The *Income Statement (Profit and Loss Statement)* reports, within a specific time period, what revenue came in, what expenses occurred, and the difference between these two figures. The most common use for this statement is the "bottom line"—or net profit, for tax purposes. Net profit usually does not equal cash flow. Noncash conventions, most notably depreciation, that are required by the IRS almost always make the "paper" profit different from the "checking account" profit.

While important, the limited goal of tax compliance can diminish the income statements use for internal managerial evaluation. Since this is the most important accounting statement to the average practitioner, it deserves more discussion than the other two reports.

The most common significant limitation of the accountant rendered income statement, even with trained interpretation, is poor classification and categorization. For tax purposes, many types of expenses can be grouped together and still render a correct net-profit figure.

For example, $500 in seminar tuition that is misclassified as medical supplies expense still renders the correct bottom line but states expenses in two very different categories. Budgeting and cash-flow forecasts may be adversely affected.

It is common to see income statements that categorize expenses into illogical groups. For example, all forms of insurance expense may be grouped together. Yet auto insurance probably belongs with other auto expenses. Workmen's Compensation insurance is actually a payroll expense. Building liability insurance probably belongs with the figures of the other premise(s). Using a single insurance category essentially understates all these other expenses, and there may not be time, interest, or ability to reallocate the insurance expenses more logically.

Illogical categorization may occur because (1) the accountant does not understand your practice, (2) cannot or will not customize the accounts, or (3) the accountant is only interested in the tax implications, or (4) the accountant has encountered a lack of proactive input from the practitioner. Furthermore, if you have the accountant enter your checks into a software program, additional blending of categories can occur as low-level employees incorrectly key in your information. Such "blending" of categories negates an opportunity to objectively see where all the money goes.

Over time, an income statement, set up with intuitively obvious expense categories and consistent data entry, yields an aggregate bird's eye view of cash flow. Gradually, spending patterns emerge. Commonly, if the only attempt to control expense has been on a check-by-check, best effort basis, significant savings can be achieved without becoming neurotic after an appropriate database is built. This is often not a single dramatic thing, but more often $10 a month here, $200 a year there. These things add up. Even a 1% savings on a $300,000 per year practice puts an extra $3,000 back in your pocket with no additional work or liability. Remember, if your expenses (exclusive of physician salary) run 33% of the gross money taken in, every $1 of expense saved has about the same affect on the practice as generating $3 of income. With contractual write offs (the amount a third-party payer forces you to deduct from your gross fees), each dollar in saved in expenses can easily have the same affect on the practice as $4 of services rendered.

The best way to build such a tool is by doing the accounts payable yourself using an electronic check register program, like *Quicken-R* or *QuickBooks-R*. Once this accounts-payable program is operational, a properly trained staff member can generate most of the checks in house and maintain proper categorization. Here, you produce a true cash-flow statement, which can be easily modified by your accountant into tax format. Such programs allow for customized categorization of expenses that can be a powerful managerial tool. The trick is to think of how you will ultimately use these categories. Who else is better qualified to determine that but the practitioner? In some practices, income classifications can also be useful, although the specialized accounts receivable programs generally do a good job on this.

Balance Sheet

The balance sheet gives a "snapshot" of the practice at a specific point in time. This timing is different from the income statement that uses a period of time. The balance sheet uses the following formula: *Assets* (what you own) equal *Liabilities* (what you owe) plus *Owner's equity* (what you have left).

Statement of Cash Flows

The third type of financial statement is the *statement of cash flows*. This statement reconciles the change in financial position between two balance sheets. Opinions vary, but it is the least useful to the average practitioner.

UNDERSTANDING FINANCIAL CONCEPTS

Even with great accounting, financial statements can be difficult to interpret. Let's start with the net income statement (NIS). The main interpretation issue here is depreciation, and its relative, *amortization*. *Depreciation* merely takes the cost of a tangible asset, like equipment, and divides this expense into the successive time periods over which the asset is expected to help produce income. Logically, if you're trying to figure up true practice costs, a piece of durable equipment often helps produce income long after it was purchased. Amortization is the same concept as depreciation but applied to intangible assets, like goodwill.

There are several methods of depreciation. Generally, practice financial statements use the deprecation methods and time frames allowed by the IRS. These have no relationship to the true life span and productivity of the item. For example, purchases of furniture, fixtures, machinery, equipment, and other personal property are not expensed, or deducted, when purchased. Rather, the medical business entity is required to capitalize and depreciate these assets over their useful lives. The Internal Revenue Code of 1986 provides asset lives to be used for tax purposes. The listing below is not all-inclusive but is representative of the most often used modified accelerated cost recovery system (MACRS) asset class lives.

Type of Asset	MACRS Depreciable life in years (in general)
Computer software purchased	3
Computers and peripherals	5
Office machinery and equipment	5
Furniture and fixtures	7
Leasehold improvements	39
Real office property, non-residential	39

For internal managerial purposes you can assign your own type, and duration, of depreciation. The dual bookkeeping is often worthwhile. The actual cost of the equipment is reflected on the balance sheet.

Internal Revenue Code (IRC) Section §179*

IRC § 179 allows a business entity to expense a certain amount of asset purchases each year that would otherwise have to be depreciated over their tax lives. This deduction is available for tangible personal property only, not real estate or leasehold improvements, and is a big benefit to most medical practices. This election is available for qualified asset acquisitions up to $200,000 during the year.

   The deduction is reduced dollar-for-dollar for each dollar of acquisitions in a year over the $200,000 threshold. Also, the depreciation expense created by this election cannot create or increase a tax loss for the practice. Any amount unable to be used in the current period can be carried forward to future periods to offset income in those periods. The amount of the expense election was $25,000 in the year 2003.

   There are various tricks to use in choosing the equipment to elect for IRC §179 depreciation. For instance, if the medical entity is adding assets in excess of the yearly limit, it would be wise to make the expensing election on those assets the entity fully intends to hold for that asset's entire tax life. Otherwise, the practice entity will have to recapture (i.e., pick up as income) the unused portion of the depreciation deduction that was taken early via the use of the election. Recapture can mitigate the tax benefit of this planning opportunity and should be avoided whenever possible.

Example: Simple IRC §179 Depreciation

Let's say you bought a piece of office equipment 3 years ago for $10,000 cash. For tax purposes, the government forces you to deduct this expense equally over five years. Thus, for the last three years you depreciated (write off/deducted) $2,000 on your taxes, each year (10,000/5), despite the fact you paid the whole $10,000 long ago. In the next two years, you also can take a $2,000 deduction each year to obtain, belatedly, the entire deduction for the initial expense. The original $10,000 is entered on, and accounted for, in the balance sheet. The government does allow a certain amount of depreciation expense to be deducted in the current year, if desired by the taxpayer, under Section 179. Thus, if other assets purchased during the year 2003 do not exceed the limit ($25,000), the practice could deduct the entire $10,000 expense of the equipment in a single year.

Example: Complex IRC §179 Depreciation

An obstetrics practice purchases four exam-room setups for $20,000 along with an ultrasound machine for another $20,000. The practice makes the expense election

---

*The Jobs and Growth Tax Relief and Reconciliation Act of 2003 increased the Section 179 expense amount to $100,000 for property placed in service in tax years 2003 through 2005. In addition, the $200,000 limitation on qualifying Section 179 property was increased to $400,000.

on the ultrasound machine because it is easier to take the deduction on one asset. After being in practice one year, the physicians agree that they don't like their current ultrasound machine. They opt to sell it and buy another one they all prefer. In the year of sale, the practice must recapture 80% ($16,000) of the expense election they made when they purchased the first ultrasound machine. This adds $16,000 to their current year's taxable income. Had they used the expense election on the four-exam room setups (that are not likely to be changed), they would be much better off for tax purposes.

New Developments in Office Depreciation

The Job Creation and Worker Assistance Act of 2002 signed into law on March 11, 2002, by President George W. Bush created significant additional depreciation deductions for assets purchased after September 10, 2001 (The Act). The Act, in general allows for an *additional* first year depreciation allowance (deduction) equal to 30% of the adjusted basis of personal property (or certain sale and leaseback, but not real property, i.e., buildings or land) acquired or placed in service after September 10, 2001. This additional first-year allowance will continue for qualified property placed into service through September 11, 2004.

The Act covers rebuilding or reconditioning of owned property; however, it does not include the purchase of used or reconditioned property. In addition, should a practice not want to take advantage of this additional depreciation allowance, there must be an election made to opt out.

IRC Section §197: Amortization of Goodwill

In many cases, the hard assets (furniture, fixtures, and equipment) obtained in a medical practice purchase make up only a small portion of the total purchase price. At least part of the price will be allocated to goodwill. Goodwill, or "blue sky" as it has also been called, is a premium paid for the reputation of the doctor or the practice entity or other intangible assets (restrictive covenants) identified within the medical entity. This goodwill, along with most other intangible assets, is amortizable over 15 years using the "straight line" method (IRC Section §197). The straight-line method is a ratable method calculated by dividing the asset's value by 180 months (15 years × 12 months). The importance of the asset allocation between asset classes becomes evident at this point, since most other assets can be depreciated over much shorter periods of time, thus providing larger annual deductions to the practice. It is preferred to allocate as much of the purchase price as reasonably possible to assets that can be depreciated over shorter periods of time.

But beware, since an unreasonably high allocation of a purchase price to assets is likely to be challenged by the IRS. When making the allocation, be sure to document the reasoning behind the allocation. Keep any documentation or research that supports the allocation methodology. The IRS has three years from the date the return (including the allocation) is filed to challenge the allocation.

Phantom Net Income

Many practitioners wonder where all that net income his account says they made actually is. Most times a true "cash" net profit never existed; it was only a phantom accounting artifice for tax purposes. Depreciation often causes discrepancies between "check book" profit, which is how much cash you actually have left over after paying the bills, and taxable income.

Initial financing of the asset also confuses matters. A standard installment loan payment, like a mortgage, has two components in it: principal, the amount actually put towards the face value of the loan, and interest, the expense of borrowing the money. Initially, the percentage of each payment constituting interest is high, and this decreases during the course of the loan. Conversely, the percentage of principal repaid with each payment increases. An extreme example of this "cash flow" profit and taxable-interest discrepancy, is buying equipment with a loan, but depreciating it completely through the use of Section 179 in a single year. This is wonderful for that first year. However, in the following years, only the interest component of the loan is deductible, and your taxable income exceeds your true cash flow because the principal, though paid that year, is unavailable to reduce it. This discrepancy is greatest in the last year of the loan, where the bulk of the loan payment is principal.

Other income statement translation problems include different accounting methods:

1) *Cash method.* Here, money is counted only as you deposit it, and "spent" only when write a check. Simplistic, but intuitively obvious, this resembles your check register. Unfortunately, the true cash-flow method is seldom seen. Most accountants use a tax-modified version of the cash flow method, as required by the IRS for tax reporting purposes.

2) *Accrual method.* Here, income is counted as you earn it, so your accounts receivable is counted as income when you treat patients, despite your receiving no cash for it as yet. Expenses get entered as you incur them In other words, you enter a supply order as an expense as it's placed, not just when you pay for it. This method affords logical treatment of a wider variety of accounting issues than does the cash method, and the IRS requires it once certain criteria are met.

3) *Modified cash (tax) method.* This is the cash method modified by depreciation and amortization as required by the IRS.

The following balance sheet problems sometimes arise:

1. *Asset valuation.* Commonly, balance sheets reflect "book" or "tax" value of assets. This is the historical value (what you paid), minus what you wrote off (depreciated or amortized) for tax purposes. Let's use the same piece of equipment, used in a previous example, bought three years ago for $10,000. Again, for tax purposes, the government forces you to deduct this expense over five years. Thus for the last three years you depreciated (wrote off/ deducted) $2000 on your taxes [10,000/5], for a total of $6000 [(10,000/5) × 3]. The current book or tax value reflected on the balance sheet is $4000

(10,000 – 6,000). Note this probably does not match the current market value of the equipment.

2. *Assets* are usually combined into groups, so that a single asset can be evaluated only by examining the accountant's work papers. Second, these groupings originate to suite the accountant's software which results in categorization different than the way the practitioner thinks of the assets.

3. The *Book (tax) value* is not immediately apparent because the historical price is listed in the asset section, followed by an entry labeled "accumulated depreciation." Sometimes the math is a little harder to follow than just the $10,000 – $6000 of our example. The book value and historical value may have no relation to the true current market value of the asset. A piece of land you paid $100,000 stays on the books as $100,000 despite the fact the neighborhood has eroded it to $75,000, or conversely, escalated it $125,000. The resulting $25,000 gain or loss is never reflected in the balance sheet. A 20-year-old building may have a book value of $49,000 ($100,000 purchase price minus accumulated depreciation of $51,000), but is really worth $110,000 in the current market. With buildings, improvements are not listed in the value of the building, making interpretation even more difficult.

4. Some assets are intangible. Lets consider goodwill, for example. Goodwill is basically the value of the practice as a going concern minus the book value of the assets. In a mature practice, where accumulated depreciation has decreased the book value of the assets below true market value, and the reputation of the clinic allows selling it for a premium price, goodwill can be considerable but will not reflected in the balance sheet.

BENCHMARK YOUR PRACTICE WITH FINANCIAL RATIOS

Financial ratios are figures or percentages derived from components of the financial statements. Even with the inherent limitations, financial ratios are the cornerstone of interpreting financial statements. They are being increasingly used by external sources to value and evaluate practices. Thus, it behooves you to understand them. Some financial ratios are valuable in the managerial report: a time series of certain practice financial ratios helps reveal its trends, strengths and weaknesses. All practice information, including financial ratios, should be integrated into the "big picture"; undue emphasis on a single facet may skew interpretation.

These financial ratio values are "benchmarked" to values obtained by surveys that become "industry standard." As described earlier, the average practice's financial statements have some inherent problems, making the derived financial ratios suspect. The government regulates, and the accounting industry strongly guides, the accounting principals used to generate a publicly held company's financial statements. This makes them more uniform and accurate than the average financial statements of a health care practice. Even here, Enron type scandals occur. Note that benchmark figures in publicly held companies are based on published financial statements. Surveys add another level of unreliability in using financial ratios for health care practices.

Financial ratios fall into four main classifications: (1) liquidity and solvency, (2) asset management, (3) debt management, and (4) profitability ratios.

LIQUIDITY AND SOLVENCY FINANCIAL RATIOS

The two most useful ratios are the: current ratio and the current liabilities to net worth.

Current Ratio

$$\frac{\text{Current assets}}{\text{Current liabilities}} = \text{Current ratio}$$

The *current ratio* measures short-term solvency. Unfortunately, practice financial statements often do not segregate out current and long-term assets and liabilities accurately. Current assets include cash on hand, the percentage of accounts receivable you can reasonably expect to collect, and short-term investments like a three-month CD. Current liabilities are notes payable and loans due within one year. This ratio should be at least one, preferably higher. A banker or venture capitalist probably wants to see this be in the range of about 1.3–1.5.

Short-term solvency has an impact on the ability to pay current obligations, which dramatically affects credit, which is an essential tool to controlling practice expenses. Thus, it is an important figure to track internally over time. Establish your definitions that allow consistent calculation of the current ratio.

For example, if you enter gross fees into accounts receivable and then adjust off for contractual write off and bad debt, use the last six month's figures of these adjustments to establish the true eventual cash value of your accounts receivable.

Current Liabilities to Net Worth

$$\frac{\text{Current Liabilities}}{\text{Net Worth}} = \text{Current Liabilities to Net Worth}$$

This should be low, probably beneath 0.5, but not zero. Net worth, or owner's equity, is often distorted on the financial statements, as most practitioners take out all the money "left over" as salary or distributions. This can be especially true if the practitioner holds major assets personally, like the building (a common scenario), and "leases" them to the practice. Bankers circumvent this by evaluating the practitioner and practice simultaneously.

ASSET MANAGEMENT FINANCIAL RATIOS

The four most important *asset management financial ratios* are the (1) average collection period, (2) fixed assets utilization, (3) fixed assets to net worth, and (4) total assets utilization ratio.

Average Collection Period

$$\frac{\text{Total Accounts Receivable}}{\substack{\text{Average Daily Charges (those not} \\ \text{collected on the day of service)}}} = \text{Average Collection Period}$$

The acceptable figure depends on the type of practice. A practice that handles a lot of personal injury cases has a higher number than an one that deals mostly in cash. Note that the total accounts receivable is inherently over valued if it includes eventual contractual write off and bad debt. Average daily charges would very on the time period sampled and can be difficult to obtain. This is a vital practice parameter, however, and, it is well worth setting up the process to obtain and track the required figures. Tracked over time (see the later section on trend graph analysis), it provides essential monitoring of the entire collections and billing process. For internal managerial purposes, the top dollar third-party payer components should be tracked individually, as the aggregate figure may not immediately detect a rapid change in a single insurance company.

Each extra day of this parameter means someone else is enjoying the float or interest on your money for an additional day. Ten extra days of $50,000 in accounts receivable means at least an additional loss of income to you of $120 a year if you could have banked this at 8% annual percentage rat (APR). Since a practice with protracted collections usually has cash-flow problems, this probably translates out to $270 if you are borrowing money at 18% APR.

Fixed Assets Utilization

$$\frac{\text{Net Revenue}}{\text{Net Fixed Assets}} = \text{Fixed Assets Utilization}$$

This shows how productively a practice utilizes its assets. Obviously, you would like any asset you invest in to render as much as possible in additional revenue. Asset evaluation issues (like accumulated deprecation described above) and true practice assets being held by the practitioner for tax purposes make the managerial use of this figure marginal.

Fixed Assets to Net Worth

$$\frac{\text{Fixed Assets}}{\text{Net Worth (Doctor owner's equity)}} = \text{Fixed Assets to Net Worth}$$

A higher ratio indicates a greater investment in fixed assets, which, conversely, may indicate low working capital. This is a great concept in publicly held companies with strict accounting but less useful to the average practitioner. See the potential problems of fixed asset evaluation (and ownership) and net worth described earlier.

Total Assets Utilization

$$\frac{\text{Net Revenue}}{\text{Total Assets}} = \text{Total Assets Utilization}$$

This is similar to fixed assets to net worth (described above) but eliminates some of the asset evaluation problems. If the proper definitions are consistently employed, this is a good figure to track internally over time. An example of an appropriate definition might be any asset originally costing over $250 that is in current use, including any held "artificially" by the practitioner for tax purposes. While a "soft" figure, it has value as an indicator of productivity.

DEBT MANAGEMENT RATIOS

The two most common are (1) total debt to total assets, and (2) total liabilities to net worth.

Total Debt to Total Assets

$$\frac{\text{Total Debt}}{\text{Total Assets}} = \text{Total Debt to Total Assets}$$

Obviously, less debt is generally preferable, so this ratio should be low. Remember, debt can be a useful managerial tool if used wisely, and a total debt to total assets figure of zero might have negative implications. A banker looks for a low figure since he is being asked to provide more debt and wants to ensure his investment.

Total Liabilities to Net Worth

$$\frac{\text{Total Liabilities}}{\text{Net Worth}} = \text{Total Liabilities to Net Worth}$$

This can be a useful figure if appropriate definitions are used and some practitioners track this internally. Generally, lower is better.

PROFITABILITY RATIOS

These include (1) profit margin, and (2) return on investment ratios.

Profit Margin

$$\frac{\text{Net Income}}{\text{Net Revenue}} = \text{Profit Margin}$$

Generally expressed as a percentage, this figure reflects how much profit the practice makes on each dollar of revenue, usually gross fees. When the practitioner's salary encompasses "what's left over," this is zero. For internal purposes, it can be considered as potential practitioner salary over gross fees. Obviously, higher is better.

Return on Investment

$$\frac{\text{Net Income}}{\text{Total Assets}} = \text{Return on Investment}$$

This reflects how well assets are used to generate net income. Again, one would strive to make the most money with a given asset, making this figure as high as possible. This concept appears in a breakeven analysis, wherein the expected return on investment on an individual asset is calculated before buying it. Sometimes it makes sense to refer potential gross fees to outside sources, despite inherent clinical expertise, because of the equipment cost involved. Other times, traditionally out sourced services now performed in house help the practice.

Other Ratios

Other useful financial ratios can also be correlated to help show practice efficiency. For example, staff gross salary as a ratio of gross fees and/or collections helps monitor the amount of revenue produced by each dollar of staff salary. This is analogous to the asset utilization financial ratios explained earlier. And, the current ratio can generally be derived without the financial statements. Tracking it may help keep the important topic of short-term liquidity in mind.

Your practice needs hands on management. A managerial report made of financial ratios is a good tool for managing your practice in a time efficient manner. It is a valuable exercise that can help you spot both negative and positive trends earlier than they would otherwise become apparent.

How to Waste Money

Despite monitoring financial ratios, there are still many ways for your medical practice to lose money:

1) *Have no consistent billing policy.* Design appropriate controls and implement monitoring so all services get billed, bills are accurate, bills are sent in a timely fashion, and accounts receivable gets checked for potential problems regularly.

2) *Have no consistent collections policy. Your chances of getting paid erode progressively with time.* Collect cash up front when possible. Don't be afraid to institute phone reminders of past due balances. Become familiar with your county's small claims process, especially the techniques available, for example, writ of execution, to have the sheriff seize property for you.

3) *Have no internal controls.* (See the sidebar on this.) Proper controls help insure good things happen consistently, and minimize chances of bad things such as embezzlement happening.

4) *Bounce checks.* Each incident can cost up to $50 in bank and vendor fees along with time and stress to remedy the situation, more if attorneys get involved. Criminal charges against you are also possible. Use an electronic check program like Quicken, get online service that helps you calculate the checking balance daily, and arrange with the bank to set up overdraft protection at a reasonable cost.

5) *Run up a lot of employee overtime.* Whenever possible, have a schedule that makes paying time-and-a-half unnecessary.

6) *Fail to claim all legitimate deductions for tax purposes.* Let's say you spend $1,000, out of your own pocket every year on legitimate business meal expenses instead of running these through the clinic. Remember, meal expenses are only 50% deductible, making this a dramatic example. Maybe you think the relatively small amount of each meal is too trivial to track, or, the hassle of tracking meals is too cumbersome. At your marginal tax rate, plus payroll taxes, the clinic has to pay greater than $1500 up front for you to net the $1,000. It gets this extra $500 back in tax savings eventually. If the practice pays directly, it only costs $1,000 up front and produces a $500 deduction (half the cost of the meals), making the eventual cost around $750. Let Uncle Sam pick-up the tab occasionally.

7) *Don't have the most advantageous business entity for the practice.* This decision depends on the state you practice in, the goals of the clinic, and your own personal tax position. For example, if the practice needs to save money for a down payment on a building, it may make more sense to be a C corporation than an S corporation. While the C corporation pays "double taxes," it probably does so at a lower rate then the marginal tax rate of the practitioner to whom this money would flow with an S corporation. But, since health care professionals practice within many different legal structures, there are various differences in tax planning techniques, depending upon how the entity or entities you practice within are structured.

The various entities and types of returns that are filed for business entities are as follows:

Entity	Type of Return
Sole proprietor	Schedule C, Form 1040
C corporation (inc., corp., PA or PC)	Form 1120
S corporation (inc., corp., PA or PC)	Form 1120S
Professional corporation (PC)	Form 1120, or 1120S
Professional association (PA)	Form 1120, or 1120S
Not-for-profit-corporation	Form 1120
General partnership	Form 1065
Limited partnership	Form 1065
Limited liability partnership (LLP)	Form 1065

Limited liability company (LLC)	Form 1065, Form 1120 or 1120S
Foundation Model	Form 990
Tax Exempt, Not for Profit Corp.	Form 990

Each state is responsible for enacting its own legal statutes on the organization of physician corporations. Therefore, if a practice entity is a corporation, it could be an inc., corp., PA, or PC, depending on the state in which the practice entity is organized. In addition, almost every state has enacted legislation to create limited liability entities that provide the liability protection afforded a corporation, while having the attributes of a partnership. These entities have become very popular with professional practices (physicians, lawyers, accountants, engineers, architects, etc.) because they allow more flexibility with regard to buy-ins and buyouts, and in the allocation of income and deductions. For federal income tax purposes, these entities are viewed as partnerships, unless an election to be treated as a corporation is made. The election is made on Federal Form 8832 and is also known as a "check the box" election. Three other entities are described:

BUSINESS ENTITIES

Corporations

Within the C Corporation status, there is a distinction between entities providing personal services and those that provide goods and services that are not personal in nature. A physician corporation (C corporation) is considered to be what is called a "personal service corporation" for federal income tax purposes. A personal service corporation pays federal income tax on every dollar of taxable income at a rate of 35%.

All other C corporations follow a progressive tax rate structure that taxes corporate income below $100,000 at lower tax rates (15% on the first $50,000, 25% percent on the next $25,000 and 34% percent on the following $25,000). The IRS believed that professionals had too much ability to manipulate their year-end income and, therefore, the tax they paid. The IRS asked Congress to close this loophole. Congress created the personal service corporation designation to remove this tax planning opportunity. This is now one of the disadvantages of being organized as a C Corporation for those providing personal services.

The difference between a C corporation and an S corporation is strictly a federal tax consideration. The S corporation was created by Congress to allow small business corporations the flexibility of a partnership while retaining the limited liability advantages of the corporate structure. Therefore, for federal income tax purposes, the S corporation reports its income, deductions, expenses, and credits to its shareholders more along the lines of a partnership. This is important to note since C corporations are taxpaying entities, while all of the other entities are generally considered to be tax reporting, or pass-through, entities. S-corporation status is achieved by filing Form 2553 with the IRS either within 75 days of when the practice is incorporated, when business is actually started, or within 75 days of the beginning of a corporation's fiscal year. This election can be made even if an entity has been a C corporation for many years; however, there are potential tax traps (known as the "built-in gains" tax) in a C corporation conversion to an S corporation for those unaware of the law. This is an area where the assistance of a qualified tax professional would be well worthwhile, since the tax cost of falling into the traps can be very significant.

Pass Through Entities and Favored Tax Status

Partnerships, S corporations, and limited liability entities (LLPs or LLCs) are all generally considered to be pass-through entities. The term "pass-through entity" is based upon the way in which the tax attributes of the entity (e.g., income, expenses, deductions, and credits) flow through to the owners and are taken into account in the owners' individual tax returns. This treatment allows owners to avoid the potential of double taxation that exists in C corporations.

Sole Proprietorships

A sole proprietor is an individual physician owner whose medical practice is accounted for on a separate schedule of the owner's individual income tax return. Typically, physicians filing their business returns via the use of Schedule C of Form 1040 have the lowest level of reporting requirements and also (in general) do the poorest job of keeping good records of business activity. There is only one level of tax for the sole proprietor. The net profit (or loss) from the Schedule C business is reported on page one of Form 1040 and is combined with all of the other income items reported to arrive at gross income. Different from interest and dividend income, or investment income that is typically considered passive in nature, self-employment income is income considered generated by ones own actions. There is "self-employment" tax to be paid on virtually all self-employment income reported in the tax return. Many doctor sole proprietors get into trouble because they neglect to take this tax into account when estimating their tax liability for the year; this tax is significant, as noted below.

Self-employment tax is paid on 92.35 percent of all self-employment net profits. This tax is the equivalent of the combination of the employer's and employee's Social Security tax and Medicare tax. Social Security tax is 12.4% of the first $87,000 (in 2003) in net income, and Medicare tax is paid at the rate of 2.90% of net income, without any upper-income limit. The Social Security income limit is indexed and adjusted (upward) annually. The sole proprietor is allowed to deduct one half of the self-employment tax against income; however, this deduction is worth far less than the actual tax.

Tax Entity Example

Dr. Smith is a sole proprietor with a self-employment tax liability of $11,500. She gets to deduct $5,750 (50% of $11,500) against her income. Now, she is in the 31% tax bracket. Therefore, her deduction is worth $1,782.50 in actual income tax dollars ($5,750 × 0.31). The discrepancy between one half of the self-employment tax, $5,750, and the self-employment tax deduction is $3,967.50 in tax. Therefore, although Dr.

Smith received a 50% deduction for her self-employment tax, she actually pays $9,717.50, or 84.5 percent of the self-employment tax. This is not the bargain that the Congressional spin-doctors made it out to be when it was being sold to the general public. However, it is still better than paying the entire $11,500 in self-employment tax.

8) *Don't make timely payroll and unemployment tax deposits.* Cascading penalties on late 941 payments start a viscous cycle with the IRS, often increasing the eventual cost by 15% or more, excluding additional accounting fees. The government feels you are holding employee's money in trust, and that not depositing it is criminal embezzlement. Imagine that.

9) *Don't pay off the practice's credit card bills in full each month.* This starts an expensive cycle of paying expensive interest on expensive interest. Credit cards are a great tool, but abuse of them costs big money.

10) *Pay vendors late.* Most vendors charge 18% interest on unpaid balances. A habit of late payments inevitably makes itself known in your Dunn and Bradstreet report, and this erodes your credit.

11) *Don't take advantage of vendors "early pay" discounts.* A 2% discount, even at 30 day net terms, is a substantial reward for having adequate cash flow and paying responsibly.

12) Don't have a Certified Financial Planner©(CFP©) and/or Certified Medical Planner© (CMP©) to help you do investment planning, retirement planning or estate planning, or a managerially astute medical accountant for general and office tax planning. Proactive planning often nets significant tax savings.

WHAT CAN YOUR ACCOUNTANT DO FOR YOU?

Your financial accountant can do more than just compile your bookkeeping into tax format. For someone who works to live, instead of living to work, health care practitioners have more power to control their own destiny than most of America. Many people work as hard as they can and adjust their life style accordingly: life happens to them.

Instead, try imagining what you want life to be like at a certain point in the future. "I want a house in X neighborhood, with a full recording studio and indoor/outdoor pool, vacation three weeks a year," and so on.

If you can't dream it, it probably won't happen. Proactive planning sometimes makes such dreams more affordable too. Have your accountant help you "back in" to what your practice has to be doing to support that lifestyle. This will probably result in a spreadsheet that you can play "what if?" scenarios with.

Also consider asking about the following:

1) If your current business entity is a **S** or **C corporation** for the practice and state where you live. Is a C corporation for example, the most advantageous for your practice? The answer depends on your long-range plans.

2) If you're taking all the legal deductions allowable, professional and personal. It is surprisingly common for people to under-claim deductions. Remember, most accountants only look for "red flags," that is, expenses that are present

but shouldn't be. They may not think about the converse: what is not there, but should be.

3) Proactive tax planning is not the same as retroactive restructuring in March.
4) Performing a breakeven analysis before completing a major purchase.
5) Different ways to finance major purposes. Issues include cash flow, immediate tax ramifications, and long-term tax implications.
6) Setting up a cash-flow projection system that you can perform yourself on a regular basis.

BANKERS VS. MEDICAL PRACTITIONER'S (A CASE OF PERSPECTIVE)

Consider a banker evaluating you and your practice for a loan. Bankers sometimes get a bad reputation. Aphorisms like, "banks won't loan money unless you don't need it," typify this perception. Bankers are different from practitioners in the following ways:

1) Bankers are well trained financially. Practitioners usually are not. In fact, medical professionals have earned a stigma of being poor business people by, historically, over paying for products and services. Some of us are even disdainful about the business aspects of the practice. Anticipate this perception by the banker. A bit of homework on the practitioner's part, along with prudent use of an accountant or business manager, can ameliorate this potential disadvantage.
2) Bankers tolerate risk less than the average practitioner. This stems from the practitioner's belief in his own intangible strengths, like skill and dedication along with the inherent risk in entrepreneurship.
3) Bankers want to cover their assets, of course, but don't really want a loan going bad. Conversely, a practitioner may feel that it is no concern of the banker's how a loan is handled, since the underlying collateral more than covers the loan should adverse conditions ensue. A bad loan signifies poor judgment and makes the banker look bad to their superiors. Second, they are generally not in the business of seizing collateral, like medical equipment, and trying to resell it. Red tape makes this a hassle while limiting their profit. They much prefer you living up to the loan agreement.
4) Bankers generally do not understand the current trends and dynamics of your profession. Bankers have to justify their decisions to superiors. Educating them on what it is you do, and the business environment you do it in, helps them "sell" a loan to the bank.

Now, consider your banker's reaction after you improve practice performance by 1% through trend analysis in three key parameters: gross fees, contractual write-offs, and overhead expenses.

CONCLUSION

The appropriate use of financial ratios and the managerial accounting techniques outlined in this chapter are not familiar to most physicians, today. They will become more important in the future as physician/executives seek to achieve maximum profits and economic efficiencies from their new or ongoing medical practice operations.

ACKNOWLEDGMENTS

Thanks to Dr. David Edward Marcinko, MBA, CFP©, CMP©, Hope Rachel Hetico, RN, MHA and Thomas P. McGuinness, CPA, CVA, for technical assistance in the preparation of this chapter.

CHAPTER 16

Return on Medical Practice Investment Calculations

David Edward Marcinko

> In recent years, the phrase *maximizing shareholder value* has become a battle cry for (medical) managers and directors of both public and private companies throughout North America. This has often led to drastic changes, such as a major restructuring or the divestiture of one or more of its business (practice service) segments. But do those initiatives actually create value for (physicians) shareholders?
>
> —Howard E. Johnson
> www.Workopolis.com

eturn on investment (ROI), residual income (RI), and medical enterprise value added (MEVA) calculations are important managerial accounting concepts for physician executives. These three key parameters must be high enough to warrant continued existence of the medical office or the practice will eventually cease as capital flows to profitable business endeavors and away from unprofitable ones.

RETURN ON INVESTMENT CALCULATIONS

To enhance understanding of this concept as well as facilitate its pragmatic use, the ROI equation may be decomposed into its three individual component parts:

- net operating income
- practice revenue
- average operating assets

These parts may then be mathematically stated as follows:

$$\frac{\text{Net operating income}}{\text{Practice revenues}} \times \frac{\text{Practice Revenues}}{\text{Average operating assets}} = \text{ROI}$$

Example: Dr. Miller reports the following office data:

Practices Revenues $500,000
Avg. Operating Assets 200,000
Net Operating Income 30,000

$$ROI = \$30,000/500,0000 \times 500,000/200,000 = (6\%) \times (2.5) = 15\%$$

Using the above example, it is intuitive that there are three ways in which Dr. Miller can improve her ROI: (1) reduce expenses, (2) increase revenues, and (3) reduce operating assets.

Approach 1: Reduce Expenses

Assume that Dr. Miller is able to reduce expenses by $10,000 per year, so that net operating income increases from $30,000 to $40,000. Practice revenues and operating assets remain unchanged.

$$(\$40,000/500,000) \times (500,000/200,000) = (8\%) \times (2.5) = 20\% \text{ ROI}$$

Expense reduction is the simplest parameter of office ROI to adjust, and the recent downsizing of corporate America is an example of the social tumult it can produce. Many believe that in a mature market or HMO environment, there is more leverage for increasing profits by cutting costs than by increasing revenues (Revenues = Price × Volume). In fact, the smaller the HMO contract's profit margin, the greater the leverage achieved through cost reduction, in the short term (the inverse also applies).

For example, general surgery has the lowest median overhead operating costs among selected specialists and surgical cardiology has the highest (as listed in Table 16.1) for single specialty practices.

Moreover, in a reduced or discounted fee environment, there is far more leverage for increasing profit by reducing expenses (costs), than from increasing revenue.

There are many items whose costs can be reduced through innovative purchasing and volume buying. These include: printed material, super-bills, and stationary; telephone, travel; car rental and airline reservation costs; computer and copier equipment; maintenance and supplies; durable medical equipment (DME) and laboratory fees; staff salary, benefits, and overtime pay reductions; and bulk purchases (economies of scale) by pooling with other groups to obtain discounts.

The increasingly popular professional employee organization (PEO) outsourcing strategy represents another industry transforming the way small- and medium-size medical offices are run, giving them many advantages previously available only to

TABLE 16.1 Median Total Operating Costs per Full-Time-Equivalent (FTE) Single Specialty Group According to Specialty*

- Cardiology: $377,644
- Family Practice: $245,661
- Ob/Gyn: $294,238
- General Surgery: $216,699
- Orthopedic Surgery: $354,963
- Urology: $359,196

*Aventis Managed Care Digest Series, 2003.

very large group practices, clinics, hospitals, MSOs, or IPAs. This innovative approach assists doctors to concentrate more time and economic resources on treating patients and less on running and/or growing their practices.

Advantages include cost reductions associated with no longer having to deal with administrative services such as: payroll processing (2.5%), tax administration (3%), employee benefits (2.5%), claims and audits (3%), and insurance and human resource management (3%). In fact, it has been estimated that these services are the equivalent of about 14% of the typical gross office payroll.

Still, the cost reduction strategies noted above may be merely a temporary fix since some baseline cost of business will always remain. Such a "slash and burn" costing mentality also does not foster future growth, expansion, innovation, research, or business development. Remember, you can be cost conscious without being too neurotic.

Approach 2: Increase Revenues

Again, assume the Dr. Miller is able to increase revenues to $600,000 because she is in a growing market. Net operating income increases to $42,000, and the operating assets remain unchanged.

$$(\$42,000/600,000) \times (600,000/200,000) = (7\%) \times (3.0) = 21\% \text{ ROI}$$

An increase in office revenue is a bit more difficult to engineer than simple cost cutting efforts, but the results are also more worthwhile. Growth is again emphasized in this model. with corresponding profit increases (i.e., 21% > 20% ROI).

Approach 3: Reduce Assets

Finally, assume that Dr. Miller is able to reduce her average operating assets from $200,000 to $125,000. Revenues and net operating expenses remain unchanged.

$$(\$30,000/500,000) \times (500,000/125,000) = (6\%) \times (4.0) = 24\% \text{ ROI}$$

Now, it can be seen that asset reduction is the most profitable economic course to pursue in search of increasing practice ROI (24% > 21% > 20%). Growth is favored over downsizing and is augmented by asset reduction; as variable or virtual costs are increased only on an as needed basis.

Criticism of ROI Calculations

Although physicians are just beginning to use the ROI approach in evaluating medical office performance, it is far from being a perfect profitability analysis tool. The ROI method is subject to the following criticisms:

- Like traditional financial ratio analysis, ROI tends to emphasize short-term performance rather than long-term profitability. In an attempt to protect or increase ROI, a physician may become motivated to accept of reject an otherwise good investment opportunity.

- ROI is only controllable by physician owners and not employed practitioners, associates, or HMO physician employees. This inability to control ROI not only leads to personal frustration—it can make it difficult to distinguish between performance of the practice and performance of the physician.

RESIDUAL PRACTICE INCOME CALCULATIONS

Residual Income (RI) is the net operating income that a medical office is able to earn above the minimum ROI. In fact, some physician executives believe that residual income is a better measure of performance than is return on investment. The residual income approach encourages physician managers to make profitable investments that would be rejected under the ROI approach

Example

Dr. Ray, a medical executive, owns two large office complexes, A and B. Complex A has $1,000,000 in operating assets, and Complex B has $3,000,000 in operating assets. Each complex is required to earn a minimum of 12% on its investment in operating assets.

	Complex A	Complex B
Average operating assets	$1,000,000	$3,000,000
Net operating income	200,000	450,000
Required return		
(12% × average operating assets)	120,000	360,000
Residual income	**$80,000**	**$90,000**

Example

Dr. Ray's Medical Complex A has the opportunity to make an investment of $250,000 that would generate a return of 16% on invested assets (i.e., $40,000/year). This investment would be in his best interest, since the 16% rate of return exceeds the minimum required rate of return. However, the investment would reduce the complex's ROI.

	PRESENT	NEW PROJECT	OVERALL
Average operating assets (a)	$1,000,000	$250,000	$1,250,000
Net operating income (b)	200,000	40,000	240,000
ROI: (b) / (a)	20.00%	16.00%	19.20%

On the other hand, the investment would increase the complex's RI.

	PRESENT	NEW PROJECT	OVERALL
Average operating assets	$1,000,000	$250,000	$1,250,000
Net operating income	200,000	40,000	240,000
Minimum required rate return	120,000	30,000	150,000
(12% × Avg. operating assets)			
Residual income:	**80,000**	**10,000**	**90,000**

Thus, informed physician executive realizes that profits are made by pursuing a triad of decreasing costs, increasing revenues, and decreasing operating assets.

Criticism of Residual Income Calculations

The major disadvantages of the RI approach to practice profitability analysis is that it can not be easily used to compare the performance of different sized offices, as appreciated above. Economies of scale and other efficiencies are not considered, nor are the intangible goodwill attributes of the personal patient-physician relationship. This last objection is increasingly less important, as medicine becomes commoditized, by producing a standardized HMO medical service product.

(MEDICAL) ECONOMIC VALUE-ADDED CALCULATIONS

It is not unusual for a medial practice to incur extraordinary expenses by investing in technology or equipment. There are two methods of evaluating these capital expenses.

- The older generally accepted accounting principles (GAAP) removes them from the income statement that is used to evaluate enterprise profitability.
- The newer economic value added (EVA) approach treats them differently by considering both capital expenses and operational expenses when calculating profit.

The concept of EVA was developed by New York City–based consultants Stern Stewart. MEVA is a riff off this distinction applied to medical-practice capital investments by distinguishing between illusory profits and real economic gain. The concept is useful to keep physician executives from weakening the balance sheet by chasing profits. It may also better reflect enterprise value, since to have a positive MEVA, practice revenues must exceed operating costs, taxes, and a charge for the cost of capital (debt interest rate charges, or the risk of saving/conserving capital rather than spending/investing it).

In other words, the benefits of major equipment must be weighed against the financial drain of purchase. In addition, taxes are also left out of a GAAP analysis of operating profit, but MEVA expensing includes them to keep operations as lean as possible. Nevertheless, the MEVA formula may be expressed, as follows:

$$\text{MEVA} = \text{net operating profit after tax (NOPAT)} - (\text{cost of capital} \times \text{capital})$$
$$\text{Or}$$
$$\text{MEVA} = (\text{operating profit}) - (\text{a capital charge})$$
$$\text{Where: NOPAT} = (\text{taxable income} - \text{income tax})$$
$$\text{Where: cost of capital} \times \text{capital}) = \text{depreciation} \times (\text{beginning book value})$$

As seen in the MEVA equations, there are two key components. NOPAT and the capital charge, which is the amount of capital times the cost of capital. NOPAT is the profit derived from operations after taxes but before financing costs and noncash bookkeeping entries. In other words, it is the total pool of profits available to provide cash return to the physician executives who provided capital to the practice.

The cost of capital is the minimum rate of return on capital required to compensate physician debt and equity owners for bearing risk—a cut-off rate to create value. On the other hand, capital is the amount of cash invested in the practice, net of depreciation.

Simple Example

The Mackenzie Medical Group (MMG) invests one million dollars, which is a capital expense amortized over several years, for a new PET scanner that produces $100,000 in revenue each year. The scanner adds $50,000 in operating costs, while operating profit is $45,000 after taxes. So, MMG is a clear winner, correct?

Step 1: Net Operating Profit after Taxes (NOPAT)

A.	How much revenue did the scanner produce?	**$100,000**
B.	Annual expenses to run and maintain the scanner	**$50,000**
C.	Operating profit (&100,000 − $50,000)	**$50,000**
D.	Tax effects @ (5% × $100,000)	**$5,000**
E.	NOPAT = C − D ($50,000 − $5,000)	**$45,000**

Step 2: Weighted (Average) Cost of Capital

F.	Cost of PET scanner	**$1,000,000**
G.	Rate of return investing elsewhere (opportunity cost)	**10%**
H.	Weighted Cost of capital ($1,000,000 × 10%)	**100,000**

Step 3: The Economic Value Added Difference

EVA:	Subtract E − H ($45,000 − $100,000)	**($55,000)**

The picture changes if the project is modeled using adjusted return or a MEVA that seeks hidden costs. There is really a $55,000 loss, or (−) ROI compared to GAAP analysis.

Advanced Example

In a more complex scenario, suppose your practice buys a piece of medical imaging equipment (MIE) equipment for $345,000, which is expected to have a useful life of 6 years. The government allows you to depreciate the equipment using a Modified Accelerated Cost Recovery System (MACRS) with a 5-year schedule. The equipment vendor estimates revenues of $120,000/year during the years of operation, and estimates that after its useful life, the MIE equipment will have a market value of $120,000. However, in order to keep the equipment running properly, you are required to spend $8,000/year in maintenance costs. Assuming that your practice requires a minimum rate of return (MARR) of 10%, and assuming that you are subject to a tax rate of 50%, calculate the MEVA for the investment for each of the years of operation.

MIE Investment Intermediate Values ($)

Year	Gross Revenue	Book Value	Depreciation Deduction	Taxable Income	Income Tax (0.50)
0	−345,000	—	—	—	—
1	120,000 − 8,000	345,000	69,000	43,000	21,500
2	120,000 − 8,000	276,000	110,000	1,600	800
3	120,000 − 8,000	165,600	66,240	45,760	22,880
4	120,000 − 8,000	99,360	39,744	72,256	36,128
5	120,000 − 8,000	59,616	39,744	72,256	36,128
6	120,000 − 8,000	19,872	19,872	92,128	46,064
6	120,000	0	—	120,000	60,000

Economic Value Added Calculations for MIE ($)

Year	Taxable Income − Tax = NOPAT	MARR*(BOY Book Value) = (Cost of Capital × Capital)	EVA
1	43,000 − 21,500 = **21,500**	(0.10)*(345,000) = **34,500**	−13,000
2	1,600 − 800 = **800**	(0.10)*(276,000) = **27,600**	−26,800
3	45,750 − 22,880 = **22,880**	(0.10)*(165,600) = **16,500**	6,320
4	72,756 − 36,128 = **36,128**	(0.10)*(99,360) = **9,936**	26,192
5	72,756 − 36,128 = **36,128**	(0.10)*(59,616) = **5,962**	30,166
6	92,128 − 46,064 = **46,064**	(0.10)*(19,872) = **1,987**	44,077
6	120,000 − 60,000 = **60,000**	0	60,000

Source: http://filebox.vt.edu/users/ovalero/eva/definition.html

Criticism of MEVA Calculations

It is important to note that these calculations only represent one of the many ways to define MEVA. In reality, the definition of MEVA should be tailored to the specifics of the practice that uses it. Also, in reality, there are adjustments that may change the way a practice defines MEVA. These equity-equivalent (EE) adjustments are to both NOPAT and the capital employed to reduce noneconomic accounting and financing conventions on the income statement and balance sheet. EEs are adjustments that turn a practice's accounting book value into an economic book value, which is a more accurate measure of the cash that physician owners have put at risk and upon which they expect to accrue some returns. Equity equivalents turn capital-related items into more accurate measures of capital, and they include revenue- and expense-related items in NOPAT, thus better reflecting the practice's base (upon which owners expect to accrue their returns). Furthermore, equity equivalents are designed to address the distortions suffered by traditional financial ratio measures that change depending upon the generally accepted accounting principles adopted or the mix of financing employed.

Moreover, the basic formula for MEVA tends to produces a more conservative picture of ROI and medical practice profits or losses. Therefore, MEVA should not be used too rigorously for fear of excessive risk aversion and the paralysis of analysis.

CONCLUSION

Although bewildering to the uninitiated, a careful analysis of ROI, RI, and MEVA calculations will assist the physician executive develop the most economically profitable service, financial, and office operational flow process. This will result in improved profits, decreased stress, and improved patient care, which is the ultimate successful outcome in any medical practice.

CHAPTER 17

Creating Practice Equity Value

David Edward Marcinko and Charles F. Fenton, III

> Many (medical practices) struggle with the task of executing their key (equity building) strategies. In fact, strategy execution (or lack thereof) has been referred to as the single biggest obstacle to success. Far too many well-formulated strategies are wasted by a practice or organizations' inability to execute them.
>
> —Cam Scholey, CMA
> —Howard Armitage, CMA, FCMA

The bad strategic news is that there are about 15–25% too many physicians in this country, which means hypercompetition. A surprising fact is that a minority of small group practices control the majority of assets and managed-care contracts. This trend will undoubtedly continue as the process of consolidation takes place in the profession. The clear message is that you are going to have to build value into your medical practice just to compete.

The good strategic news is that there is an almost geometric growth potential possible for doctors, but you are going to need the following:

- executive management skills
- hospital, clinic, outpatient facilities, and health system synergies
- information systems technology with ASP partners
- significant capital resources
- ability to build transferable equity into your medical practice

Determinants of Practice Equity

There is no magic rule of thumb to build equity into your practice; it is not that simple. However, the following suggestions are offered for their value, regardless of the practitioner's specialty or degree designation.

1. Use the appropriate legal entity status for your practice, since it is important for taxation and liability reduction purposes that are often not available to the sole physician proprietor or general partner:
   (a) *Sole Proprietor.* This business form eliminates corporate taxes, as income is only taxed at the owner level. The sole proprietor physician, however, is

personally responsible for all debts and liabilities of the medical practice. Capital may be difficult to raise with this entity.

(b) *General Partnership.* Enjoy the advantages of establishment ease, management flexibility, and "pass through" tax treatment. On the other hand, partnerships have the disadvantage that each partner has unlimited personal liability for each partners liabilities, debts, and malpractice obligations.

(c) *S Corporation.* Recent tax law changes have made some S corporations eligible for employee stock ownership plans, which is a change from past policies. Certain restrictions however, limit the eligibility of this corporation to 35 shareholders. Liability avoidance is available in this corporate entity.

(d) *Professional Corporation.* This business entity has limited liability but is not transferable to nonprofessional entities. May be either an S or C corporation.

(e) *C Corporation.* A publicly traded company, such as a PPMC, has to be a C corporation and will have too many shareholders (> 35 doctors) to qualify as an S corporation. The four characteristics that define a corporation are (1) centralized management (less than all doctor owners have decision making authority), (2) transferability of ownership (substitution through assignment, gifting or sale), (3) limited liability (no personal responsibility), and (4) continuity of life (notwithstanding certain "trigger events" such as retirement, bankruptcy, and/or death of the owner). Capital is easier to raise under this business structure.

(f) *Limited Liability Corporation/Partnership.* LLCs, LLPs, and limited partnerships are cousins of the S corporation that combine the corporate and partnership forms of business, limit partner liability, are size neutral, and, as flow-through entities, avoid the burden of double corporate taxation. Moreover, if they are properly structured to have two or fewer of the four corporate characteristics, they will be taxed like a partnership and thus avoid corporate taxation. Cautious physicians recognize the relative scarcity of case law to help judge how the law will be applied through established legal principles to these new business entities.

Tax consequences are important considerations, since there are many creative strategies for doctors to minimize state and local taxes. For example, a C corporation is its own tax paying entity, as opposed to an elected S corporation, in which net earnings are passed directly to the owner shareholder(s) (conduit). When an owner dies, the C practice corporation may have to pay an unexpected *alternative minimum tax (AMT)*. As a way to avoid the AMT, the practice may wish to alter its officer's life insurance into the form of a cross-purchase agreement. In this case, the owner's have life insurance on each other, and the agreement provides that, should an owner die, the other owners have the right to acquire the deceased owner's shares.

2. Maintain good financial records including all three consolidated financial statements, according to Financial Accounting Standard Board (FASB) rules: (a) balance sheet, (b) statement of cash flows, and (c) net income statement (profit and loss statement). Keep them for at least the last three years. There is nothing

that will kill the purchase, sale or merger of a practice quicker than not having these important documents. Consultants are often amazed if one in 10 doctors can produce even simple monthly reports of what they've budgeted, what was actually spent, or what was at variance.

3. Continually monitor key financial ratios, such as profitability ratios, creditor ratios, long-term debt management ratios, and medical-economic-value-added (MEVA) considerations:

    *   **Profitability ratios** include profit margin, *return on assets ratio* (net income + [interest expense × 1 (1 − tax rate)], *fixed/total assets utilization ratio* (gross charges/net fixed practice assets), and *fixed assets/net worth ratio.*
    *   **Creditor (solvency) ratios** include *working capital ratio* (excess of current assets over current liabilities), *current ratio* (current assets/current liabilities), *acid test ("quick") ratio* (current ratio net of inventory), *accounts receivable turnover ratio* (noncash revenue/average AR balance), and the *current liabilities to net worth ratio* (current liabilities/equity).
    *   **Long term debt management ratios** include *total debt to total assets ratio, total liability to net worth ratio, times interest earned ratio* (net operating income/ interest expense), and the *debt to equity ratio* (assets provided by creditors per owner assets). Other considerations include managed-care organization (MCO) contracts under management and free cash flow. Try to benchmark them with other comparable practices, and monitor them at least quarterly. Intervene immediately when necessary.
    *   **Medical economic value added ratios** distinguish between illusory profits and real economic gain. They are a good reflection of practice value, since to have a positive MEVA, practice revenues must exceed operating costs, taxes, and a charge for the cost of capital (debt interest rate charges, or the risk of saving/conserving capital rather than spending/investing it). In addition, MEVA expensing includes taxes to keep operations as lean as possible.

4. Be profitable, since you are in practice not only to help your patients, but also to make money. No one is going to buy a dying practice for more than a few pennies on the dollar, and you can't help anyone if you are not in business. Charity work is fine, as long as you realize that it is pro bono, but real value is a function of the amount and timing of discretionary cash flows, when it is—

    *   withdrawn from the practice in the form of dividends, a bonus or doctor remuneration above market rates (common in privately held medical offices;
    *   retained for growth investment opportunities or held as a redundant asset, like cash to increase value; and
    *   used to reduce the outstanding interest-bearing debt and increasing the equity component of total practice enterprise value.

Discretionary cash flow to doctors is normally calculated as follows: earnings before interest, taxes, depreciation, and amortization (EBITDA) less income taxes on EBITDA, capital expenditure requirements (net of the related income tax shield), incremental working capital requirements, and debt servicing costs (interest expense net of tax and changes in principal). Equity value is created when the discretionary cash flow that is generated from practice equity exceeds the required rate of return on equity.

Of course, large medical groups have certain advantages over solo or independent group practices. These include: access to capital, avoidance of "vendor" status, elimination of redundancy, and control and potential physician ownership in an organization larger than the sum of its individual practices. Financial managers and other corporate health care professionals possess the business acumen lacked by most physicians. Remember to think long-term profits versus short-term transactions. Also realize if you consolidate your practice, you are still going to be expected to work hard, perhaps even as though you never merged it in the first place. Be prepared for this eventuality. A practice purchase, merger, or even sale is not always a retirement plan or exit strategy Philosophically, larger groups often separate the *"individual current income"* approach to wealth building from the *"organizational future growth"* approach by focusing on maximizing equity value, by retaining capital and generating a return. This *value differential* is illustrated in Table 17.1.

5.   Obtain Workers' Compensation insurance to provide coverage for lost income due to on-the-job accidents or work-related employee disability or death. Benefits vary by state. Its purpose is not only to provide these benefits but also to reduce potential litigation. Employees accepting the benefit payments from a Workers' Compensation claim generally forego the right to sue their employer. Workers' Compensation rates are established by job descriptions and commercial rates for the medical professional's office are some of the lowest available. There are three methods of providing Workers' Compensation coverage:

- private commercial insurance
- governmental insurance funds
- self insure

There are, however, seven "monopolistic" states—Nevada, North Dakota, Ohio, Washington, West Virginia, and Wyoming—that do not permit private commercial insurance. The medical professional may be inclined to the third method, especially in the larger offices. As weekly benefits are typically below $500, this would seem to make sense. Since in larger groups, the owners can

TABLE 17.1   Economic Objective

	Individual Wealth	Group Wealth
End of Year Five		
Present Value Compensation (1)	$500	$500
Present Value Group Equity	1,000 (1,2)	6,200 (1,3)
TOTAL VALUE	**$1,500**	**6,700**
DIFFERENTIAL VALUE	**$1,500**	**$5,200**

Assumptions: (1) 10% Discount Rate (2) Net Book Value (3) 1X revenues.

elect not to be covered, it is usually more convenient for the medical professional to cover this risk with personal disability income insurance. Larger offices that wish to take more direct control of costs and benefit management should consider self-insuring only after receiving expert advice. This is one form of coverage that truly requires a knowledgeable insurance advisor.

6. Obtain practice business insurance that is offered on a simplified package basis. Similar to homeowner policies, it contains both property and liability coverage. Property coverage is available on either an actual value or replacement value basis and it can be purchased for named-perils or on an all-risk basis. Also, like homeowner policies, the medical professional should compile a basic inventory of property to be covered. Medical records and important papers are typically covered for a flat amount. Don't forget to allow for supplies, instruments, and leased equipment.

    Liability coverage protects the physician owner from claims arising from bodily injury or property damage while the claimant is on the premises. Liability insurance not only pays the damage awarded to the claimant but also the attorney fees and other costs associated with any defense of the suit. Coverage under a business owner policy is typically very broad and can be tailored to fit almost any practice. Since coverage can often be coordinated with other practice related insurance, it may be provided by the same company.

7. Have a practice continuation plan or buy/sell agreement that stipulates upon the death or disability of a business partner or sole proprietor, how the business must be sold, or how the practice is to be continued. In a typical buy/sell agreement, the sole proprietor, or partner is the insured of a life insurance policy, which can create the funds to complete the agreement. There are a number of keys to creating a successful buy/sell agreement:

    *   It must be decided who will buy the practice from the disabled proprietor or partner or from his or her heirs. It may be the remaining partner(s), the practice entity itself, or, in the case of a sole doctor proprietor, a key physician employee.
    *   The buy/sell agreement must be stipulated as mandatory. According to the IRS, if the agreement is not mandatory, the value of the practice is not considered fixed. As a result, the IRS might not consider the agreement binding in determining the value of the practice for estate tax purposes.
    *   Be specific as to what is to be purchased. This can include land, buildings, inventory, licenses, and even goodwill and other intangible (but valuable) assets.
    *   The most important key is determining the correct value for the practice or share in question. The IRS will rarely challenge a value for being set too high but will challenge those deemed valued too low. Valuation should not be taken lightly; it can be a fixed dollar amount or it can be based on a formula. The usual recommendation is to use a formula rather than a fixed dollar amount.

    There are a number of different forms of buy/sell agreements. The following is a quick overview of four different variations.

    a. **Sole Proprietor Buy/Sell Agreement.** Since sole proprietors do not have partners (other than a spouses), they usually must look elsewhere for buyers. Therefore, the sole proprietor is likely to turn either to a valued physician employee to continue the business. In this case, a life insurance policy is purchased on the life of the proprietor and the agreement is signed between the current and the future owners providing the guidelines for the future practice transfer. In addition to being the owner of the policy, the future doctor/owner typically names himself or herself the beneficiary as well.

b. **Cross Purchase Buy/Sell Agreement.** This type of buy/sell is normally used for any practice with multiple owners, although it is best used for agreements with only two owners. In this arrangement, each owner purchases insurance on each of the others lives. Again, the owner of each policy names him/herself beneficiary as well. Upon the death or disability of one partner, the remaining partner(s) are provided the funds to purchase a pro rata share of the deceased or disabled individual's practice interest.

c. **Entity Purchase Buy/Sell Agreement.** This form is used for multiple owners, and/or when the owner(s) of the practice wants to use the assets of the business to fund the insurance policies. In this arrangement, the practice owns the policies on each partner or shareholder and is also listed as the beneficiary of each policy. Upon the death or disability of the physician partner, the business would be able to purchase the shares from the disabled partner or from the deceased's heirs.

d. **Optional Purchase/Wait and See Buy/Sell Agreement.** This type of agreement allows either the practice or the individual partner(s) the option of purchasing the deceased or disabled partner's interest in the practice. Normally, if the practice does not initially exercise its option to buy within a set period, the remaining partner(s) would then have a period in which to exercise their option. If they do not buy the outstanding interest, the practice would then be forced to purchase the shares.

Often, a trusteed agreement is advisable. It is not unusual to find situations where the practice partners work together smoothly and efficiently. Their spouses, however, are another story.

In order to remove personalities from the transfer of ownership interests for money, especially at a very stressful point in their lives, it is often a good idea to let a disinterested third party (a trustee) conduct the transfer.

Example. Dr. May has been the sole owner of The Family Physician Group, which includes 6 other physicians and 12 other employees, for over 10 years. He has often thought about who will continue this successful practice. In the past month, he has decided that Dr. Roy is the best candidate for the job. She has also expressed an interest in becoming the successor to Dr. May. As a result, they have decided to set up a trusteed sole proprietor buy/sell agreement that would provide for the mandatory transfer of the practice in the case of the death or disability of Dr. May. Once the practice is correctly valued, she plans to purchase a life insurance policy on the life of Dr. May, which will be owned by a third-party trustee, who will also be the beneficiary. Upon the death or disability of Dr. May, the agreement is executed by the trustee, and Dr. Roy becomes sole owner of The Family Physician Group.

8.   Do not forget to obtain key-person (doctor) insurance. In this case, the practice would purchase and own a life insurance policy on the key doctor. Upon the death of the doctor, the life insurance proceeds could be used to

- pay off bank loans,
- replace the lost profits of the practice, and
- establish a reserve for the search, hiring, and training of a replacement physician.

Example. Local Eye Clinic has gained national recognition in innovating a new procedure for laser eye surgery. Not only has the practice invested an enormous sum of money in the equipment used, but it is very dependent on the talents and continued employment of Dr. Mackenzie, who helped design the equipment and procedure. Fearing the economic consequences if Dr. Mackenzie were to die, they have purchased an insurance policy on his life to help pay for the immediate replacement and the training of another specialist.

9.   Develop a forward thinking valuation business plan, since all doctors should plan to sell their practices at some point in the future; whether to retire, merge, or acquire another practice. By understanding how practices are valued and designing sales value into your plan, you can create tremendous value for yourself. For example, according to IRS guidelines, the three most common methods of practice valuation include (a) discounted cash flow analysis (DCFA), (b) the multiplier (comparable sales) method, and (c) the replacement cost method (RCM).

(A) Discounted Cash Flow Analysis

The DCFA, or income method, is the discounting of a dollar's value today by some factor to estimate its future value. DCFA is used to establish the present value of these future practice cash flows, using mutually agreed upon financial assumptions, such as time frame, interest rates (discount rate), lump sums, periodicity (annuitization), and equality or inequality of actual funds received.

The discount rate depends on prevailing interest rates and risk factors (more risk means a larger discount). For a physician thinking about a capital partner, sales, or merger, the appropriate rate in 2005 might be between 7 and 15 percent, as calculated in Table 17.2.

To compute the present value of future cash flows, the net income (profit and loss sheet normalization) statement must be analyzed to recast it, if necessary, to eliminate expenses not related to running the practice (i.e., payroll salary expense for absent wife/secretary), project future after tax cash flow, and develop a rate of return, as indicated earlier.

The second part of this economic model is to calculate the present value of future net income without merging with the capital partner (large group, hospital, venture capitalist, etc.) and remaining independent. In some cases, staying independent requires the application of a higher rate, since it may be a more risky endeavor. Therefore, the discount rate might even be higher, likely in the range of 12%–20%. The difference between the present value of the baseline scenario and what can be

TABLE 17.2   Medical Practice Discount Rate

Risk Factors	Rate Impact
Risk Free Rate (Treasuries/CDs)	5.00%
Business Risk Rate (Specialty)	3.00%
Competition Risk	2.00%
Medicare/Medicaid Risk	2.00%
Management Risk	2.00%
Commercial Managed Care Risk	1.00%
Capitalization Rate:	**14.00%**

expected from taking a capital partner is the best measure of economic consequences to physicians and medical groups.

(B) Replacement Cost Method (RCM)

The RCM seeks to replace tangible assets or certain intangible assets (trained and assembled workforce, patient records, etc.) at current or fair market value prices. It assumes that a prudent buyer will pay no more for an existing practice than the cost of creating a similar new practice.

It merely represents the actual cash value (ACV) of the practice, less its liabilities, plus the depreciated value of those assets; expressed mathematically by the equation: RCM = ACV + depreciation. In other words, it is the cost to reproduce or replace appraised property less allowances for deterioration and functional or economic obsolescence. This method is most applicable in cases of land ownerships and improvements (i.e., physician medical-building ownership), special purpose buildings (i.e., ambulatory surgery centers), and other special instruments. The approach is static and provides only a snapshot of the value of a practice as of a certain date. It does not take into account attributed to good will and ignores your practice's past and future ability to generate income.

Alternatively, the cost method for the "ongoing concern" practice may be the cost avoided by not having to start a practice from scratch and grow its operation to a breakeven point. For example, the going concern value is inclusive of all practice assets as shown in Table 17.3.

TABLE 17.3

Ongoing Concern Practice Value	$$$
Working Capital (current assets less current liabilities):	W
Tangible Assets:	X
Intangible Assets:	Y
Goodwill:	Z
Total (going concern value):	WXYZ

TABLE 17.4 **Case Study Example: (ABC Medical Practice)**

A medical practice (ABC) was valuated using the two methods just discussed. The results are given below. *What price should the practice sell for?*

DCFA Method:	**Valuated @ $500,00**
Replacement Cost Method:	**Valuated @ $200,00**

Using the cost method, one would expect that a book value of $200,000 is at the bottom of the market range for this practice, since goodwill and ongoing concern estimates were not considered. On the other hand, the DCFA method of analysis did consider these factors. Therefore, the price range of the practice would be $200,000–500,000, but $350,000 or so might be a more reasonable number to consider in a sales situation.

Thus, this fair market value cost approach is simply the estimated amount at which the practice might be expected to exchange between a willing buyer and a willing seller, neither being under a compulsion to buy or sell, and each having reasonable knowledge of all relevant facts. Often, both the cost and income methods are used to appraise a practice; the resulting information serves as a cross-reference to develop a valuation *range* rather than a specific price.

(C) Multiplier (Comparable) Sales

Although DCFA is probably the most precise method of practice valuation today; the comparable sales method in which gross EBITDA or net profits are multiplied by some established industrial norm may occasionally be used.

The gross revenue multiplier is most appropriate for a market share gaining strategy, while an EBITDA multiplier might be generally more reliable if earnings are an important concern. A net-profit multiplier is probably most unreliable, since many income tax machinations are possible to alter this number.

Unfortunately, this multiplier market approach is also difficult to use because of the limitations of data relative to similar practice sales and the lack of full transparency in private business transactions. Key information that might drive valuations and market price might include fee schedules, payer mix, cost structures, physician compensation, collection rates, productivity, and prospects for future practice growth. Thus, the use of the comparable method is limited by the constraint of information on practices sold.

Above all, realize that the value of a medical practice today is not always a function of its gross revenues but of net income; and that net income applies more to the purchaser's ability to perform rather than the seller's. In addition, it is not unusual for a practice sold on the open market to experience some attrition of patients and managed care plans upon the change of ownership.

10. Brand your practice and recapture youthful dreams of success by building value into your business. But, brand recognition is not going to come from just adding more managed-care patients, shifting your markets or demographics, or specializing in surgery or sports medicine. You may already be doing that, and that's very good. The real paradigm shift, however, will come from creating

value inside your office. You do that by making your business worth buying to someone else. In other words, a group "brand" identity, rather than an individual physician identity, is the hallmark of increased practice value in the future.

In fact, most authorities opine that in today's medical marketplace, bigger is better and size matters. We are now in an environment of large group practices, where cachet value matters, not individual practitioner accomplishment. Hot medical groups; not individual doctors, will flourish going forward. Even if you are a young practitioner and not interested in merging your practice, you still want to build it up as if you were going to sell it at some point in the future because this strategy will maximize value. The secret is to create the best transferable medical system around. Transferable operations not only make your practice profitable and build value, but also do right by your personal, corporate, or private investors.

Of course, building a transferable patient base is increasingly more difficult with all of the managed care contracting today; but it still can be done. If you build a system that revolves around either a single (few) MCO contract(s), yourself, or another key man or key woman, it is difficult to transfer the business to someone else, and so key person insurance is also important. And, realize that if you project yourself as the medical guru for your area, patients will have a hard time accepting a new doctor or consolidated group. By focusing on something larger than yourself, such as group practice, you will begin to develop a business that others can operate easily.

11. Use proper management information systems (computer hardware, software, and peripherals) and the Health Insurance Portability and Accountability Act of 1996 (HIPAA) specifications, without spending too much money on information technology gadgetry. You do not necessarily need to become an early adopter of the newest or untested information technology systems, but do become an adopter of mature products, nevertheless.

12. Absent a covenant not to compete, if a physician leaves the practice and immediately competes against it, the departing physician will probably take revenue away from the original practice and potentially decrease its value—significantly and abruptly. Therefore, have a covenant to specify the procedures to follow should a departure occur. For example, the covenant may require either a-time bomb, distance-bomb, or buy-out discount in the case of a departing partner, precluding the new practice or practitioner from achieving a monetary gain. Although covenants may have many different inclusions, such contracts depend on the laws of the sate in which the practice is located. Moreover, many believe that the covenant is not worth the time and money necessary to enforce; however, its existence will add equity value to the existing practice, to the benefit of the remaining practitioners.

13. Obtain an extension of the above noncompete agreement, also known as a nondisclosure agreement, for practice techniques, information, and so on.

Sample: Nondisclosure Agreement

The undersigned acknowledges that "The Practice" has furnished to the undersigned potential "New Associate," either directly, indirectly, or by way of "normal office operations and business practices," certain proprietary data, economic information, insurance contracts, patient names, contact information, medical records, charts, paperwork, authorizations, agreements, and disclosures, material safety data sheets (MSDSs), MCO contracting, OSHA, Patriot Act (PA), Sarbanes-Oxley Act (SOA), HIPAA, and other information relating to the business affairs and operations of "The Practice," for study and evaluation by the "New Associate" for possibly working/ investing in "The Practice."

- It is acknowledged by "New Associate" that the information provided by "The Practice" is confidential; therefore, "New Associate" agrees not to disclose it and not to disclose that any discussions or contracts with "The Practice" have occurred or are intended, other than as provided for in the following paragraph.
- It is acknowledged by "New Associate" that information to be furnished is in all respects confidential in nature, other than information which is in the public domain through other means and that any disclosure or use of same by "New Associate," except as provided in this agreement, may cause serious harm or damage to "The Practice" and its owners and officers.
- Therefore, "New Associate" agrees that "New Associate" will not use the information furnished for any purpose other than as stated above and agrees that "New Associate" will not either directly or indirectly by agent, employee, or representative, disclose this information, either in whole or in part, to any third party; provided, however that (a) information furnished may be disclosed only to those directors, officers and employees of "New Associate" and to "New Associate" advisors or their representatives who need such information for the purpose of evaluating any possible transaction (it being understood that those directors, officers, employees, advisors, and representatives shall be informed by "New Associate" of the confidential nature of such information and shall be directed by "New Associate" to treat such information confidentially); and (b) any disclosure of information may be made to which "The Practice" consents in writing.

At the close of negotiations, "New Associate" will return to "The Practice" all medical records, reports, x rays, documents, insurance contracts, and memoranda furnished and will not make or retain any copy thereof.

14. Maintain services, responsiveness, and consistency with your patients, referring doctors, fellow physicians, and supply vendors. And, be flexible. For example, start a pharmacy services program if you do not have one. Or, consider limiting laboratory services if they no longer remain cost effective for you.

    This is critical, because if you do not build strong relationships with these local players, premium value just isn't there, since a new doctor will not be able to rely on those established relationships going forward.
15. Use life insurance correctly to benefit your practice in the following three ways:

A. Physician Executive Bonus Plan

A physician executive bonus plan (or §162 plan) is an effective way for a larger medical practice or clinic to provide to valued, select doctors an additional employment benefit.

One of the main advantages to an executive bonus plan, when compared to other benefits, is its simplicity.

In a typical executive bonus plan, an agreement is made between the employer and physician/employee, whereby the employer agrees to pay for the cost of a life insurance policy, in the form of a bonus, on the life of the physician employee. The major benefits of such a plan to the employee doctor is that he or she is the immediate owner of the cash values and the death benefit provided. The only cost to the doctor employee is the payment of income tax on any bonus received. The employer receives a tax deduction for providing the benefit, improves the moral of its selected employees, and can use the plan as a tool to attract additional talent.

Example: Dr. Smith is a sole practitioner in rural Wyoming. Among his employees is Nurse Jones, who has been with him for over 10 years. She is the single parent of two boys. Although he pays well and provides additional benefits, he has been looking for a way to selectively reward Nurse Jones for her years of service and hard work. Recently, Nurse Jones has expressed a concern for her children if she were to die prematurely. Dr. Smith chooses to provide an executive bonus plan by allowing Nurse Jones to purchase a life insurance policy on her life. Dr. Smith will provide the premium payments in the form of a bonus to her. Nurse Jones must simply pay the tax on this additional income. Dr. Smith's practice will get a tax deduction for the premium and improve the morale of an important employee. Nurse Jones will get needed protection for her family.

B. Nonqualified Salary Continuation

Commonly referred to as deferred compensation, this is a legally binding promise by a doctor's employer to pay a salary continuation benefit at a specific point in the future in exchange for the current and continued performance of its doctor employee. These plans are normally used to supplement existing retirement plans.

Although there are different variations of deferred compensation, in a typical deferred compensation agreement, the employer will purchase and own a life insurance policy on the life of the physician employee. The cash value of the policy grows tax deferred during the employee's working years. After retirement, these cash values can be withdrawn from the policy to reimburse the company for its after-tax retirement payments to the doctor employee. Upon the death of the doctor employee, any remaining death benefit would likely be received income tax free by the employer. (Alternative minimum taxes could apply to any benefit received by certain larger C corporations.) The death benefit could then be used to pay any required survivor benefits to the employee's spouse, or provide partial or total cost recovery to the employer.

In a typical plan, the terms of the agreement are negotiated as to the amount of benefit received by the physician employee, when retirement benefits can begin, how long retirement benefits will be paid, and if benefits will be provided for death or disability. The business has established what is commonly referred to as "golden handcuffs" for the doctor/employee.

As a result, the benefit will only be received if the employee continues to work for the company until retirement. If the physician/employee is terminated for cause or quits prior to retirement, the plan would end and no benefits would be payable.

Example. Dr. Olde has been working for Northeast Orthopedics for almost seven years. His employer knows that he has been approached by a number of other orthopedic practices in regards to joining them in the future. Northeast Orthopedics wants to keep Dr. Olde on its staff for a few more years and needs to create an incentive program for Dr. Olde to want to stay. They have agreed to enter into a deferred compensation plan with Dr. Olde. According to the agreement, Dr. Olde will agree to continue to work for Northeast until normal retirement age. In exchange for his continued services, the company will provide him, or his surviving spouse, an additional $50,000 per year starting at age 65 and lasting for 20 years. In order to fund this plan, Northeast has astutely decided to purchase a life insurance policy on Dr. Olde. As the cash value grows tax-deferred, it will eventually be available to provide the company reimbursements for the after-tax additional retirement benefit. Should Dr. Olde die prematurely, the policy's death benefit would be available to provide the agreed benefit for his surviving spouse. It has also been designed to provide some key person coverage.

C. Split Dollar Plans

Split dollar arrangements can be a complicated and confusing concept for even the most experienced insurance professional or financial advisor. This concept is, in its simplest terms, a way for a practice to share the cost and benefit of a life insurance policy with a valued employee doctor. In a normal split dollar arrangement, the doctor employee will receive valuable life insurance coverage at little cost to them. The practice pays the majority of the premium but is usually able to recover the entire cost of providing this benefit. Following the publication of IRS Notices 2002-8 and 2002-59, there are currently two general approaches to the ownership of practice split-dollar life insurance: employer-owned or employee-owned. (In addition, Proposed Regulation 164754-01, if finalized in present form, would substantially change split-dollar arrangements even further. The practitioner should research this area thoroughly before making any recommendations.) Regardless of the method used, a written agreement must be prepared to spell out the rights and obligations of the parties.

Employer-Owned Method

In the employer-owned method, the employer is the sole owner of the policy. A written split-dollar agreement usually permits the doctor employee to name the beneficiary for most of the death proceeds. The employer owns all the cash value and has the unfettered right to borrow or withdraw it as necessary.

At the end of the formal agreement, the practice can generally (1) continue the policy as key doctor insurance, (2) transfer ownership to the insured doctor and report the cash values as additional income to the insured, (3) sell the policy to the insured doctor, or (4) use a combination of these methods. This is commonly referred to as "rollout."

Note: Practitioners should be careful not to include rollout language in the split-dollar agreement. Many plans are set up with the intent—although not in writing—to transfer the policy to the insured after a certain number of years. The reason the rollout should not be included is that if the parties formally agree that after a specified number of years—or following a specific event—related only to the circumstances surrounding the policy, that the policy will be turned over to the insured, the IRS could declare that the entire transaction was a sham and that its sole purpose was to avoid taxation of the premiums to the employee. If that happens, the IRS may deem that the premiums paid should be considered income to the employee when they were paid. If this comes up in an audit years after the inception of the agreement, it may generate substantial interest and penalties in addition to the additional taxes due.

The death proceeds available to the doctor's insured employee's beneficiary is considered a current economic benefit. Also called reportable economic benefit (REB), it is an annually taxable event to the employee. If an individual policy is involved, the REB is calculated by multiplying the face amount times the government's annual Table 2004-05-06-07 (etc.) rates or the insurance company's alternative term rates, using the insured's age. If a second-to-die policy is involved, the government's PS38 rates or the company's alternative PS38 rates will be used. Any part of the premium actually paid by the employee is used to offset any REB dollar-for-dollar.

The employer-owned method is primarily used when the employer wishes to maintain as much control as possible over the life-insurance policy or for physician executives of publicly held corporations. This doctor employee perquisite can be used to reward key physicians with current inexpensive death protection and simultaneously provide a potential handcuff for them by informally funding a deferred compensation agreement.

Employee-Owned Method

With the physician employee-owned method, the insured doctor/employee is generally the applicant and owner of the policy. Any premiums paid by the practice are deemed to be loans to the employee, and the employee reports as income an imputed interest rate on the cumulative amount of loan based on Code § 7872. A collateral assignment is made for the benefit of the practice to cover the cumulative loan amount. In some cases, the assignment may allow the assignee to have access to the cash values of the policy by way of a policy loan. This method is unavailable for physician/officers and executives of publicly held corporations because of the current restrictions on corporate loans (the Sarbanes-Oxley Act).

The employee-owned method is somewhat similar to the older collateral assignment form of split-dollar. The benefits for the employee are both the ability to control large amounts of death proceeds as well as developing equity in the policy.

Whether or not this new method catches on will depend greatly on the imputed interest rate published by the IRS every July. If set low enough, this may be an excellent opportunity for the doctor employee to use inexpensive practice dollars to pay for life insurance. In the fall of 2003, for example, the rate was about 1.99%.

Example. Dr. Tyler is a valuable member of a team of surgeons at St. Mary's Hospital. He has recently developed a new technique for treating heart aneurysms. The hospital would like to keep him on staff for years to come. Dr. Tyler is married and has one small child—and his wife is pregnant. He has requested that the hospital provide him with more life insurance. The hospital's board of directors meets with a number of financial advisors to review their options and they settle on an employer-owned method split dollar arrangement. As a result, they will purchase and pay for a life insurance policy on Dr. Tyler, providing him the bulk of the death benefit for his family, as long as he is a member of their hospital staff. They have also agreed to bonus Dr. Tyler the amount equal to the reportable economic benefit in order to keep his insurance cost at a minimum.

16. Identify the right buyer, seller or merging partner, be it another physician, larger group practice, or multidisciplinary medical operation, Make sure that the buyer has the necessary capital and that you are not taking all of the risks in the transaction. You want to risk financial share with the buyer and have faith that he or she can pull off the sale. You also want a good intangible heuristic match, since your lifeblood probably went into building the practice and you should want it to flourish going forward.

17. In addition to selling or buying a practice, it is often important to know its value—during your lifetime or at death—when making a gift ($11,000 individual annual exclusion and $22,000 tax free with spouse) of your of practice interest, planning your estate, or for other practice succession needs; whether to physician offspring or to practice outsiders. If you don't know its value and the IRS determines its fair market value to be higher than the value set under your buy-sell agreement, for example, your estate could be required to pay estate taxes (37%–55%).

It is also important to be aware of the exclusion amount, or the amount of property that can be passed to your heirs without estate taxation. In 2004 and 2005, this amount was $1,500,000. So, for a married couple, both spouses can pass $1,500,000 free of estate taxes. Under current law, the unified credit and exclusion amount will increase as follows:

Year	Unified Credit	Exclusion Amount
2002		
2003	$345,800	1,000,000
2004–2005	555,800	1,500,000
2006–2008	780,800	2,000,000
2009	1,455,800	3,500,000
2010	Estate tax repealed	

The escalation of unified credits and exclusion amounts with the ultimate elimination of estate taxes in 2010–11 has a potential wealth benefit for future generations of medical professionals. Skepticism is always a part of new tax legislation, and several pundits are predicting that estate taxes will not be eliminated, although there are those who believe the exclusion amount will be permanently increased.

18. Assist the transfer but don't think you can sell your practice in a couple of months. The average timeframe is about 1–2 years. So, if you become sick or disabled, you may lose your practice or have to sell it for a fraction of its value. Make sure you have an ample capital surplus during the sales period with contingency plan and timetable if you can't sell. If you provide owner

financing to the buyer, make sure that you purchase an insurance policy on his or her life. After retirement, you probably won't want to suddenly return to practice if your income stream abruptly stops because of the premature death of the buyer.

Finally, get professional assistance if you can't, or do not want to, go it alone. Align yourself with a trusted MBA, CPA, CMP©, CFP™, JD, or practice management (specialty specific) firm, or continue practicing as a corporate employee.

CONCLUSION

Contemporary physicians still have a huge opportunity to build equity value into their medical practice for sale or consolidation. Whether or not this becomes a reality depends on the creation of maximum equity value as if a transaction was possible. Then, design your office to enhance its value and achieve everything dreamed about when the practice was first begun many years ago.

ACKNOWLEDGMENTS

Thanks to Gary A. Cook, MSFS, CLU, ChFC, CMP©, CFP™, for technical assistance in the preparation of this chapter.

CHAPTER 18

The Science and Art of Medical Practice Valuation

David Edward Marcinko

> The value of a business (medical practice) represents a tremendous investment for both the buyer and seller, and it's shortsighted not to have a professional appraiser, working with both the buyer and seller so they understand the valuation issues involved. It's very easy in the emotion and passion of buying a business to make a mistake. And competent professional business appraisers bring a dispassionate view of value that should be important to all buyers and sellers of businesses.
>
> —Steven F. Schroeder, Esq.
> American Business Appraisers

The health care industry continues to undergo major revisions in its form of health care delivery. Market evolution has been described as revolutionary, fraught with continual organizational changes. Recent years have been marked by significant and increasing politically sensitive industry consolidations, although the frenzied rate of previous merger and acquisitions activity has abated. This occurred amid the bankruptcy of noted private organizations and practices, as well as the alleged and massive fraudulent activities of a highly visible publicly traded healthcare company. All despite the passage of the Sarbanes-Oxley Act in the winter of 2002, which required corporate executives to sign financial reports attesting to their veracity.

Today, the major industry segments grabbing the headlines are physician-to-physician consolidations. Other industry segments, such as long-term care, medical devices; pharmaceutical and supply distribution, PHOs (physician hospital organizations), and PPMCs (Physician Practice Management Corporations) are no longer setting record levels in terms of volume and dollar value of business combinations. The macroeconomic health care merger and acquisition fervor, as seen on the grand scale of several years ago, is virtually absent.

So, why is there this urge to buy, sell, or merge in the private clinical and microeconomic practice arena? Medical practice consolidation is being fueled by the rapid growth of managed care and the continuing squeeze on the health care dollar.

Aging physicians are retiring, midlife doctors are getting divorced, and newly minted physicians are desperately seeking to retain one last vestige of business autonomy.

The health care market is over $1 trillion dollars, with physicians controlling 85% of total health care spending. According to the Health Care Financing Administration (HCFA), the government agency that administers the Medicare and Medicaid programs, direct spending on physicians has grown from $5.3 billion in 1960 to nearly $500 billion in the year 2005. Figure 18.1 illustrates this explosive growth trend in physician spending.

STRONG IMPETUS TO CONSOLIDATE

The federal government is the largest single payer in the United States, accounting for approximately one third of all of health care expenditures. With the aging population, legislative efforts to control health care spending can only escalate. Further accelerating the urge to merge, many insurers are increasingly basing provider payments on some level of Medicare reimbursements. Medical practices are continually attempting to offset declining revenues by controlling costs and offering broader services. With market forces squeezing the health care dollar, continual change and industry consolidation is eminent, and this is the reason for many public debates.

THE REGULATORY CLIMATE

Federal and state fraud and abuse laws, self-referral laws, tax-exempt entities prohibitions on inurement and private benefit, and a host of other federal and state laws and regulations have significant impact on what medical practices can acquire and how those acquisitions are structured.

The IRS and the *Office of the Inspector General ("OIG"), Department of Health and Human Services* are scrutinizing the formation of integrated delivery systems ("IDS"), with major focus on physician transactions. The impact to the health care industry has been

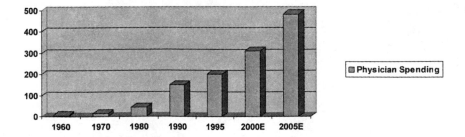

FIGURE 18.1

Source: Health Care Financing Administration, 2003.

- increased scrutiny by regulators,
- the need for greater understanding of regulations and their impact on determining value, and
- the need for greater documentation in rationale and support of underlying value conclusions.

Current health care policy issues are likely to address four broad areas: Medicare, Medicaid, access to care, and managed care. With Medicare and Medicaid taking up significant portions of the federal budget, efforts to bring revenues in line with spending will require painful reductions of provider payments. Under previously enacted Medicare reform legislation, provider-sponsored organizations (PSOs), that are groups of hospitals, physicians, and other providers, are allowed to contract directly for Medicare capitation. This legislation also has significant negative impact to physician payments and, in particular, to specialty practices. Medicare, Medicaid, access to care, and antimanaged-care legislation will continue to be hotly debated topics.

THE ECONOMIC CLIMATE

Other legislation negatively impacting traditional physician economics and independence include the following risks:

- Health Insurance Portability and Accountability Act (HIPAA)
- Patriot Act,
- Balanced Budget Amendment
- Sarbanes-Oxley Act,
- antitrust
- Federal False Claims Act
- civil asset forfeiture
- Material Safety Data Sheets requirements,
- OSHA and Clinical Laboratory Improvement Amendments (CLIA)
- Drug Enforcement Agency
- Environmental Protection Agency
- managed care contractual
- ERISA
- business and employee
- systemic economic
- workplace violence and terrorism

PHYSICIAN MERGER MOTIVATION

There are approximately 850,000 allopathic physician practitioners (i.e., MDs) in the United States, and, according to the American Medical Association, slightly over 210,000 are organized in groups of three or more.

In addition, there are more than 225,000 dentists (DDS, DMD); more than 160,000 optometric physicians (OD); 125,000 chiropractors (DC); 55,000 osteopathic physicians (DO), and about 13,000 podiatric physicians (DPM).

This huge fragmentation of medical practitioners has allowed for the proliferation of managed care organizations commanding significant reductions in provider payments.

Declining incomes and increasing administrative challenges have motivated a significant number of physicians to sell their practice assets and join hospital systems, align with corporate partners, or decide to merge with larger medical groups to form even larger regional groups. There are countless acquisition and physician management models, some successful and many unsuccessful. Undoubtedly, there will be more models evolving as there will always be organizations that think they have built a better mousetrap. And the truth is, these affiliations must be flexible and evolving to adapt to an ever changing health care market.

Small medical group acquisitions continue at a steady clip despite the past collapse of behemoth corporations, like MedPartners, PhyCor, and FPA Medical Management. Investors have increasingly abandoned the industry since MedPartners and PhyCor called off merger plans and FPA Medical Management filed for Chapter 11 bankruptcy protection (in 1998). The publicized financial difficulties of many physician practice management corporations (PPMCs) are well known, as is the accounting debacle of Health South in 2003–2004.

In the past five years, the industry has lost substantial macroeconomic value in the public equity markets. Fourth generations PPMCs are now small, locally directed, privately held, and physician owned. Many that have not met earnings expectations are reinventing themselves once again as virtual Internet educational portals or retail sales sites. Initial public offerings are nonexistent; analysts have been fired and venture capitalists have gone into hibernation.

Why all this market uncertainty? Generally, the September 11, 2001, incident, depressed domestic economy, the continued threat of international terrorism with weapons of mass destruction (WMDs), and the SARS (sudden acute respiratory syndrome) epidemic, among other events, have all been funneled into a vortex to create the current conundrum.

Economically, no one knows precisely the best formula for physician practice microintegration. The move from a traditional fee-for-service environment to capitation and other fixed-fee reimbursements are shifting financial risks from payers to providers. In addition, physicians are faced with ever increasing needs for negotiating clout, capital for expansion, and administrative and management burdens in a time of declining incomes. All market forces continue to motivate private practitioners and physician consolidation.

THE NEED FOR MEDICAL PRACTICE VALUATIONS

Physicians are entrepreneurial by nature and take great pride in the creation of their businesses. Market pressures are motivating physicians to be proactive and to make informed decisions concerning the future of their businesses. The decision to sell, buy, or merge, while often financially driven, is inherently an emotional one.

Other economic reasons for a practice valuation include changes in ownership, determining insurance coverage for a practice buy-sell agreement or upon a physician-owners death, establishing stock options, or bringing in a new partner. Practice appraisals are also used for legal reasons such as divorce, bankruptcy, breach of contract, and minority shareholder complaints. In 2002, the Financial Accounting Standards Board (FASB) issued rules that required certain intangible assets to be valued, such as goodwill. This may be important for practices seeking start-up, service segmentation extensions, or operational funding. Other reasons for a medical practice appraisal, and the considerations that go along with them, are discussed here.

Estate Planning

Medical practice valuation may be required for estate planning purposes. For a decedent physician with a gross estate of more than $1.5 million, his or her assets must be reported at fair market value on an estate tax return. If lifetime gifts of a medial practice business interest are made, it is generally wise to obtain an appraisal and attach it to the gift-tax return.

And, realize that the following price discounts/price premiums may apply in any case:

- **Practice Appraisal Discounts.** A discount may be applied to a medical practice valuation when there is no ready market for such interest, as in the case of a small-town community, specialty provider, or niche market. If the interest is not a controlling one, then a minority discount or lack-of-control discount may be appropriate. Two appraisals may even be used; one to valuate the practice, the other to valuate the discount.
- **Control Premiums.** A control premium occurs when majority practice ownership provides a physician executive with the ability to: set practice business strategy, hire and fire employees, accept and reject managed care contracts, and determine compensation and perquisite levels, among other things.
- **Reverse Practice Appraisal Premiums.** On the other hand, the IRS may disallow a minority interest discount and instead apply what is known as a swing-vote premium (SVP). Let's say that if a 20% interest in a three-doctor practice is being valuated, and there are two other physician shareholders each owning 40%, the fair market value of that 20% may have significant and valuable controlling aspects, suggesting the SVP.

Buy-Sell Agreements

The ideal situation is for physician partners to put in place a buy-sell agreement when practice relationships are amicable. This establishes the terms for departure before they are required, and is akin to a prenuptial agreement in the marriage contract. Disagreements most often occur when a doctor leaves the group, especially if the doctor leaves acrimoniously. Business operations of the practice decline, employee and partner morale suffers, feuding factions develop, which spills over into the office, and the practice begins to implode creating a downward valuation spiral. And so, valuations should be done every two to three years, or as the economic circumstances of the practice change. Independence and credibility are provided, and emotional overtones are purged from the transaction.

Physician Partnership Disputes

Medical practice appraisals are often used in partnership disputes, such as breach-of-contract or departure issues. Obvious revenue declinations are not difficult to quantify. But, revenues may not immediately fall since certain current procedural terminology (CPT) code reimbursements may actually increase. Upon verification however, lost business may be camouflaged as the number of procedures performed, or number of patients decrease after partner departure.

Divorce

Physicians getting divorced should get a practice appraisal. Either side may hire the appraiser, although occasionally the court will order an expert to provide a neutral valuation. Such valuations should be done in light of both court discovery rules and IRS requirements for closely held businesses. Generally, this requires the consideration of eight elements:

- practice specialty and operating history
- economic and healthcare industry condition
- estimates of practice risks and future returns
- book value and financial condition of the practice
- practice future earning capacity
- physician bonuses, dividends, and distributions
- intangible assets
- comparable practice sales

Sometime, the nonphysician spouse may even desire a lifestyle analysis by a forensic accountant, or appraiser to evaluate the potential for under-reported income. A family-law judge is often the final arbiter of different valuations, and because of varying state laws, there may be 50 different nuances of what the practice is really worth.

Additive Value and Organic Growth Ingredient

Sometimes, medical practice appraisals can add value where little actually exists or add value where not apparent. For example, mature doctors may believe their practice is worth more than it actually is in the modern climate. Upon appraisal, they are devastated and can't understand the reasons for its minimal value. So consultants, business advisors and financial planners can work to leverages practice assets to greatest advantage. Tasks may be identified that require less labor, human resources may be outsourced, service line segments dropped according to CPT code reimbursement, paraprofessionals utilized as substitutes, and office processes automated to increase practice bottom line profits. Sans the appraisal epiphany, these changes may never have occurred.

Moreover, even successful practices can use periodic valuations as an ingredient to future organic and nonorganic growth. Some basic concepts to grow a medical practice through appropriate mergers and acquisitions include the following.

Establish Goals and a Time Frame

When considering a merger, knowing where you want to go makes getting there more likely. And, although merging practices to achieve economies of scale may seem perfectly logical, be sure to have other objectives, as well. Set revenue and profitability goals, and leave time to digest the acquisition.

Have a Strategic Plan

Make sure the new practice acquisition fits into your current medical service offerings as a complementary line in a hot sector, or as an alternate to a service you do not currently provide. Complementary services that require little continuing education might include botox injections for dermatologists and internists, as well as plastic or cosmetic surgeons. Counter-intuitive and alternative services might also include them for gynecologists and oral surgeons.

Other synergies include orthopedic surgeons teaming up with podiatrists, ophthalmologists joining optometrists and opticians, and chiropractors merging with osteopaths. A formal written business plan is an even better idea.

Address Financial Issues Early

Lending vast sums of money to buy medical practices is a new business for bankers, who are very conservative by nature. And, many venture capitalists have been burned in recent years by the PPMC implosion. Both may not fully understand new concepts, such as managed care, fixed reimbursement rates, or boutique medical practices.

The bureaucracy will cause much frustration, but getting the paperwork done early will provide an advantage over other potential buyers.

Be Flexible

With a preponderance of sellers, over buyers, in the medical marketplace today, the more accommodating you can be to the buyer, the better you chance to consummate the deal.

Purpose of the Practice Valuation

Therefore, it is critical that physicians fully understand the purpose of their valuation and how their assets will be valued. Estimates of value can be markedly different dependent on the purpose of the appraisal. Some of the many questions to ask when valuing a medical practice include the following:

- What is the value of the medical operating business for purchase or sale?
- What is the value of a medical practice for merger with other medical groups?
- What is the value of practice assets for joint venture with a corporate partner?
- What is the value to establish the buy-in or buy-out arrangements for partners?
- What is the value of certain practice assets for purchase or sale apart from the ongoing business operations?

To arrive at an appropriate estimate of value, qualified appraisers will also will ask the following:

- What is the purpose of the valuation?
- What assets require valuation?
- Who will perform the valuation?
- Who will pay for the appraisal?
- What is your timeline?

The answers to these questions will guide the appraiser to select the appropriate definition of value and appraisal methods to value your practice.

UNDERSTANDING VALUATION DEFINITIONS

Most practice valuations for mergers and acquisitions use fair market value, as the criterion. This is the standard term used to derive a reasonable value for the medical practice. As a key definition of value, this is important, as it guides the appraiser's choice of methods to apply in determining the appropriate value. *Fair market value* means the appraiser will value your medical practice assuming an arm's length transaction of "any willing buyer and any willing seller" scenario, and without synergies of a specific buyer.

Synergies common among the most likely hypothetical (any willing) buyers, however, are appropriately considered in valuing medical practices.

If you are selling your medical practice as a going-concern business, inclusive of all the medical practice's underlying assets, then you should understand the term business enterprise. The business enterprise of a medical practice equals the combined values of all practice assets (tangible and intangible) and the working capital of a continuing business. Stated another way, the business enterprise value is equal to the combined values of owner's equity and long-term debt, also referred to as the "invested capital" of the operating business.

The value of the *owner's equity* of a medical practice equals the combined values of all practice assets (tangible and intangible) less all practice liabilities (booked and contingent). In essence, the equity value is the net worth of the business (after deducting debt). The business enterprise value is the total sum for the business including the owner's net worth plus the long-term debt.

The business enterprise value and the owner's equity value definitions are relevant when you are contemplating a sale of your ongoing medical practice, inclusive of all medical practice assets. In transactions involving the sale of medical assets separate and apart from the ongoing business operations, other value definitions and methodologies will apply.

Many medical practices are acquired without working capital. The *working capital* of a medical practice equals the excess of current assets (cash, accounts receivable, supplies, inventory, prepaid expenses, etc.) over current liabilities (accounts payable, accrued liabilities, etc.). When working capital is not a part of the transaction, the business enterprise value is adjusted for the buyer's post acquisition buildup of practice receivables and the associated delay from the collection of those receivables.

Other less formal terms and definitions include the following:

- The *asking price* is often an arbitrary and difficult to substantiate price which is typically reduce 25%–50% after negotiations.
- The *realistic price* is one that both buyer and seller believe is fair.
- The *"friendly price"* is usually used for associates, partners, or other colleagues.
- The *creative price* involves what is derived by creative financing. For example, the practice may actually provide the down payment in this case.
- The *emotional price* may involve either a motivated buyer or seller who pays an under- or over-inflated price for the practice.

WHICH MEDICAL PRACTICE ASSETS HAVE VALUE?

The medical practice's tangible and intangible assets can be grouped into four broad asset categories. Medical practice assets typically valued for merger and acquisition include the following:

Tangible (physical) Assets

- real estate or leasehold improvements
- medical equipment and furnishings
- accounts receivable

Intangible Assets

- Goodwill

The tangible assets of the medical practice include medical office building furnishings, medical equipment, and practice receivables. Depending on the facts and circumstances, intangible assets include professional goodwill and may also include favorable leasehold improvements, location, patient relationships, a trained and assembled work force, and restrictive covenants, among others. The combination of all the intangible assets of a medical practice is collectively referred to as *goodwill*.

Medical practices can be valued in their entirety as an operating business, often referred to as the *business enterprise*. The business enterprise value includes all of the underlying assets employed in the medical practice's business operations. The business enterprise analysis is the more cost-effective way of estimating practice value. Practice assets can also be valued apart from the operating business or in addition to the operating business. Which assets can be acquired and the deal structure will determine whether there is a need to separately value the practice assets only, or in addition to the business operations.

Medical practices are dependent on the highly specialized skills of the physician providers. With the exception of practices that own real estate, typically the majority of practice value lies in intangible assets, or goodwill.

Defining the Standard of "Value"

In addition to fair market value, medical business appraisers generally refer to three other standards of value.

- **Investment value** focuses on value to a specific physician buyer rather than value to a hypothetical buyer. For example, let us examine the physician owner of an ambulatory surgery center who is considering the acquisition of a competing ambulatory surgery center (ASC) that operates in the same geographic market. The owner might calculate value based upon the knowledge that the combination of the two ASCs will create economies of scale and less competition. This would result in greater profitability per dollar of revenue. Therefore, such a buyer, all else equal, may assess a greater value to the company than a buyer who would expect to operate the ASC in its current free-standing situation, without the expected cost saving and corresponding expectation of increased cash flow.
- **Intrinsic value** is similar to investment value; however, the practice is typically viewed in a stand-alone mode as a going concern. That is, value is based upon the expected cash flows of the practice based upon its current operating configuration. However, changes in operating policy, such as changing its financial structure can have an impact on its intrinsic value.
- **Going concern value vs. liquidation value.** A medical practice or any business cannot be worth less than its liquidation value. Thus, liquidation value sets a floor for value. Liquidation value assumes that a practice's operations cease and assets are sold either piecemeal or in groups and obligations are satisfied. Liquidation value is generally based on an "orderly liquidation," process wherein assets are sold in a manner that will realize the greatest possible value for them. In contrast, a "forced liquidation" process refers to occasions when assets are sold as quickly as possible, often through an auction. *Going concern value* views a medical practice as a holistic combination of tangible and intangible assets, in which the sum is often greater than its parts. This synergistic view of the practice is typically what is being valued.

Health Care Regulations—What Doctors Needs to Know

Federal and state regulatory oversight is increasing. The trend of not-for-profit community hospital conversions into for-profit groups is generating business for appraisers to perform *fairness opinions* to calm community benefit fears. A number of industry regulations must be considered, regardless of the buyer's tax status, when organizations acquire or affiliate with physicians. These regulations include the following:

- Medicare fraud and abuse legislation makes it a criminal offense to offer, pay, solicit or receive payment for patient referrals for business covered by a federal health care program
- Anti–self-referral legislation (Stark I and II) makes it illegal for physicians to refer Medicare patients for certain identified services if the physician holds an ownership interest in the business of the service provider. The legislation identifies health services such as lab work, radiology, magnetic resonance imaging, ultrasound, home health services, durable medical equipment, computerized axial tomography, and hospital services.
- Section 501c(3) of the Internal Revenue Code makes it illegal for not-for-profit organizations to pay more than or receive less than fair market value in physician and other transactions.

- Intermediate Sanctions allow the IRS to impose tax penalties on individuals in tax-exempt organizations as well as those physicians who benefit from excessive compensation.
- Antitrust laws protect against combinations that may preclude market competition
- Patriot Act (PA) fiscal reporting constraints
- The Sarbanes-Oxley Act was signed into law in 2002

Health South is the first major corporation to be prosecuted under the Sarbanes-Oxley Act, which requires that corporate executives sign financial reports attesting to their accuracy and truthfulness. This law will result in valuation, criminal precedents, and case law reports for years to come.

Valuations Regulations That Impact Practice Value

Both the buyer and seller need to understand how industry regulation impacts practice value and also have an appreciation for accepted appraisal definitions and methodologies used by qualified appraisers to estimate value. *The Uniform Standards of Professional Appraisal Practice (USPAP)* are promulgated standards, which provide the minimum requirements to which all professional appraisals must conform. *USPAP* requires the three recognized approaches to value (the income, market, and cost approaches) be considered to estimate value.

In the fall of 1994 and 1995, the *IRS* first issued training guidelines pertaining to the valuation of physician practices. These guidelines suggest that appraisers consider all three of the general approaches to valuation as required by the *USPAP*. Specifically in transactions involving physician organizations, the *IRS* implied:

1. The discounted cash flow (DCF) analysis is the most relevant income approach.
2. The DCF analysis must be done on an "after-tax" basis regardless of the tax status of the prospective buyer.
3. Practice collections must be projected for the DCF based on reasonable and proper assumptions for the practice, market, and industry.
4. Physician compensation must be based on market rates consistent with age, experience, and productivity.

THE PUBLIC VALUATION PROCESS

The market value of a publicly traded company's equity can be calculated at a point in time by multiplying its share price by the number of shares of common stock outstanding. The share price is determined in the public marketplace by buyers and sellers who trade the stock.

Buyers of publicly traded company shares, such as the medical IT outsourcing firm, Superior Consultant Company, Inc. (NASD-SUPC), expend money now (invest) for the right to receive uncertain future economic benefits. The price (value) an investor pays for a share is based upon his or her assessment of the size, timing and certainty of receiving future economic benefits. Likewise, a seller of SUPC equity is willing to forego his or her expectation of future economic benefits if the investor believes that the benefits given up are worth less than the proceeds (value) from selling the ownership position. Thus, the share price of SUPC at a given point in time represents the value of future economic benefits as perceived by buyers and sellers of SUPC equity at a point in time. This value is observable through transactions in the marketplace.

THE PRIVATE VALUATION PROCESS

Valuation of securities is, in essence, a prophecy as to the future and must be based on facts available at the required date of appraisal.

IRS Revenue Ruling 59–60

In contrast to the above, closely held businesses, such as medical practices, clinics, and surgery and wound-care centers also produce economic benefits for their owners, but the value of those companies cannot be directly observed by activity in traded markets. And so, valuation professions estimate value by applying valuation theory. The value of financial assets, whether traded or not, is generally based upon the following:

- The level of expected distributable future cash flows.
- The timing of those expected distributable cash flows.
- The uncertainty in receiving expected future cash flows.

Valuing your medical practice will require consideration of many other factors that influence value. A thorough valuation analysis will include a study of the economics of the health care industry, reimbursement trends, competitive market conditions, and historical earnings trends, as well as management experience. These factors, collectively considered, influence the future prospects of your medical practice and, ultimately, its estimate of value as a going concern.

The appraiser will want to gain an understanding of the history of your practice, its operations, and local competition and payer contracting issues. The business and management fundamentals studied are patient retention and potential for new patient growth, providing services efficiently and cost effectively, timely collections for services, and maintaining competitive equipment and facilities.

After the need for an independent valuation is determined, here is what you can expect:

- Who pays the bill? An independent valuation appraiser may be engaged by the buyer, or seller or, in some cases jointly by both buyer and seller.
- Make sure the appraiser understands the health care industry and, most important, educates both the buyer and seller in the conduct of an appraisal. All too often, values are misunderstood and may result in deals unnecessarily falling apart.
- The appraiser will request financial information, operating statistics, and other information in advance of a site visit.

- The appraiser should visit your medical practice to conduct key interviews and review the physical condition of the facilities and medical equipment.
- The appraiser will review historical practice patterns and financial and operating performance as a basis for forecasting future operations.
- The appraiser will adjust, or normalize, historical financial data to eliminate one-time, nonrecurring expenses, adjust for excessive or below normal expenses, and eliminate expenses not expected to be a part of future practice costs. The rationale for adjusting practice costs is to estimate the fair market value price of the business that is transferable.
- The appraiser should work with you to assist with the development of key assumptions concerning future reimbursement trends, physician productivity, practice cost structure, and physician compensation for use in financial projections.
- The appraiser should review valuation assumptions and forecasts with you.

APPROACHES TO MEDICAL PRACTICE VALUE

As discussed earlier, industry regulations will govern how a deal will be structured and which medical practice assets can be acquired; this will, in turn, determine which assets require appraisal and which appraisal methods should be applied.

In most cases, a significant amount of practice value lies in the business operations as opposed to the physical assets. The value of a going concern medical practice is directly linked to the value of the practice's ability to generate economic benefits to its owners, as measured by future cash flows. As a result, the development of a reasonable forecast of future operations is crucial to determining a meaningful practice value. And, the three valuation approaches will be discussed here.

INCOME APPROACH

Since medical practice value correlates directly with the measurement of economic benefits to owners, earnings or cash flow methods are the best tools for estimating practice value.

Capitalization of (Excess) Earnings Method

The *excess earnings method* estimates or adjusts value by dividing normalized historical or current earnings by an appropriate rate of return for the buyer.

Net Income Statement Adjustments

When analyzing a set of financial statements, adjustments are generally needed in order to produce a clearer picture of likely future income and distributable cash flow. This normalization process usually consists of three types of adjustments to a medical practice's net income (profit and loss) statement.

1. Nonrecurring Items.

   Estimates of future distributable cash flow should exclude nonrecurring items. Proceeds from the settlement of litigation, one-time gains/losses from the selling of assets or equipment, and large write-offs that are not expected to reoccur each represent potential nonrecurring items. The impact of nonrecurring events should be removed from the practice's financial statements in order to produce a clearer picture of likely future income and cash flow.

2. Perquisites.

   The buyer of a medical practice may plan to spend more or less than the current doctor-owner for physician executive compensation, travel, and entertainment expenses and other perquisites of current management. When determining future distributable cash flow, income adjustments to the current level of expenditures should be made for these items.

3. Noncash Expenses.

   Depreciation expense, amortization expense, and bad debt expense are all noncash items that impact reported profitability. When determining distributable cash flow, the link between noncash expenses and expected cash expenditures must be analyzed.

   For example, annual depreciation expense is a proxy for likely capital expenditures over time. When capital expenditures and depreciation are not similar over time, an adjustment to expected cash flow is necessary. For example, a practice may have radiographic equipment with a useful life of 14 years that are depreciated over seven years for tax and financial reporting. Depreciation expense will likely overstate the funds needed to maintain the equipment as the useful life exceeds the depreciable life and distributable cash flow. In determining distributable cash flow, one must add back the annual noncash depreciation expense and subtract an estimate of funds needed to fund medical equipment replacement. In this way, the cash flow available for distribution to owners will be more properly stated.

   Some practices reduce income through the use of bad debt expense rather than direct write-offs. Bad-debt expense is a noncash expense that represents an estimate of the dollar volume of write-offs that are likely to occur during a year. If bad debt expense is understated, practice profitability will be overstated. A close examination of accounts receivable to see if any past due accounts need to be written off is generally part of the due diligence a buyer of a practice will undertake. The calculation of distributable cash flow avoids this problem, because the actual monies received from patients and payers, rather than just the revenue generated by patients, is measured.

Balance-Sheet Adjustments

Adjustments can also be made to a practice's balance sheet to remove nonoperating assets and liabilities and to restate asset and liability value at market rates, rather than cost rates. Assets and liabilities that are unrelated to the core practice being valued should be added to or subtracted from value depending on whether they are acquired by the buyer.

Examples include, the asset value less outstanding debt of a vacant parcel of land, and marketable securities that are not needed to operate the practice. Other nonoperating assets such as the cash surrender value of officer life insurance are generally liquidated by the seller and are not part of the business transaction.

Thus, CEM can provide a reasonable estimate of practice value in situations where limited information is available, or when the practice is likely to maintain stable cash flows. The main advantage of this method is it does not require assumptions regarding future forecasted operations for the medical practice.

DCF Method

DCF method is favored by the IRS and is considered more relevant, given the changing nature of health care. DCF is a sophisticated analysis requiring assumptions of forecasted practice operations regarding future reimbursements and physician productivity, practice efficiencies, and competitive market conditions. An estimate of practice value is developed by discounting future net cash flows to their present worth based on market rates of return required by an investor physician.

In other words, the discounting process converts future expected distributable cash flows to arrive at their present value, according to several core valuation principles.

- The discounting process is one of converting expected future practice cash flows into a present value.
- The value of an investment is based upon the level of expected future practice cash flows, the timing of those cash flows and the risk or uncertainty attached to those cash flows.
- The discount rate represents the purchaser's (investor's) required rate of return.
- The discount rate or required rate of return is based upon a purchaser's (investor's) other opportunities to invest in alternative investments whose cash flows have similar risk and duration.

Thus, the value of your medical practice is primarily dependent upon future practice earnings that will provide an adequate return on an investment for the buyer. An informed buyer will not pay more than the present value of all anticipated future economic benefits of ownership. Supportable practice values are entirely dependent on realistic financial and operating assumptions about future practice operations.

Key DCF Assumptions

A DCF analysis includes a financial forecast projecting net cash flows for the business operations for usually a period of three to five years or until the practice achieves stable operations. In estimating practice value, key variables and assumptions used can have a significant impact to your value. The key DCF elements include these:

1. Reasonable supportable projections of future practice revenues based on historical practice patterns and with consideration of future physician productivity, reimbursement trends and shifts in payer mix.

2. Reasonable supportable projections of future practice cost structure based on expected normal levels of practice expenses.
3. Projected physician compensation based on market rates for physicians with comparable age, experience, and productivity.
4. DCF model calculates after-tax cash flows regardless of the tax status of the buyer. The tax rate is based on a blend of federal and state rates.
5. Reinvestment in the business are necessary for funding working capital needs and capital expenditure requirements to replace and acquire new equipment or other medical assets.
6. Terminal value represents the going concern value at the end of the projection period. Stated another way, it is a residual value for the expected remaining practice value at the end of the forecast period.
7. Discount rate is applied to the future net cash flows to arrive at the present (cash equivalent) value for the medical practice. The discount rate must be based on the industry's weighted average cost of capital that takes into consideration the specific risks for the practice.

The DCF analysis consistently produces higher values than other methods of estimating practice value because there may be supportable reasons to forecast improvements in future practice performance. Understanding the key DCF variables and assumptions used in the income method will assist in producing a meaningful estimate of practice value.

Determining the Required Rate of Return for DCFA

A physician's required rate of return takes into account that monies received sooner have a greater value than those received later, the greater the risk in receiving future cash flows the lower their current value and one must always keep in mind returns that can be earned on alternative investments.

The process of selecting an appropriate required rate of return begins with an assumption that all investors will require, at a minimum, the riskless rate of return offered by government securities. Government securities with maturity similar to that of the duration of the investment in a private company are selected, and normally, a duration of 10–20 is used. Because of the minimal default risk associated with government securities, the rate is referred to as the risk-free rate.

Physician investors typically require returns greater than the risk-free rate. The additional return (in excess of the risk free rate) is called the risk premium. Risk premiums are generally calculated through an analysis of historically realized rates of return segmented by varying levels of risk. This analysis illustrates that higher historical rates of return occur in situations of higher risk. For example, securities issued by the U.S. government have lower rates of return than do securities issued by large corporations. Returns on the equity of large corporations are greater than those of debt securities issued by the same firms. Thus, historical rates of return are generally used as a proxy for future required rates of return.

When valuing a practice, one must compare the risk of the expected cash flows of the firm being valued to the risk of the cash flows of publicly traded securities and to determine an appropriate required rate of return based on that assessment.

It is generally assumed that the expected cash flows from an investment in a closely held business are at least as risky as those of large publicly traded firms. The combination of the large firm equity risk premium and the riskless rate of return provide an indication of the required rate of return for an investor in a large public firm. Beyond that, additional risk premiums related to firm size, proportion of debt, industry conditions, and many other possible company specific risk factors may be appropriate. When valuing a small medical practice, appraisers generally employ required rates of return 15%–25% percent beyond the current long-term risk-free rate. However, this rate may vary greatly.

Market Transaction Approach

The market transaction method is a useful gauge in setting a valuation bottom and top range for comparison with the income approach. Market multiples are ratios developed by correlating market sale prices of guideline practices to key practice performance measurements. Common physician practice market multiples include comparisons of sale price to revenues, sale price to earnings before interest and taxes (EBIT), sale price to earnings before interest, taxes, and amortization = A, depreciation (EBITDA), and sale price to number of physicians.

Market transaction multiples are typically limited to serving as a benchmark for testing the reasonableness of the income approach. To apply the market approach, information on the guideline practices such as size of practice, specialty, number of physicians, growth potential, cost structure, payer mix, and profitability are necessary for determining comparability to the medical practice being valued. Often, information concerning transaction specifics and practice particulars is either insufficient or not available for direct comparison with the practice being valued.

Cost Approach

The cost approach to estimating value calls for the identification and separate valuation of all the practice assets, including goodwill. Also referred to as Sum of the Assets, this approach is more labor intensive and costly than using the business enterprise analysis to estimate practice value. Generally this approach is not very useful for estimating going concern value.

Although rarely used to estimate going concern value, another cost approach method may be used to estimate the costs that would be incurred to start-up a medical practice and develop to the current level of practice operations. The costs of establishing a new medical practice typically include the expenses involved in the recruitment of physicians, acquisition of space, office furnishings, patient treatment equipment, computer software, medical records; advertising for staff; and losses incurred during the start-up period.

This estimate of *replacement cost or cost avoidance* value represents an upper limit (or ceiling) of value. It has limited use as an accounting artifice, and no prudent buyer would pay for an existing medical practice a price equivalent to what it would cost to build and develop a new medical practice.

The most appropriate application of the cost approach involves the valuation of medical practice tangible assets. However, valuing only the tangible assets used in a profitable, medical practice is not representative of the business value of the company. Since the intangible assets typically represent a significant portion of practice value, the cost approach is generally not considered useful in estimating the value of a going concern medical practice.

UNDERSTANDING CORPORATE DEAL STRUCTURES

Although now less common than a few years ago, corporate deal structures often acquire substantially all of a medical practice's assets, excluding the working capital, and then enter into employment agreements with its physicians. In this scenario, the selling physician is left with the accounts receivable, cash, and the practice liabilities. Most of these asset purchases are cash deals. When the sale price is based on an enterprise value, this usually provides the physician with the ability to settle the practice debt.

Stock Purchase vs. Asset Purchase

There will be some variation in appraisal methods dependent on whether the transaction is structured as a stock purchase or an asset purchase. Due to corporate practice of medicine laws in some states and desires of buyers not to assume practice liabilities, most practice acquisitions are structured as asset purchases. In an asset transaction, the buyer will receive a tax amortization benefit associated with the intangible value of the business. This tax amortization represents a noncash expense benefiting the buyer. In this case, the present value of those future tax benefits is *additive* to the business enterprise value.

Corporate Partner Transactions

PPMCs historically acquired medical practice assets, excluding real estate, and entered into management service agreement (MSA) with physicians. There were a myriad of MSAs involving fees based on a percentage of revenue, compensation based on a percentage of practice profits, and some fee arrangements that varied with managed-care enrollment levels. The negotiated MSA fee depended on the scope and level of services provided, such as practice management, administrative services, contract negotiations, and marketing. The past market of a few years ago saw fees drop to 5%–18% of relevant revenues, dependent on the level and menu of services provided. MSAs are now no longer in vogue, except for very large corporations and health systems.

Practice management agreements with physician organizations are coming under closer scrutiny as well, particularly when the agreements are fee-based revenue arrangements for management services. The OIG is concerned when compensation arrangements for management services based on a percentage of net revenues include business from managed care contracts arranged by the PPMC. The OIG may imply that such activities violate anti-kickback statutes because the compensation will, in part, be for marketing services.

Market uncertainties since 1998 have resulted in downward pressure on prices paid for physician groups by physician practice management companies. It has been estimated that prices for multispecialty groups fell by as much as 25% in 1998 and even more in 1999 and 2000.

For example, in 1998, some PPMCs paid as high as 8–10 times EBIT to secure a strategic practice. Since the industry fallout however, those sale prices have fallen to a range of 2–4 times EBIT, or lower. The deals usually involve a combination of cash, common stock, notes receivable, and possibly assumption of liabilities. When common stock is used as payment, considerable premiums are included in the sale price to compensate for the risk of receiving stock instead of cash. The use of equity adds a premium of as much as 50% or more to the sale price.

Restrictive Covenant Value Is Goodwill

Restrictive covenants for physicians usually involve *covenants not-to-compete* related to the sale of a medical practice or other assets. The value of covenant-not-to-compete lies in the protection it affords the buyer from potential loss of income due to competition from the selling physicians (Figure 18.2).

To estimate the value of a covenant-not-to-compete, the income approach is considered to be the most appropriate method. The cost to secure the agreement is irrelevant to the value of the protection afforded the buyer. The sales comparison approach requires sales of similar or like assets; because each medical practice is unique and public data are unavailable for transactions of physician's noncompete agreements, the sales comparison approach is not useful. Generally, an income approach includes the value associated with a noncompete agreement as part of the intangible asset value. As such, the noncompete agreement value is *not additive* to your business enterprise practice value. Instead, it is a component of practice good-will, which can be separately valued if desired.

Buyer Mistakes (Caveat Emptor)

Significant federal funding has been provided targeting physician transactions with penalties potentially imposed on both the physician and individuals in the acquiring

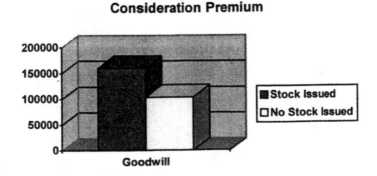

FIGURE 18.2
Source: Adapted from CHIPS, 2002

organizations. Recently, there were several federal investigations of for-profit hospital systems alleging those systems deliberately overpaid for physician practices as inducement to receive patient referrals (a violation of the anti-kickback statue). When selling your practice beware of the following buyer blunders:

- **No Outside Appraisal Performed.**
  If the buyer is a tax-exempt entity *or* participates in federal healthcare programs, ***get an independent third-party valuation from a qualified appraiser.*** There are too many stories of hospitals and health systems that bought practices with no appraisal. BIG MISTAKE!
- **Overpaying Physician Practice Value.**
  Some buyers obtain a business enterprise value and will also obtain separate values for the medical equipment and noncompete agreements. These values can be useful in allocating the overall purchase price. The business enterprise value, however, represents an estimate for a 100% ownership interest in the medical practice. The separate values for the assets are *not additive* to the business enterprise value, but, rather, are components of the total value of the business. Some buyers have overpaid for physician practices by adding these separate asset values to the overall business enterprise value to determine the sale price. BIG MISTAKE! Not understanding values can be misconstrued as overpaying in exchange for patient referrals.
- **Overpaying for Physician Compensation.**
  Industry surveys have reported that more than 75% of practices acquired fall short of the projected productivity used in the valuation. This fact coupled with exposure to IRS audit and intermediate sanctions has increased the need to value practices based on reasonable appropriate projections of practice collections and market rates for physician compensation.
- **Not Buying Insurance on the Physician.**
  Much of the value to an investor rests with the physician's skill and talent to remain with the practice after acquisition. The buyer expects to achieve a return on the investment in the medical practice based on future cash flows and to eventually recoup the purchase price. Since most practice acquisitions are cash deals, the buyer is at significant financial risk due to a business interruption associated with an unexpected loss of life or permanent disability.

FINDING QUALIFIED MEDICAL PRACTICE APPRAISERS

Finding a qualified medical practice appraiser is not always an easy task. Your office accountant or a general business valuation expert may not be familiar with the current managed care environment, nor the specifics of your medical specialty. So, consider the following guidelines:

- Make sure appraisers use generally accepted IRS methods and have a proven track record with the government for medical appraisals.
- Make sure the valuation is written and that it substantiates the medical practice value, provides details to support conclusions, and is signed by the appraiser.

- Avoid conflict of interest or self-dealings. Seek an unbiased and independent viewpoint.
- Make sure the appraiser will qualify as an expert witness and is presentable on the witness stand, if needed.
- Request references and examples for previous medical practice appraisals.
- Inquire about experience in publishing, speaking, and teaching medical practice valuations techniques.

Organizations that accredit business, but not necessarily medical practice appraisers, include:

- Institute of Business Appraisers: (www.go-iba.org), awarding the certifications of Certified Business Appraiser (CBA), Master Certified Business Appraiser (MCBA), and Business Valuators Accredited in Valuation (BVAL).
- National Association of Certified Valuation Analysts (www.nacva.com), awarding the designations of Certified Valuation Analysts (CVA), Accredited Valuation Analyst (AVA), and Certified Forensic Financial Analyst (CFFA).
- American Society of Appraisers (www.appraisers.org) offers the ASA (American Society of Appraisers) designation for business appraisers.
- American Institute of Certified Public Accountants (www.aicpa.org), providing the Accredited Business Valuation (ABV) for CPAs only.

Since some appraisers feel that certain organizations set the bar for certification significantly higher than others, the American Society of Appraisers (ASAs) website at www.apraisers.org offers a comparison of the accreditation criteria required by all four major organizations.

Well-known medical practice and healthcare system appraisers include the big 4 consulting firms for larger healthcare organizations. The impression that "bigger is not always better" may be confirmed by the Arthur Andersen debacle.

Medical practice niche players include Health Capital Consultants, Inc. (www.healthcapital.com), who provide medium sized practice valuations, software and Certificate of Need (CON) economic determinations. And the Institute of Medical Business Advisors, Inc., specializes in small practice valuations, and confers the designation Certified Medical Planner© (CMP©), on its related independent consultants and advisors (www.MedicalBusinessAdvisors.com).

HOW MUCH MONEY IS YOUR MEDICAL PRACTICE REALLY WORTH?

Now that you have a background of what factors influence value, the need for valuation, a general understanding of appraisal theory and how industry regulations impact value, and the valuation process itself and the methodologies employed, we will get to the heart of the matter.

Understanding Your Value

Understanding value is crucial to a successful negotiation. Both buyers—and sellers, too—often misinterpret the value conclusions of appraisers, which strains buyer/seller relationships and unnecessarily jeopardizes deals.

How to Maximize Medical Practice Value

There a few critical areas you can review for opportunities to maximize your practice value:

- Use the DCF method to estimate practice value. This method consistently produces higher values than others—but recall the USPAP edicts.

Practice Revenue

- Can the practice and local market support adding additional providers such as physicians or midlevel providers? Providers usually take two to three years to ramp up their practice before they begin to significantly contribute to the bottom line. Generally, adding a midlevel provider will produce a greater impact to value, as their compensation levels are lower than physicians.
- What future provider productivity is expected?
- Does the practice plan to offer new services?
- Is the current practice fee schedule at market rates? Is there an opportunity for fee increases?
- Is there an opportunity to improve payer mix?

Review Practice Costs

- Eliminate any unnecessary practice expenses. Identify any unusual nonrecurring costs.
- Eliminate any physician-related costs not likely to be paid by a buyer.
- Eliminate any special perks of business ownership.
- Adjust for any over-inflated salaries of relatives and eliminate any unnecessary salaries.

Physician Compensation Inverse Relationship to Value

- Although physician compensation must be based on market rates, fair market value is a range. Practice value correlates directly with the net cash flows available after all practice expenses including physician compensation. As a consequence, the higher the compensation, the lower the practice value, and conversely, the lower the compensation, the higher the practice value. As little as a $10,000 swing in salary can have significant impact to value, and as physician compensation rises, practice value falls.

Completing the Transaction

Depending on whether the likely buyer is a health system or a corporate partner, the deal structures will vary. From the physician's perspective, deal negotiations are based on consideration of personal and financial planning goals. Some of the key negotiations considered in the "art of the deal" include the following:

Working Capital—In or Out

Including working capital in the transaction will increase the sale price.

Stock versus Asset Transaction

Structuring the deal as an asset purchase will increase practice value due to the tax amortization benefits received by the buyer for intangible assets of the practice.

Common Stock Premium

The sale price can be as high as 50% more than a cash equivalent price for accepting the risk of common stock as part of the payment.

Physician Compensation

If your personal financing planning goals are to maximize practice value, negotiating a lower salary within a range you feel comfortable with will increase the sale price.

UNDERSTANDING PRIVATE DEAL STRUCTURE

Now, assuming a practice sale is a private transaction, deal negotiations are based on the following discount-and-premium pricing methodologies, as presented below:

Seller Financing

Many transactions involve an earn-out arrangement wherein the buyer puts money down and pays the balance under a formula based on future revenues or gives the seller a promissory note under similar terns. Seller financing decreases a buyer's risks—the longer the terms, the lower the risk. Longer terms demand premiums, while shorter terms demand discounts. Premiums that buyers pay for a typical seller-financed practice are usually more than what you would expert from a simple time value of money calculation, as a result of buyer risk reduction from paying over time, rather than up front with a bank loan or all cash.

Down Payment

The average down payment for a modest solo medical practice is about 20%–25%. This increases the buyer's risk: the greater the amount, the greater the risk. Consequently, sellers who will take less money up front can command a higher than average price for their practice, while sellers who want more down usually receive less in the end.

Seller Involvement

The key to practice purchase success boils down to how many of the selling doctor's patients and managed care contracts, can be transferred to the new doctor/owner. The most important factor in transitioning patients is the involvement of the selling doctor. The system of seller financing and earn out arrangements can work well if the seller continues to be involved in the practice and can create an incentive for the seller to make the transaction work. Sellers typically remain at least for six months, and usually for not more than a year, to ensure a seamless transaction. When a deal fails, it is usually due to lack of seller commitment.

Location

Variations between the value of a practice in a major metropolitan city and one in a small town can be as much as 20%, just for the location. Usually, practices in a small town have a larger, but less affluent, basis. Managed care penetration is another factor to consider.

Profit Margin

Determining medical practice profitability is distinctly different from determining a practice's value. It is not unusual for selling doctors to run every expense imaginable through their practices in order to reduce profit and hence, taxes. In many cases, however, a practice with high overhead can be sold for the same price as one with low overhead, because all expenses are not transferable, as we have seen when the Net Income Statement (NIS) becomes normalized.

Taxation

Tax consequences can have a major impact on the price of a medical practice. For instance, a seller who obtains the majority of the sales price as capital gains can often afford to sell for a much lower price and still pocket as much or more than if the sales price was paid as ordinary income. In a usual deal structure, 70% of price value is in the seller's patient list, medical records, name brand, and goodwill and files, all of which qualify for capital gains treatment. Then, 20% is paid for the selling doctor's continuing assistance after the sale, and 10% goes to a noncompete agreement, both of which are taxed at ordinary income. But, a buyer willing to allocate more for items with capital gains treatment, or a seller willing to take more in ordinary income, can frequently negotiate a better price.

CONCLUSION

The above discussion solidly presents the reasons for, and methodology behind, acquiring a professional appraisal when contemplating the sale, purchase, or merger of any medical practice.

ACKNOWLEDGMENTS

The first edition of this chapter was written by Bridget Bourgeois, CPA, CVA.

REFERENCES

Cimasi, R. J. (2003). A guide to consulting services for emerging healthcare organizations. St. Louis: Health Capital Consultants. ASA, CBA, AVA, FCBI, CMP.

Hinchcliff, D. (May 2003). Small business, big stakes. *Financial Advisor.*

Contemporary Aspects of Medical Practice

CHAPTER 19

Medical Information Systems and Office Business Equipment

Carol S. Miller

> Patient care is fragmented. It doesn't focus on prevention issues surrounding getting patients to comply with their treatment. Medicine still largely is practiced in firms of two, three, or four doctors. It is still a cottage industry. This is an industry that is years behind in information technology. This adds cost—and inefficiency—to the health care system. There are many things that, if put in practice tomorrow, would mean better health outcomes for thousands of patients.
>
> —Kenneth E. Thorpe, PhD
> Emory University
> Rollins School of Public Health

A new or established, single, multispecialty, or multi-office site physician's practice whether operated individually or are linked via a network, are faced with hardware, software, and other office-equipment decisions. Even though the competitive marketplace provides a large selection of information systems and equipment for the office practice, the physician's office is straddled with selecting the best system that not only meets their needs today and in the future, but also efficiently integrates the data with the various technology applications. Coupled with these decisions, the offices want to make sure that the choices contribute and support the operational and financial viability of the practice. Physician practices face not only the cost decisions related to new or upgraded software and equipment, but also the impact from the Health Insurance Portability and Accountability Act (HIPAA) regulations, continual reimbursement changes from insurers, escalation of malpractice insurance rates, state and regulatory compliance issues, and day-to-day operating expenses of the practice.

Practices changed on April 14 and October 16 in 2003 to an electronic automated, Web-based back-and-forth transmission process of data that provides instant communication of clinical and nonclinical data, financial transactions, and other relevant information amongst peers, hospitals, insurers, and other business associates. Today's technology advances must accommodate the continual changes of e-health solutions, making it more secure, faster, and more economical to the physician.

One of the biggest objectives of 2004–2006 is more streamlined compliance with those HIPAA requirements affecting the electronic transmission of medical data. The following is an abbreviated summary of the HIPAA requirements that affect the physician's practice as well as examples and time frames.

HIPAA

HIPAA is a comprehensive federal law that addresses data transmission and protection, fraud and abuse, and insurance data portability. In addition, the Administrative Simplification section contains provisions governing the transmission and protection of health data and addresses the confidentially challenges created by the complexity and speed of new technologies used for gathering, storing, and disseminating health data. The Administrative Simplification section is designed to promote two goals:

- electronic data interchange uniformity that will streamline information exchange
- electronic health data confidentiality

The integral aspects of the Administrative Simplification rule include the following:

Electronic Transaction and Code Sets

This area addresses the technical standards, formats, and data content when electronically submitting patient-specific medical information to insurers or requesting insurance eligibility verification. Physician compliance for this requirement was October 16, 2003. Those providers who completed and submitted a Center for Medicare and Medicaid Services (CMS) Compliance Extension Request Form had a one-year extension.

Privacy Standards

The privacy rule creates federal protection for individuals prohibiting physician practices from using or disclosing protected health information unless authorized by patients. The only exception to this rule is that information can be shared if withholding it interfere with access to quality of health care, if the information was for public benefits, or if restriction of patient information interferes with efficient payment of the health care service.

The deadline for compliance for the confidentiality policies and procedures governing the use and disclosure of protected health information was April 14, 2003. Physician practices must provide a good faith effort to obtain the patient's acknowledgment of the notice. As part of the final amended change, written consents for the release of protected information is optional for the purposes of treatment, payment and health operations.

Treatment is defined as the provision, coordination or management of health care and related services among health care providers or between health care providers and insurers. This includes consultations and referrals between providers and includes the sharing of information between nurses, providers, and other members of the team to determine the correct treatment as well as document and review the actions and observations of staff.

Payment is defined as the activities performed by a provider's office to obtain payment for services, diagnoses, and procedures rendered and, on the other side, the responsibility of the insurers to reimburse providers for covered services. Payment activities include such items as determining the charge and adjudicating claims, billing and collection, reviewing of claims for medical necessity, coverage and benefits, and justification of charges.

Health Care Operations is defined as certain administrative, financial, legal and quality improvement activities of the physician's practice that are necessary to effectively run its business operations and support the core functions of treatment and payment. Examples include the following: evaluating provider and health plan performance, training staff, accreditation, certification, conducting medical review, legal and audit services, and business activities including those related to implementing and complying with the privacy rule and the Administrative Simplification rule.

Patient data from a physician's office *may* be provided without patient authorization in the following examples:

- Health information on a patient as part of a claim for payment to a health plan.
- Copy of a patient's medical record from a primary care physician to a specialist.
- Information on the patient's health insurance plan to an independent lab or diagnostic/therapeutic radiology service in order for that entity to bill.
- Disclosure to family or person identified.
- Patient health information to the Health Education Data and Information Set (HEDIS) as long as the plan had a relationship with the patient.
- FDA in regard to adverse events with respect to food or drugs.
- Workmen's compensation.
- Public health for control of diseases.
- Administrative proceedings (only for specific conditions).

Disclosures are not to be considered violations if the physician's office have met the requirements for reasonable safeguards and "minimum necessary." Therefore, sign-in sheets in a physician's office may be acceptable as long as they are concealed from public access, patient telephone messages are acceptable as long as they are placed on the physician's desk away from public view, and schedules listed on computer screens are acceptable as long as they are not visible by the patients.

As part of the minimum necessary requirements, a physician's office must (1) develop policies and procedures that reasonably limit its disclosures to the minimum necessary, and (2) assess and determine which staff people need to have access to protected patient information.

Finally, any patient has the right to restrict how the physician's office will use or disseminate protected health information for treatment, payment, and health care operations; the physician's practice does not have to agree, but if the practice does agree with the patient's restrictions, they are bound.

Limited data sets can be used by the provider's office in providing patient health care information for research or to public health. These data sets are "stripped" of individually identifiable information and an agreement must be done between the physician's office and the intended user of the data that the recipient would only use the information for its intended purpose.

- *Unique identifiers.* The deadline for unique identifiers for medical providers, small health plans, and others was April 14, 2004.
- *Security standards.* Includes safeguards for the physical and technical storage and transmission of protected health information. The security compliance deadline is April 21, 2005.
- *Electronic Digital Signature.* Has been proposed by HIPAA but is not mandated.

Compliance with each of these mandates will require significant changes to the physicians' medical practices. Patient confidentiality, whether it is written, electronic, or verbal, will be an element that will affect each physician and each staff member. To maintain this confidentiality while rendering patient care, systems and processes will need to be instituted in each physician's office for the following matters:

- Training staff on the regulations.
- Handling and documenting privacy complaints.
- Verifying fax numbers and e-mail addresses before transmitting patient information to an outside source.
- Restricting staff access to patient data on a "need to know" basis.
- Developing a process to handle patient privacy and security on those individuals terminated.
- Identifying a person in the practice who will be responsible for implementing the HIPAA related policies and procedures.

In summary, each physician's office is required to—

- Provide any existing or new patient a Notice of Privacy. Elements include a description to the patient of the related treatment, payment and health care operation, a description of the authorization and revocation ability, any intentions by the physician's office to send appointment reminders or other health care information, physician duties, the ways to register a complaint, and the date.
- Have existing or new patients sign an authorization form indicating the uses and/or disclosures of their patient data to outside organizations or entities. This includes employers, schools, research facilities, and others. Key elements include a description of the information to be used and by whom, an expiration date, the purpose of the request, and space for the patient signature and date.
- Develop and/or update business associate agreement with vendors, contractors, billing services, lawyers and others that legally and contractually bind them to insuring that all patient data is properly utilized. Physician practices have been granted up to an additional year to bring existing contracts with business associates into compliance.
- Develop a HIPAA policy and procedure manual addressing all the aforementioned changes to the day-to-day business process.

According to HIPAA consultants, the one time cost to small physician practices for HIPAA electronic compliance could range from $5,000–$20,000 for technology instruction or upgrades and staff training.

Practices need to focus first on the electronic transaction sets and codes with your software companies and/or clearinghouses and, secondarily, focus on privacy regulations.

Health care providers who transmit any health information in electronic transactions (billing, eligibility verification, referral authorization, or financial transactions, any health plans, and any health care clearinghouses) must comply with the HIPAA regulations. Electronic is the key word in this regulation. Practices who do not perform any electronic transactions (those providers submitting manual hard copy claim forms to the insurer), need not comply. However, there are two exceptions: (1) if the practice uses a billing company to bill insurers, the billing company is an extension of the practice and therefore the office must comply with the HIPAA regulations; and (2) after October 16, 2003, a federal law signed by President Bush that requires providers to submit electronic format claims in lieu of paper claims to Medicare became effective. An exception can be granted if the practice has less than 10 full time equivalent employees or has no method for electronic submission of claims available.

Reference sites to HIPAA follow:

- AMA HIPAA link. A subscription fee is required; however, provider offices will be given (1) a *gap assessment* to help practices evaluate gaps between current process and procedures and regulatory requirements, (2) a policy generation tool for customized HIPAA-compliant policies, and (3) online training and periodic regulatory updates
- American Medical Association Web site at www.ama.assn.org
- Centers for Medicare and Medicaid (CMS) Web site at www.cms.gov/hipaa
- www.hipaa.org
- www.hipaadvisory.com

EQUIPMENT/FUNCTION OVERVIEW

"The IT [information technology] systems in which doctors are practicing medicine in the 21st century needs to be changed. We know how to treat patients better, but we are not practicing in organized systems to do that very well." (Stephen M. Shortell, PhD, Dean, School of Public Health, University of California, Berkeley.)

As an overview, a physician's office will need the following:

- Equipment to communicate internally within the office as well as externally to hospitals, other providers, insurers, and patients.
- Depending on the size of the office practice or practices, multiple workstations to provide registration, scheduling, billing, posting, accounting, and contact management functions.
- Billing software that provides electronic billing to insurers.
- Electronic capabilities directly with insurers or with a clearinghouse to verify eligibility and medical necessity, such as state Medicaid access system or Web MDEnvoy.

- Standard word processing and spreadsheet capabilities for letters and reports.
- Internet service to correspond via e-mail with peers, hospitals, managed care organizations, and patients; obtain clinical communication updates such as lab or x-ray results and schedule online; and provide educational patient information to the patient via a separate portal. For the physician's practice, the Internet represents a communication tool that will continue to expand as the office adds access and one that will improve the efficiency of the operations as well as expediting information to other resources.

As physicians determine potential upgrades to their existing office equipment or begin to select information systems for their new practice, they should keep an important point in mind: The applications and tasks drive the software selection, which in turn drives the hardware suited to the software. Electronic sophistication in one or multiple practices—for example, wireless communication, Internet capabilities, multiple office networking, and others—is expensive. The functions of the electronic world need to be weighed against not only what the physician wants but also the realistic comparison of cost versus revenue. Cost relates to the actual cost of the hardware, software, and full time equivalents and the additional cost of implementation man-hours and training time, as well as ongoing support and maintenance. Some physicians may want to have all of these functions done internally or centralized at one of their offices, or they may want to outsource various aspects of the business process such as billing, collection, or accounting to firms specializing in these processes, thereby eliminating the need for specific equipment internal to the office.

For these reasons, it may be wise to engage an experienced, unbiased outside firm to evaluate the practice, determine the workflow process, develop a task and function matrix, evaluate the cost impact, and provide recommendations based on actual needs of the practice. The assessment should focus on the following five areas:

Workflow Process

The office manager and physician need to assess the existing workflow for the main and ancillary offices not only pertaining to the staff, but also as it affects the patients. This type of assessment, many times, determines the actual need of additional or upgraded systems. The best evaluation tool is to follow the flow from the initial point of entry (registration) through and including the account reconciliation process. The following represents a key list of items to address:

Single Physician Office

- Is any activity duplicated in the process?
- Does your staff have immediate access to computer systems to update data to electronically verify insurance and medical necessity during the registration process while the patient is still present?
- Do you have an adequate number of staff to—

- Efficiently manage the registration process?
- Answer telephone calls in a timely manner to include responding to patient's medical problems, pharmacy refills or billing and insurance inquiries?
- Provide after hours emergency access to physicians?

- What do the physicians and office manager want the practice management system to do?
- What do you want outsourced versus what do you want done at the office?
- What can be done to reengineer the process to be more direct, organized, and efficient?
- Does the staff need to be trained?

Multiple or Networked Physician Offices

- Are there duplicative functions at each office that could be consolidated at one site?
- Are physicians considering a decentralized or centralized business operation? As an example, the "back office" could be centralized at one office site if an identical or interfaced system existed. In this instance, *back office centralization* would refer to billing, follow up, collections, and account reconciliation.
- Will the practice management system be the same for all offices, sharing the same patient demographics and clinical data, or will the each office have its own management system but still be provided with a "view" capability in case the same patient is seen at another office?
- Will the scheduling system support multiple physicians and/or multiple practices?
- Will the scheduling system be part of an ASP Internet model?
- Are there sufficient telephone lines to not only support each staff members and physicians, but also to provide direct connectivity between each office site?

Practice Management Software Systems and Hardware Platform

This process includes a review of the various systems available in the marketplace, the programs included in the packages, their capabilities, and configurations.

Projected Revenue, Cost, and Return on Investment (ROI)

As with any business, the cost outlay and depreciation of any new equipment needs to be evaluated compared to the projected revenue. A ROI is an important quantifiable measurement that needs to be developed as part of any evaluation for new technology or application. It includes a comparison of all the direct cost (software, hardware, printer, staff) and indirect cost (training, installation, utilities, administrative oversight) compared to projected revenue (from insurance and patient payment). It also evaluates the time it takes to recover the cost of the initial investment. Therefore, will the office be able to obtain a return on investment during the viable life of this system, or will the office before a ROI is realized have to purchase additional systems and upgrades to maintain its functionality? What is the projected net revenue for the office practice? Is it realistic to support a new system and package or would a modified version be acceptable?

Other Factors

Other factors to be considered in making selection decisions include warranties, guarantees, replacement and data loss insurance, data backup, regulatory issues, initial HIPAA cost compliance changes, legal and liability issues, office expansion or decline, market growth in area, and future performance and enhancements.

Task and Function Matrix

With the workflow needs assessment, evaluation of various hardware and software systems, a review of various cost and revenue projections, and a determination of incidental costs, the physician's office will have the needed data to accurately assess the full scope of the project and determine what is wanted and then see more clearly what is really needed. The final step in the assessment exercise is for the consultant, along with the office manager, to develop a "task and function matrix" that includes each of the management systems' functions compared to the tasks or required needs of the office. This activity quickly will sort out what equipment can or cannot perform the tasks, whether a new system is needed, or whether replacement components will suffice. In addition, the matrix will be a valuable tool in determining if new functionality, such as an ASP Internet connection, different software programs, or different interfaces, would be a better avenue for the office. Finally, it will enable the physician and outside vendors to communicate more succinctly with each other on exact requirements and configurations for both short-term and long-term business needs, and whether the hardware or software can support those needs.

The ensuing sections contain summary information that should provide baseline data for physician managers with a single- or multiple-office practice.

HARDWARE SELECTION

The first consideration in regard to hardware selection is to determine the number of offices as well as the number of workstations needed to support the practice. Will each office function independently or be linked as a network? The latter refers to several offices being linked to each other via a wide area network (WAN) so that clinical records are accessible at any location. Needless to say, the network will be more complex and more costly.

The second and perhaps even more important consideration is that many software programs will dictate the type of hardware to support the system. However, the correct configuration of software and hardware will result in better utilization of the system and an enormous improvement in return on investment by consolidating labor-intensive activity (by reducing unnecessary staff-hours spent attending to system problems). The cost of hardware can vary depending on what is included in the package or what is purchased al la carte.

Hardware options are outlined in the following section. This information will be relevant in the selection process for a new office practice, an additional office site, or upgrading existing hardware in the existing office.

Operating Speed

The central processing unit (CPU) is the clock speed recorded in megahertz (MHz) or gigahertz (G). Most office practices purchase at least a Pentium IV, with the speed of one G+ and/or up to 2 G+ to support the practice management system and other software. System speeds nearly double every 6 months; however, current applications will run very well on 900 MHz or better, except for the Windows XP based system. XP needs at least 1 G+, with more random access memory (RAM) than was required for previous Windows operating systems. It is almost impossible to purchase or even warrant slower systems today.

RAM

RAM is measured in megabytes (MB), and 1 MB is equivalent to one million instructions in memory. Today's operating systems, such as Windows Office 2000 or Windows XP Professional 2000, require a minimum of 384 MB to perform in a stable manner. With more RAM, office systems should have at least 512 MB and at least 1 gig of RAM for graphics and imaging such as review of digital imaging and communications in medicine (DICIM) radiology. With RAM, more is always better.

Floppy, Zip disk drives, CD-ROM, CD-RW, and DVD

A 3.5″ floppy diskette can store 1.4 MB of data, whereas a Zip diskette or high intensity floppy can store 100, 200, or up to 750 MB. In addition, the new combination DVD/CD drives, priced under $300, support up to 5 gigs per disk for offline storage while being compatible with current CD technology. With this new drive, it is best to choose multiprotocol. This enables the physician's office to store and retrieve data from another storage means instead of the hard drive. However, if offline storage is dense and important, the system should consider CD-ROM drives capable of "burning" 450–750 MB of both permanent and rewritable data. CDs are relatively inexpensive at approximately 50 cents a disk, whereas read/write diskettes are a little more, about $1.50 per diskette. Most contemporary machines offer CD read/write (RW) function as a low-priced option or as standard equipment.

Nearly all the systems offer tutorials recorded on a CD-ROM; therefore, it is important to the practice to purchase speakers for the auditory portion of the tutorials.

The digital video disk (DVD), the next-generation form of the compact disk, is another means to provide training and is more cost efficient if purchased initially with the system. DVD can hold far more data, and DVD players can read and process that data at far higher speeds. DVD playback drives are very inexpensive—they are only slightly more than CD drives. Read/write DVD storage capabilities, at an average cost of $500, are beginning to actively compete with the CD-R/RW. The DVD + RW provides a good backup device option and all-in-one optical drive solution. Examples include Hewlett Packard, Philips, and Sony.

Regardless of the storage method, the practice needs to have the capability of data storage other than on the hard drive for the following two primary reasons:

- Large practice management applications or large volumes of data can be stored separately from the hard drive.
- The office will be able to load additional software into the system without slowing or bogging down the system.

Hard Disk Drives

A minimum standard to consider is at least a 40-gigabyte hard drive for a small practice or even an 80-gigabyte hard drive. Both are now reasonably priced. The best choice is to select as much as you can buy for under $200; however, be careful not to exceed the capacity of the operating system to manage the big drives. Also, there is a possibility that older systems will not be able to support increased capacity—they definitely need to be evaluated.

The office practice(s) may also wish to consider the open market server with a high performance of redundant array of independent disks (RAID) that is, now, reasonably priced. This product provides a wide range of storage solutions designed to best fit your specific requirements, and it includes backup solutions and disaster recovery.

Monitors

Physician offices should consider the 20–21-inch standard monitors priced around $250–$300 or the 19-inch flat panel monitors priced around $800–$900. These larger screens provide easier readability for the staff and physicians, and the refresh rate on newer, larger monitors can be adjusted for low fatigue and good visibility in a variety of lighting situations. Many offices are migrating toward the flat screen because of space constriction—also, the flat screen is more energy efficient.

It is hard to purchase a bad monitor given the state of technology. Equally, no one should have to spend excessively. If an equipment "package" is to be purchased, it would benefit the office to inquire about the cost difference to upgrade now from a smaller monitor to the 20–21-inch or to the 19-inch flat screen instead of at a later date.

Workstations

Workstations can be "thick" or "thin." These designations describe whether the workstation is a full computer running on the Internet or a stripped-down CPU getting all of its resources from the network. There is a benefit to both. The prevailing belief is that thin workstations are cheaper in the long run; however, this is not always the case. The additional network overhead at the server level can offset any economic gain. The best benefit is that the patient data is preserved at the network location, preventing any alteration of data at the workstation location. Thick workstations cost more but can run independently of the network and demand far few resources. In today's environments, many small thick systems run without any server at all. Again, the software application should push the configuration.

Modems/Bandwidth

Most computer systems purchased today include a modem of 56K and v92 to handle e-mail, fax communication, and Internet connectivity. The speed at which data is transmitted is measured in bauds per second (bps) and is a function of the circuit and the equality of the equipment at each end. The viable limit for standard switched dial telephone circuits is 56K. Many offices have converted to a digital subscriber loop (DSL), a high-speed direct line that can be 20–100 times faster in communication over the modem, depending on the type selected. Prices for the DSL begin at approximately $30–$40 per month; this charge includes unlimited Internet access. In addition, there is a setup charge, and a network card will need to be installed into the computer. Office workstations can usually share DSL circuits over their existing local area networks (LAN).

Backup Drives/Data Storage

Most physician offices are using a Zip drive, which will accommodate the Iomega 100, 250, or 750-MB Zip diskette; a removable cartridge device, or a CD-ROM recorder/player to store data entered onto the system. Both of these options are very cost-effective solutions. The 250 and 750 Iomega Zip drive will read, write, and format files, whereas the 100 will not write to files. In addition, practice management and billing programs have built-in backup systems as part of their package offerings. Overall, practices should backup daily to prevent unexpected loss of data. Therefore, any solution that makes this process easier is the one to purchase. The Iomega Web site is www.iomega.com.

Laptop Computers

More and more physician practices are utilizing portable laptops or tablet PCs to improve the communication of data, efficiently operate the practice and improve the timeliness and quality of patient care. There are a variety of laptops available in the marketplace ranging in cost from $1,100 to $2,500. Prices vary, based on memory, system capabilities, sophisticated video, DVD and sound, size of screen and resolution, or even the latest trend (for example, the convertible tablet with screen rotation and note capabilities). Depending on the physician's choice, laptops include either a Pentium III or IV, range from 128–512 MG of RAM, usually have 30–40 GB hard-drive disk space, and are loaded with Microsoft Windows 2000, Windows XP Professional, or Windows XP Home Edition. Most laptops today include credit-card size PC card slots and 1–2 universal serial bus (USB) ports. Modems for Internet access, if not built into the laptop, will need to be purchased separately—as a card modem. The Internet connectivity charge varies from $20–$25 per month, depending on the Internet service provider (ISP).

Laptops can be purchased at a retail store, over the Internet or directly from the manufacturer (such as Dell). Brands in the marketplace are IBM, Apple Mac and iMac, Toshiba, Dell, Gateway, Sony, Compaq, Hewlett Packard, Fujitsu, and others.

WAN/LAN

Depending on whether the practice is housed in one or multiple-office locations and there is a need to connect multiple computers, either a LAN or WAN should be part of the package consideration. The LAN is a computer network that covers only a small area (often a single office or building). The advantage of a LAN (besides connecting several computers to a network system) is the ability to configure one printer for multiple stations. The same may be said for sharing administrative, clinical, financial, and operational data in real-time manner to support smooth office function. The WAN provides the ability to link data on one network for multiple office-site locations.

Printer for PC

The number of workstations in the practice and the estimated volume of potential printing will determine whether each workstation needs its own printer or whether multiple workstations should be networked with one printer. Printers can be the laser or ink-jet type and can print in black and white only, color, or color/photo quality. The best buy for under $250 is an ink-jet printer, which is a reliable, durable product. However, the office needs to be aware of the cost for replacement ink. The next best buy for an office practice is the low cost (now under $1,000) color laser jets. This product is good for many clinical applications.

In addition, today's printers offer many multiple features, such as copying, faxing, and multitrays for legal or letter-sized paper. The better printers have a print speed capacity of 6–8 pages per minute and resolutions of 600 dots per inch (dpi) or more for black and white or $2,400 \times 1,200$ dpi for color on premium photo paper. These allow printers to print clinical images for "takeaway" references for medical or family referrals. Examples include Hewlett Packard, Canon, Epson, Dell, and Lexmark. Price ranges are from $80 to $300. Professional quality printers start at approximately $500 and typically range to $1,500 or higher.

Scanner

Physician practices are scanning documents and before-and-after pictures of surgical pictures and pre- and posttreatment pictures as a means of permanent storage. Dots per inch can be as low as $600 \times 1{,}200$ or up to $3{,}200 \times 1{,}600$ optical resolution. Some scanners also include the capability to fax, copy, e-mail, or store documents. Examples of scanners include Gateway, Visioneer, Dell, Microtek, Epson, Canon, and Hewlett Packard. Depending on the need for higher resolution (for photo quality pictures), prices for scanners may vary from as low as $100 up to $1,200. In selecting a scanner, make sure it includes a USB port for linkage to your computer.

Power Protection and Circuit Capacity

An uninterruptible power supply with uninterrupted power supply (UPS) protection will save office staff unnecessary reentry of data. An American Power Conversion (APC) backup instantly switches your computer to emergency backup power and allows you to work through brief outages or be able to shut your system down. High performance suppression surge protects your computer from electrical noise and damaging power surges, such as lightning. Prices range from $80 to $150. UPS protection should be provided for the computer, networks, telephone, fax, and security systems.

Digital Cameras

Physicians in the specialties of plastic and reconstructive surgery, dermatology, oral surgery, and oncology are detailing before-and-after pictures to accurately record and archive events. In addition, these instantly captured digital pictures are used to train new physicians, share case studies in grand-round presentations, demonstrate examples in published journals, and provide body-mapping capabilities for dermatologists.

Digital pictures can be stored on the hard drive, CD ROM, or Zip disk and can then be retrieved easily when needed. Depending on the printer, photo-quality hard copies can also be produced. Most digital cameras include 3–5 megapixels, have automated and manual features, and vary in price from $350 to over $1,000. Several examples of digital cameras are Kodak, Olympus Camedia, Toshiba, Minolta, HP Photosmart, and Nikon Coolpix.

For information on feature and price comparisons of digital cameras and for on-line purchases, the following Web sites are available: www.digital-camera.com, www.kodak.com, www.pcmall.com, www.digitaldirect.com, and www.buydig.com.

In addition, reference material on various digital cameras for health care practices can be found at Canfield Clinical Systems at www.canfieldsci.com.

Deletion of Data on Hard Drives, CDs, Floppy Disks, and Zip Disks

With offices storing patient medical and billing information on their computer systems or storing this information onto CDs or disks, the office also needs to address how to permanently delete this data when selling or eliminating any of the computer equipment or storage devices. The answer is not just using the delete key or reformatting a hard drive, for any technically savvy person can and will be able to retrieve the data. Remember that destroying data is an essential part of the HIPAA compliance. Health and Human Services (HHS) has directed any covered entity (physician office) to deploy appropriate technical, physical, and administrative safeguards for patient privacy. Therefore, any organization handling patient data in health care must ensure that this data is not disseminated to anyone other than its intended recipients and that mechanisms are in place for securely decommissioning magnetic media that contains this data.

As an information note, scrambling the contents of the media into an unrecognizable mess can be accomplished with the following techniques:

- For low-density media such as disks, a degaussing technique of adequate power can be a quick and effective way of clearing data. For high-density storage, this process is time consuming and less effective and has side effects such as potentially damaging the drive.
- Data wiping is a technique where data is overwritten with new data. Depending on the method, it can make it virtually impossible to determine the previous data ever existed.
- Another more common method is just physical destruction.

For paper destruction, the answer is simple—a $90–$100 paper shredder; however, the computer and its storage devices require other ingenuity. For other media processes, there are many agencies that will format hard drives and destroy CDs and floppy disks at a cost. Examples include Cybercide—a specialized utility used to securely erase all data from storage media in a manner that can not be undone; EMag Solutions—a firm that uses degaussing that exposes storage media to extremely powerful magnetic fields; and Cascade Asset Management.

The following are some common guidelines for effectively destroying data.

Hard Drives

One of the products on the market for destroying data on hard drives is East-Tec Eraser, located at www.east-tec.com/erprod/. This product deletes all of the existing data, eliminating any trace of the old files while still allowing new data to be rewritten over it.

CDs

First you need to burn the CD. Most of the data should be eliminated if not all of the dye layer. Then, split the CD into several pieces and dispose each piece into separate trash containers, preferably in different buildings or sites.

Floppy and Zip Disks

First, crack opens the disk to expose the actual disk platter. Next, burn the platter and then split the disk into several pieces and dispose each piece into separate trash containers, preferably in different buildings or sites.

On the opposite site of data destruction, the physician offices in their system-design process need to consider processes for data recovery. Examples include (1) using the undelete key on the computer, which is a simple solution; (2) low-level reads—a technique that bypasses the operating system view of data and attempts to retrieve data from the physical media itself; and (3) magnetic force microscopy—opening the drive to access the storage media outside standard digital boundaries. Firms that the office is interviewing should be willing to discuss their process for disaster or data recovery.

Ergonomics, Lighting, Acoustics

To effectively support the new technology and systems and to provide a comfortable, useable workstation to the staff, the office manager should evaluate the supporting office environment. This includes power, temperature, lighting, floor surface, space, static charges, chair and desk height, design configuration, noise interruption or traffic patterns, and telephone circuits.

Without a comfortable work environment, staff will be unproductive, potentially develop health-related issues, increase their use of sick time, and/or resign. Office supply firms provide a wide array of workstation configurations that can be adapted to your office space at very affordable prices.

SOFTWARE

> Automated systems reduce charges in a really odd way: They take the smaller of two prices when they bundle them together. (David Rogers, MD, Texas Medical Association.)

A wide variety of individual or packaged medical office management software programs are available in the marketplace to include word processing, spreadsheet, Power Point, financial/accounting, billing and accounts receivable programs, electronic medical records, medical and digital transcription, fax software such as WinFax, and others. Many of the practice management software systems include at least the majority of the following features:

- Registration.
- Scheduling.
- Electronic insurance eligibility or medical necessity verification, through such firms as Health Data Exchange (HDX) or WebMD. Note: HDX has partnered with National Data Corporation (NDC) to form the largest processor of health care electronic data interchange for claims.
- Charge and procedure capture.
- CPT, ICD9 and Healthcare Common Procedure Coding System (HCPCS) coding database with rules based engines based on insurance criteria.
- Electronic data exchange billing for all insurers directly, through clearinghouses or specific ASP models such as NextGen or Athena Health.
- Automated accounting posting and reconciliation.
- Patient collection letters and tracking systems.
- Authorization verification for managed care.
- Numerous standard and customized management reports based on the needs of the practice, such as aged AR report, copayment tracking reports, productiv-

ity volume reports by physician, service or site/location, total and specific insurer revenue report by time period, and adjustment and write-off reports by time period.

- Referral tracking.
- Various graphs and charts based on data stored in system.
- Managed-care tracking.
- Reference guides and tutorials.
- And other features.

The office manager and physicians need to consider whether the software patient data will be totally integrated and shared by all the practice locations or whether the patient data will be segregated by physician or by office site. Decisions need to be made whether the software system will have thin-client network connectivity (a central server serving each of the sites), whether a standard Web browser application is the choice, or whether an ASP is offered by the software firm. In addition, the ease and versatility of training staff, data entry, and prompt retrieval of data needs to be actively evaluated in selecting the software program.

Typical software packages can range as low as $1,000 to over $100,000 depending on the sophistication of the software system, office network, and packages selected. For high-end solutions, there is an additional monthly cost for maintenance and service usually averaging around $500 to $2,000 per month depending on the vendor. For a midpriced solution, the average cost is around $8,000 or higher with an average maintenance cost of $500–$1,500 per month.

A partial list of companies that offer computer software specifically designed for physician practices is found in Appendix A. The categories include

- physician practice management system
- dictionary, encyclopedia, and coding software
- voice recognition software
- medical diagnosis software
- financial and accounting software
- electronic medical record software programs
- fax software

INTERNET

The Internet is a constantly evolving service that continues to grow at an exponential rate, especially in physician practices. Primarily, the Internet is used as a means to electronically and expeditiously transfer data via e-mail as well as obtain information from a variety of sites. Initially, in the physician's office, the primary use was e-mail communications with peers, hospitals, and others. Next, providers linked to hospitals and managed care organizations to obtain more direct connectivity for clinical information and benefit coverage. Today physicians are finding other beneficial avenues to expand their utilization of the Internet. Several examples include the following:

- Direct e-mail inquiries from the patient to the physician.
- Patient educational newsletters and links to other health care related educational Web sites.

- Continuing medical education (CME).
- Chat room consultations, conferences, or presentations on particular cases or research with other specialty providers.
- Nurse to patient e-mail connectivity.
- Immediate data on lab results with posted alerts for abnormal high or low values.
- Computerized purchase order entry systems(CPOEs).
- Radiology images.
- Electronic medical records (EMR).
- Monitoring of patients blood sugars or EKGs via the Internet.
- Appointment scheduling on-line by patients.
- Patient appointment reminders via the Internet.
- Secure physician portals such as Medicity, located at www.medicity.com, that allows access to pertinent and prioritized data from a wide range of sources and vendors to include, labs, imaging centers, hospitals, payers. and others.
- HIPAA compliant ASPs for dictation, recording, routing, and speech recognition and transcription services, such as Speech Machines at www.speechmachines.com.

Besides the value to the patient and the physician, the physician can utilize his or her Internet connection with software firms such as NextGen to automate the registration, scheduling, eligibility verification, billing, and "clean" claims processing via innovative Web-base solutions in real-time scenarios. All the physician's office needs is a PC, a standard Internet browser, and a connection to the Internet to take advantage of this service.

All of these resources via the Internet enable physicians to have quicker and easier access to clinical information and improve productivity. Further, these tools will quickly assist providers with accurate and timely medical decision making, thus improving patient care and outcomes.

Security and Encryption

E-mails, personal digital assistant (PDA) data, and Internet connectivity, unless encrypted, can be read by anyone. Therefore, if these items are not encrypted, physicians should be careful of what they say and how they say it, especially when discussing any patient information with other providers, vendors, or managed care organizations. In addition, just because you deleted e-mail from the system does not mean that you have deleted it from the server or from the computers that maintain copies of your server's data. The HIPAA regulations outlined at the beginning of this chapter sets forth the criteria in electronically transferring patient related data via the Internet.

If you want secure messages, an encryption program should be used. If the message is intercepted the text will be scrambled to anyone other than your intended recipient. Most physicians feel encryption is too time consuming; however, programs such as Pretty Good Privacy at www.pgp.com provides an easy and nearly seamless integration into e-mail and operating systems, encrypting the sensitive files but still allowing ease of communication. Pretty Good Privacy (PCP) software developed by MIT and endorsed by HIPAA, uses privacy and strong authentication. Only the intended recipient can read the data. If files were intercepted, they would be completely unreadable. Other software programs are available in the marketplace that will work using a private key—similar to a password. Tell the program the name of the file you want to encrypt and the private key, and the program uses a mathematical algorithm to encrypt the file. For reference material on various encryption and security software programs, search the Web under "encryption" or go to one of the following sites: www.zixit.com, www.cisco.com, www.aspencrypt.com, or www.verisgn.com.

In addition to encryption, the office needs a good antivirus program that is designed to detect and prevent viruses, such as Norton Anti Virus at www.symantec.com and McAfee VirusScan at www.mcafee.com.

Internet Service Providers

To connect with an Internet service, the office will need a computer, modem, telephone line and software. The modem, whether external via a cable connection or internal via a built-in or slot card, takes the digital signals from your computer and converts them to analog signals that your phone line uses. As a rule of thumb, the faster the better; therefore, the office should have at least a 56 bps or use a DSL line.

To access the Internet, the office must obtain an ISP such as America Online (AOL), Earthlink, ATT Worldnet, Microsoft Network Premiere (MSN), and Hot Link. The cost varies on the plan selected but usually averages in the range of $15 to $25 per month. In selecting an ISP, several guidelines need to be considered:

- The major online services often make it very easy to connect to the Internet, but they may be more expensive.
- Many low-priced ISPs may have customer service that matches their prices.
- In selecting the ISP, make sure the provider has a toll-free or local support telephone line

For a nationwide directory list of ISP providers, go to the Internet site of www.isp.com.

Besides plain old telephone service (POTS), the physician may wish to have a faster connection to the Internet. Several options are available.

Cable Modem

Cable connection is very fast, providing a lot of bandwidth (the amount of information that can be sent through a particular communication channel). As an example, in the time it takes to transfer a half page across a 56K connection, the cable connection can transfer over 25 pages. As is suggested by the name, the local cable TV provider or community antennae TV (CATV) deliver this service.

Asynchronous Data Subscriber Line (ADSL) or DSL

This is a very fast digital line provided by the telephone company. If available in your area, the ADSL provides fast connections, but generally not as fast as cable.

There are various choices, beginning around 256 kbps (about five to six times the speed of a fast modem) going up to 7 Mbps. Prices begin around $60 per month (including Internet service). There is also a setup charge, and a card needs to be inserted in your computer.

DSL is a high-speed direct line that can be 20–100 times faster in communication over the modem, depending on the type selected. Prices for the DSL begin at approximately $30–$40 per month and that includes Internet access. In addition, there is a set-up charge and a network card will need to be installed into the computer. Office workstations can usually share DSL circuits over their existing LAN.

To connect with the Internet, as a rule of thumb, the faster the better; therefore, the office should have at least 56 kbps. DSL normally runs over the same line as a basic telephone voice circuit and provides Internet access from speeds of 384 kbps all the way up to 1.54 mbps (megabits per second). The advantage of this configuration is you not only have high-speed access to the Internet, your telephone is still free to make and receive calls at the same time.

ISDN (Integrated Services Digital Network)

A digital telephone line that allows voice and data to be transmitted on the same line in a digital format—instead of analog—and at a relatively high speed, usually around 64 to 128 kbps. When reviewing this service, make sure the ISP has an ISDN connection. If not, you will be charge more by both the telephone company and the ISP. Prices for the ISDN average around $300 plus, with an extra fee to install the telephone line and a monthly service charge of $25 to $100 plus to maintain.

Wireless Network (WiFi—802.11b)

The biggest change to happen to computers in the last ten years has undoubtedly been the Internet. Close on its heels in importance may just be the adoption of the wireless network access. Wireless Fidelity, or Wi-Fi, is now cost effective and available at the computer store. It is no longer necessary to rewire buildings with Category 5 wire to provide LAN connectivity and resource sharing to multiple computers.

Wi-Fi, or IEE standard 802.11b, enables small offices to connect up to four computers to a single network for less than the cost of a single computer. This means the days of multiple analog lines to offer Internet access to every computer, or a printer on every desktop, are going away. Now a single cable modem or DSL line and a centralized printer can service four users. This can save a small business hundreds of dollars a year.

For limited connectivity, computer stores are stocked with wireless vendor products that are cost effective, easy to install, and very robust. This will push even the most cautious computer user to take the leap to wireless computing. Not only does it make the initial cost to install a network cheaper than it has ever been before, it eliminates the cost to remodel or move computers within a building since instead of requiring data wiring at each proposed desktop, all you need now is an electrical outlet to power the PC itself.

What are the costs for such a system? Prices vary by each vendor and the features required, but here is an estimate of overall cost of a four-port system:

1—Wireless 802.11b, s.4 Ghz, 11 Mbps Router	$150
(Cost for 22 or 54 Mbps are available and more costly)	
3—Wireless card adapters	$225
8—Hours of installation by a Network Engineer (estimated)	$1,000
Total Cost	*$1,375*

This assumes you have four PCs able to support this network (a typical PC, able to run Windows XP), network card in the host machine (PC where the DSL and router are connected), and all the machines are located within 1,000 feet of the router. This even means the network will work between floors of a building. Typically, if your normal cordless telephone will work at all locations where you want network connectivity, so will the Wi-Fi system.

One benefit to the practice is if you have a portable (notebook or laptop computer) you are truly mobile—nurses or physicians can roam throughout the coverage area in your office. This means moving between exam rooms or physician offices, while responding to e-mails, accessing patient data from the operating system, or printing a document.

One word of caution: Be sure to enable the imbedded encryption tool in the router, because if your users can access the network within 1,000 feet of your router, so can others. Given the benefits versus the drawbacks, wireless just may be the answer to move from a standalone computing environment to the hi-tech world of 802.11b.

Satellite

This will be the connection device of the future. Currently, satellite connections are at 400K bps or fourteen times faster than the average modem. As an example, a 2MB file would be downloaded in 30–40 seconds. Benefits of the satellite connection are as follows: The connection is always on, it is reliable, there is a secure connection, office can have multiple e-mail addresses, the Web space is free, and there is tech support coverage nationwide. Costs include around $300 for the equipment, $150 plus to install the equipment, and around $30 to $50 per month for service. Website reference is satcast.com (DirecWay Satellite Dish)

ASP

An ASP enables health care organizations to run complex software programs or applications on remote servers that can be accessed from numerous sites and by numerous devices. By installing and maintaining central, instead of on-site, services, ASPs reduce the complexity, time, resources, hardware requirements, technical support, cost of installing and distributing upgraded software (done by ASP at its host site), and cost involved in application management. In addition, ASPs provide the physician a means of low-cost entry to new applications in a very short timeframe. Upgrades are quickly deployed, and health care organizations or medical offices can experience affordable and secure business critical applications. Most ASP services are billed on a per use basis or monthly annual fee. An example of an ASP is NextGen, an Internet based enterprise and a real-time practice management system that includes an electronic medical record, appointment scheduling, connectivity with hand-held solutions, and patient indexes.

Reverse ASPs in Health care

Healthblocks (www.healthblocks.com) coined the term "reverse ASP" to signify that, as an ASP, it provides unique solutions through Healthblocks eSite, tailored to the situations and circumstances that face health care organizations and care givers on a daily basis. More formally, a reverse ASP deploys through portals; it hosts and manages access to medical applications so that offices, in a single, seamless manner, can view a patient's clinical information. The applications are delivered over networks on a subscription basis, and the reverse ASP remotely manages the packaged application over a network.

The following benefits are achieved in this model:

- Hardware and software that are located on recipient's facility can connect disparate facilities.
- User names and passwords are located on-site with extensive integration with legacy systems.
- Existing clinical data remains on-site without danger of lost data.
- Connectivity to ASP solutions is not dependent upon an ISP.

Thus, the reverse ASP model provides physicians, nurses, and allied health care providers and related personnel with rapid access to confidential clinical patient information. It can also benefit and help extend the reach and usefulness of third-party e-health solutions in a cost-effective manner.

SETTING UP A WEB SITE

Many physician practices are interested in creating their own Web sites to provide information about their practice to patients, the community, peers, and other individuals; market their practice specialty; provide ease of access to medical inquiries or scheduling appointments; and provide links to other health-related sites. There are "easy-step" programs available in the marketplace, such as the IBM home page. Web sites, such as www.Webdeveloper.com or www.homestead.com, can assist your practice with a tutorial and step-by-step process in creating and developing an initial site. Many programs include already established page templates. As part of the process, the Web site can be connected to an online service provider; however, many practices have considered using a Web-hosting company, such as www.hostdepot.com. With this process, the practice will create its own "domain" name (the name given to a host computer on the Internet). With this name in place, it will be easier for your patients to remember, easier to provide linkages to other sites, and you won't have to change your Web site's Uniform Resource Locator (URL), or Web address, each time you move your Web site. A good place to start is www.budgetWeb.com or www. e-businessexpress.com. Other reference sites are www.microsoft.com/frontpage, www.register.com to register and renew domain names, and www.verizon.net. As an example of cost for Verizon, there is a set up fee of $50–$100 for setting up the Web site, a monthly service fee between $30–$100 depending on the option selected. Web design fees are based on page count or on billable hours and range from several hundred dollars to over $1,000.

If the practice is interested in developing a more sophisticated end product, it is recommended that a Web-page designer work with the practice to design a Web site conducive to your expectations.

PERSONAL DIGITAL ASSISTANTS

Handheld personal digital assistants (PDAs), such as Palm Pilot M130, 500 or 515, Sony Clie, Visor Prism or Pro, Psion, RIM Blackberry, Zaurus, and other comparable PDA OS platforms have revolutionized the communication world. PDAs and their future counterparts are becoming the catalyst for physicians to use information technology and are becoming the intro for physicians into the world of the electronic medical record software. They are becoming the virtual office tool, enabling a provider to communicate away from the desktop as well as away from his or her office practice. The reasons for the increased utilization of PDAs by physicians are PDAs' portability; their pocket–size; and the way they provide easy access to information at point of care, regardless of location. Also, PDAs improve practice efficiency and workflow, facilitate drug related decisions, and decrease the possibility of adverse drug events.

The common uses of PDAs by physician practices are the following:

- Perform personal applications such as scheduling, telephone directories, dictionary, "to-do lists," and so forth.
- Access drug databases.
- Communicate with the clinic suite that ties into the hospital information system.
- Charge and procedure capture.
- Communicate efficiently from provider to provider, provider to hospital, provider to office, and vice versa.

Palm OS still represents the standard in handheld computing, enabling individuals to manage and access information at any time, from any location. Handhelds are easy to use. Physicians are using the Palm OS and/or compatible PDAs to access their office schedules, receive downloads of clinical information on their patients, and enter clinical services and charges when performing services at remote locations.

In selecting not only the PDA but also the software, the physician needs to answer the following questions:

- What would you like to use the PDA for—clinical reference data, patient information, nonclinical applications, personal data, and so on?
- What information do you need to know about the patient that the PDA can simplify?
- What is the connection route between the hospital, managed care, or lab and your practice? In other words, how do you get access to the data?
- What are your price considerations?

- Do you need a color or black and white screen?
- What is the system support and warranty?
- How do you plan to connect to the office or hospital?
- Do you want to go wireless or obtain information via a telephone connection?
- Do you plan to render care outside of your office practice, such as in the home, a clinic, hospital setting, and so on? If so, what would you like included on the PDA that would improve communication with the office and save time at point-of-service in documentation?

HIPAA regulations do not specifically address the specific term PDA, but the regulations do include guidelines for protecting patient information and transmission of this data, which can impact the use of PDAs. Physicians are utilizing handheld digital assistants whether they contain clinical information or just resource data, which may be or not be password protected and may or may not be officially supported by hospitals or clinics. Providers, as they prepare for future applications and usage of PDAs involving patient information, must understand the scope of the new HIPAA regulations as it impacts on patient data collected, stored or transmitted. Any application involving patient-identifiable data must be HIPAA compliant. The key issues are, first, how to protect the patient information stored on the device (what if the device is lost or stolen?), and second, how to protect patient information transmitted during a synchronization or wireless transaction. Probably the most vulnerable aspect is the inadvertent loss rate, with recent studies indicating that it is at least 30%.

Most providers using PDAs for patient data utilize an ID or password level of security. To maintain security, the provider should be required to reenter their user ID or password every time they enter the application. Likewise, each PDA should have a "time out" feature, requiring a provider to re-enter his ID or password again. This feature will not prevent individuals with technical skills from accessing this information—the only mechanism that will accomplish this is encryption.

An explanation of the differences between synchronization and wireless applications follows:

- *Synchronization* transfers information from the enterprise database to the PDA, that is, hospital lab or x-ray results, patient demographics, consultative notes, and others. It is important that the hospital or hospital system authorize and approve the physician for using and transmitting this information and, in turn, the provider authenticates and validates his agreement with the hospital before data is transmitted. In addition, for protection, an audit trail of who synchronized and what data was transmitted should be maintained by the hospital system.
- *Wireless* providers have immediate real-time access to patient data; however, this process of transmission is more vulnerable than synchronization. Wireless solutions can utilize a public or private network. HIPAA require encryption for the transmission of data over the public networks;encryption is optional for others. Sharing data from a wireless over the Internet represents potential security issues; however, more and more technical firms and providers are using a wireless virtual private network (VPN) that allows PDA users to connect securely from remote locations just as laptop users do today.

The other issues are who owns the PDA. If the provider does, he or she should be responsible for the security; however, if the hospital is the owner, the hospital should be responsible.

Future applications of Palm OS will include built-in modems for easier wireless communication, improved secure transactions, and ability of greater resolution for graphics and other Web-based services. In addition, current and future applications will include refined voice dictation. As an example, MDEverywhere's package called Everynote allows the provider to digitally record notes and in turn links with MDEverywhere's coded patient encounter.

A very versatile product is the Blackberry. It has Web-browsing capabilities, (via an embedded wireless modem) and can (1) write, send, receive, and respond to messages right from the unit; (2) access Web information; (3) has nationwide coverage with no roaming fees; (4) has voice mail message capabilities; and (5) can be the size of a pager or PDA. The next feature with Blackberry will be its text messages to cell telephones. New units start at around $150–$300, with monthly service charges of $20–$50, depending on the plan. The wireless Internet connection can be accomplished through Go.Web.

The typical cost for a PDA averages between $300 and $600, depending on whether the color option is chosen, plus the cost of additional software and accessories. For wireless connectivity, the physician will need to connect with a communication partner.

Some reference sites for PDAs are www.handheldmed.com (for clinical, reviews, and news), www.pdamd.com (PDA resources), www.freewarepalm.com (free software programs), and www.palmpilot.com, www.handspring.com. The active shopper can refer to www.zdnet.com or www.palmblvd.com.

TELEPHONE AND ANSWERING SYSTEMS

The telephone is among the most important and most frequently used communication tools in a physician's office. However, many physician offices, as they grow in patient volume, do not realize the impact on the telephone system by the increase of patient, physician, vendor, and other calls to the office complex. Configured properly, the system can be an asset to the physician and office staff, regardless of the number of office sites. Configured improperly, it can lead to frustrated and aggravated patients who may seek another physician's practice—one that will respond more quickly to messages, will not leave patients on hold for considerable amounts of time, and will immediately respond to emergencies. In addition, poorly configured systems can also result in important updates from hospitals, patients, and managed-care organizations. For a new physician, the office should be equipped with at least three or four telephone lines, with at least one left open for incoming calls and another dedicated to the fax or Internet connection. In addition, one outgoing line should always be available. At least yearly, the office should evaluate the telephone configuration and number of lines. One way to measure whether the telephone system is adequate is to seek evaluations from the patients and physician peers.

The initial telephone call with a new patient sets the basis of the doctor-patient relationship; therefore, the initial contact, professionalism, knowledge, and information gathering is crucial to a successful process. However, the initial telephone call can also establish a negative impression. Situations such as automatically being placed on hold as soon as the telephone is answered, always receiving a voice message versus a live person, being transferred numerous times, not responding to questions or returning calls, or being abruptly disconnected create negative attitudes.

Here are several suggestions to help improve communication:

- Schedule follow-up visits immediately after the visit and before the patient leaves. This will eliminate the need for an additional telephone call. In addition, provide the patient with an appointment reminder card of date and time of the future visit and call the patient the day before as a reminder.
- Obtain all demographic and insurance information at the time of the initial contact, rather than later via a letter or another call.
- Utilize the Internet as a means to have patients query the physician, nurse, or staff, read educational material on diseases or even schedule their own appointment.
- Have a dedicated line for prescription refills or nurse triage.
- Have physicians and nurses return patient calls within certain timeframes, alleviating the need for repeat telephone calls from the patient.
- Conduct reviews of your telephone system to make sure it meets demands.

In setting up an initial physician's practice, the physician and office manager need to review not only the number of staff, but also the location of the staff as well as the need for just an internal line/extension versus the need of making outbound telephone calls. It may be more economical for the practice to install a small telephone system called a key system. This allows more telephone sets to be installed in the office than telephone numbers being delivered by the local telephone company. With this configuration, there may be sets in the physician offices, reception area, examination rooms, even in the waiting room without requiring more than a couple of access lines to make or receive calls from outside the office.

One of the biggest advantages of the key system is it ensures privacy on a call. The telephone system bars access to the conversation by other extensions in the office, so there is no worry of an extension picking up and overhearing a confidential conversation.

Extensions or intercom capabilities can be used internally to communicate between the various rooms in the office. With this is mind, the office will need to evaluate the capability of being able to transfer calls and/or pick up calls at a separate location. A direct line needs to be available to the physician, triage nurse, and those individuals making external calls to insurers, patients, or other outside firms. It is recommended that checklists be created for each staff person and telephone location to determine what is actually needed versus what the individual wants. Features that should be considered in the evaluation process include: voice mail for the office only or the capability to dial an extension and leave a message for a selected individual, call forwarding, call holding, caller ID, speed dialing, three-way calling, redial capabilities, speaker phone, and others.

With voice-mail systems, the office needs to consider the use of an auto attendant that enables the caller to hear the different names or areas and press the appropriate corresponding number. Mailboxes should also be set up by group and by individual name. In addition, time-of-day call routing should definitely be considered in any practice. This technology will automatically transfer or switch the call to the answering service at a set time in the evening and then transfer the calls back to the office in the morning at the pre-programmed time. In addition, the initial voice message on the telephone should always recommend that any patient in need of emergency care either call 911 or go to the closest emergency room.

When deciding between answering machines and answering services, the physician should establish the most important criteria for service levels and make the decision based on those. Many answering machines are quite sophisticated today: They provide remote access, are able to call forward to a telephone or pager, provide a record of the call, and are inexpensive. Although human contact is provided by answering services, they are more expensive, may not offer the level of service required by the physician, and, in some cases, lead the caller to be placed on hold for long periods.

OTHER MEDICAL-OFFICE BUSINESS EQUIPMENT

The following represents an abbreviated list of general business equipment that a new office practice should consider. As with all equipment, the cost and usability need to be evaluated and periodic reviews of the equipment conducted. To evaluate and compare the various products, go to www.buyerzone.com, www.techdepot.com, or check Office Depot, Staples, or other office-equipment firms on line.

Copy Machines

Primarily, copiers are used to duplicate copies of records, insurance reports, and other documents that are not stored on the computer system. This equipment is a daily needed adjunct to the successful performance of the office staff. With the volume of copies being rendered by any given office, the copy machine(s) should be covered under a reliable service contract that will service the machine within a stipulated timeframe.

A wide selection is available in the marketplace from Canon, 3M, Hewlett Packard, Sharp, Lanier, and Xerox, among others. Physicians need to decide what capabilities they want to have for their offices: digital, color, black and white, collating, reducing and zoom capabilities, duplexer, front-and-back printing, paper-storage capabilities, multifeed or single, and-paper types (such as plain paper, letterhead, legal sized, or color). The selection of analog or digital printers also needs to be evaluated. The price difference is now minimal, but some of the benefits of digital versus analog are (1) less noise; (2) slightly better quality, especially in graphics or photos; (3) larger zoom range; and (4) multifunctional capability. In addition, depending on the size of the practice, physicians will need to determine where the printer will be located, and, based on volume, whether multiple printers (smaller/larger) are needed. Depending on capabilities, prices vary from $200 to $1,500 per printer. Average cost for optional items are: (1) multi-bin sorters (10, 15, or 20) is approximately $1000–$1500, (2) automatic stapling is $500, (3) automatic document feed (ADF) is between $100–$1500, and (4) duplexers are $600–$2,000.

Offices can buy from retail stores, a superstore, or over the Internet. Service contracts for repairs can be purchased directly from the vendor or independently purchased (which is many times cheaper). Leasing of printers is also an option, but this can be, in the long run, more expensive.

Dictation Equipment

Many practices use either the analog version such as Sony, Dictaphone, Philips, Olympus, Sanyo, Panasonic or Lanier. However, many physicians are resorting to digital telephone dictation services (voice via the telephone directly to the computer such as TrueSpeech or iDigital), voice-activated computers, and/or are typing directly into the computers. Digital dictation solutions record dictation on handheld devices, download this data onto a PC, transfer the information by LANS, WANS, or the Internet to transcribing services regardless of locations and then returns the dictated reports by the same media. For those using dictation equipment, most use a hand-held system. Dictation equipment averages from $180 to $350, depending on whether the application will be on a portable or a desktop computer. Web reference sites are www.officedirect.com or www.transcriptiongear.com.

Postage

Two reasonable options are available to the physician's practice. One is a postage meter that is leased (leasing a meter is relatively inexpensive), which dramatically speeds up the outgoing mail process. These units may be obtained with equipment that seals, weighs, and sorts. The other is downloading stamps via the Internet by using www.stamps.com. This service enables the provider to buy and print stamps online using a PC and printer. Postage can be printed to a sheet of paper, directly to the envelope or to a shipping label. The value to the latter is controlling cost and being able to efficiently manage mailing. Another Web reference site is www. shopusps.com.

Cellular Telephones

There is a host of wireless carriers available in the marketplace through AT&T, Verizon, Sprint, or your local carrier. Kyocera, Panasonic, Handspring, Samsung, Nokia, Nextel, Motorola, and Ericsson are some of the brands. Cell phones are either analog or digital or operate on a combination depending on location when making the call. The advantages of digital are better quality of service and sound, more security, ability to support the next generation of services, and stronger battery life. The disadvantages of digital are that the units cost more money than analog and traditionally have less area coverage. In addition, newer cell phones can encompass a range of products such as the telephone, PDA, or text messaging.

The cost of plans vary per month by carrier (from $30 to $100+ per month) depending on the number of projected calls during weekdays/weekends, covered service area, roaming charges for outside of the network, or the length of service agreement.

Features include call holding, three-way conference call, caller ID, call forwarding, contact telephone lists, quick one-digit dialing, list of recently dialed calls, calculator, alarm clock, voice activated dialing, speaker phone, e-mail, and connectivity to PDAs or Web. Prices range from $50–$600.

Cell phones are becoming a standard communication tool with physicians in that they enable instant two-way connections between physicians, family, hospitals, and others.

Pagers

Pagers are still actively being used along with cell phones, although the Blackberry product is gaining more notoriety. Today's pagers from Skytel, Motorola, NEC, and others have enhanced capabilities that include two-way interactive messaging, numeric and voice, emergency messaging, and message communication via Internet e-mail. A wireless service provider is needed. Activation requires a separate fee, and monthly rental and service costs between $25 and $60.

Pagers are still the preferred communication tools for patients calling the doctor after hours or for answering services.

Fax Machines

A fax machine can be a freestanding unit primarily used to transmit hard copy documents to an outside source or instantly receive copies. Most units today use plain paper or have laser capabilities. Many can be programmed, have copy reduction and enlargement capabilities, utilize the same fax and phone line, have one to two trays, have copy speeds from 9 pages per minute (ppm) up to 15, can have an auto preprogrammed dialing feature, quick scan features into memory, and/or be connected to the PC to deliver computer-generated faxes. In addition, the computer can be loaded with programs such as WinFax, Lotus Notes Fax, or Microsoft Fax, which will automatically deliver a fax via the computer. However, when a hard copy document needs to be sent, the only way to fax the document, other than scanning it into the computer, is through a freestanding fax machine. Selection criteria should include the following:

- A healthy size paper tray.
- Sufficient memory to handle those "out-of-paper" times.
- Ability to transmit at high speed—at least 14,400 bits per second (bps)—to enable lower telephone bills.
- A USB port, which is faster than a parallel port.

Communication of patient information via the fax, at this point, does not need to be encrypted. However, as a security precaution, each fax containing any information on the patient medical data needs to have a cover statement regarding the confidentiality of the information attached. In addition, the physician needs to make sure the receiving end fax is in a secure area, not just a general fax center viewable by a variety of individuals.

Brands include Sharp, Brother, Hewlett Packard, Minolta, NEC, Lanier, and Xerox. Prices range from $80 for a thermal to $180 for an ink jet and up to $400 for a laser.

CONCLUSION

Whether evaluating the information systems needs of a single small-practice office or a larger multiple-office group, physicians will need to thoroughly evaluate and make many important selection decisions regarding computers, office equipment, and software programs. With sophisticated technology available in the marketplace, combined with the powerful tool of the Internet, physicians' choices are unlimited. However, the objective of any small multiphysician or networked practice is to select the most appropriate and functional system that will meet the practice's needs today and that can easily be upgraded to serve future expansion needs.

Planning, evaluation, research, and advice from expert resources will result in an informed selection and an information systems decision that will deliver a good return on your investment.

CHAPTER 20

Human Resource Outsourcing for the Physician Executive

Eric Galtress

> Many medical practices today have found that employee leasing, also referred to as coemployment, can be an effective strategy to combat the spiraling costs of having a professional and clerical support staff. It can offer financial and administrative benefits to medical practices, which, in turn, can increase staff loyalty and reduce turnover. Many physicians will find that the personnel services of an employee leasing company will give them more time to address the efficiency of their practices and the quality of care they provide for patients.
>
> —Tony L. Sullivan,
> Journal of Medical Practice Management

As the medical community continues to seek ways to simplify and streamline their operations while increasing revenues, improvements in technology and business processes have been of enormous help. These include innovations in billing techniques to capture every earned dollar, maximize collection rates and minimize accounts receivable cycles. Meanwhile, challenges remain in the area of human-resource management. As the major expense driver of the medical practice, nursing and technical staff shortages, higher wages, Workers' Compensation and employee benefits cost increases, employee turnover, federal government compliance, and employer liabilities need constant attention. As employees and key staff members are added to the practice, you're required to comply with a plethora of specific employee-related requirements. (See Fig. 20.1). These govern the proper method of how employees must be treated and paid, as well as ensuring that their rights in the workplace are protected. For noncompliance, the practitioner/business owner can face fines, penalties, business interruption, litigation, or perhaps even business failure.

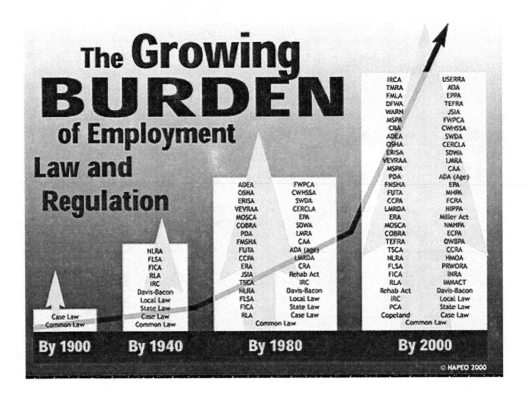

FIGURE 20.1   The growing burden of employment law and regulation.

©NAPEO 2003 – reproduced with permission of the National Association of Professional Employer Organizations

INTRODUCTION

What follows is an overview of the human resources (HR) requirements for the employer. This includes a condensed view of employment and labor laws, government compliance issues, employee related costs, and the alarming upsurge in employee litigation. The last poses a growing level of liability and distraction to today's medical executive/practitioner/business owner, second only to that of medical malpractice. As a result, many physicians without available HR expertise are finding it increasingly difficult to focus on growing their practices.

Studies show that a company needs at least 90 or more employees to justify the costs of establishing an in-house HR department, which, in most cases, must also be backed by labor attorneys, service providers, brokers, and other business consultants. The good news is that all medical practices can now take advantage of an innovative alternative: being able to delegate (outsource) most of the HR burden as well as employee-related liabilities.

Simply put, instead of the practitioner being the *employer of record* of the workplace employees, this responsibility is *outsourced* to an off-site professional employer organization (PEO) that specializes in labor management and cost control. The practitioner retains functional control of the employees, and the PEO handles the HR management issues. The PEO can provide these HR services *more cost effectively* for the practice by combining employees and servicing their needs along with the employees of the many other practices and businesses they already serve. Outsourcing is a matter of simple economics.

The PEO relationship is not to be confused with a physician practice management corporation (PPMC). The PEO has no financial interest or ownership whatsoever in the practice, but merely is there to provide valuable assistance with regard to employee-related issues.

DEFINITIONS

Outsource: To others—for example, an outsourcing organization—take responsibility and much of the liability to perform services for the business benefits all parties because people outside of your practice

- can do it cheaper and/or faster
- can do it better because of their expertise and experience
- have all of the required professional staff and/or facilities
- take all or part of the risk and the liability to do it right
- save you the time of doing it yourself or having one or more of your key staff members distracted from the priorities of the business

Human resource management. Generally speaking, HR management consists of the activities, responsibilities, and issues of any practice/business, corporation, partnership or other business entity that comes as a result of having employees (independent contractors are not considered employees). Some of these requirements are mandatory, such as paying minimum wage and providing Workers' Compensation insurance protection; other aspects and their related administrative functions can be at the discretion of the owner(s) of the business, for example, sponsoring health benefits, retirement plans for employees, or paid vacation and sick time.

HUMAN RESOURCE COMPONENTS

- *Human Resource Administration.* Employee handbook, guides and regulations, posters, procedures for recruiting, hiring, reviews, discipline, termination, and labor law expertise.
- *Payroll Processing.* Employer tax administration, record keeping, federal and state reporting and tax filings, payroll calculations/deductions, paycheck printing and distribution, check deposit, W2s, W4s, unemployment administration, management reports, time-off utilization, accruals, and payroll audit responsibility.
- *Labor and Employer Liability Issues.* Unemployment, sexual harassment, wrongful termination, employee separation (forms DE1101, DE1545) discrimination, employee rights, costs of labor disputes and litigation, personnel record keeping (I-9, W4, DE4 etc.), government compliance with Occupational Safety &

Health Administration (OSHA), Americans with Disabilities Act (ADA), Equal Employment Opportunity Commission (EEOC), Consolidated Omnibus Budget Reconciliation Act (COBRA), immigration, and a variety of other government regulations.

- *Workers' Compensation Protection,* Insurance Premium and full legal coverage, claims filings, management and administration, fraud investigation and defense, audits and loss control, communication with injured employees, return-to-work procedures.
- *Safety.* Establish and implement an illness and injury prevention program (IIPP) in accordance with the requirements of Senate Bill 198 (SB198) and OSHA. Provide all required general and specific safety training as well as all required personal protective equipment.
- *Benefits:* Administration of mandatory employee benefits such as overtime pay, work breaks, unemployment insurance, and the like as well as additional benefits and employee incentives that may be provided at the discretion of the owner(s) of the business such as health, dental, and vision insurance, tax savings, and pension plans, vacations, paid time off, sick leave, and other rewards.

EMPLOYEE-RELATED OVERHEAD COSTS

Typically, employee related overhead costs are tracked by expressing the applicable costs as a percentage of the total gross wages of the practice. Figure 20.2 provides a breakdown of the primary activities which amount to 24%–26% above gross wages, depending upon the employees' specific job function. This is a national average, including Workers' Compensation insurance for low risk job functions such as clerical, programming, outside sales, doctor's office staff, and similar positions at the workplace. This 24%–26% does not include the cost of health, dental, or vision insurance for the employees, since this varies as to whether the practice will sponsor these benefits; the age and health status of the employees; the type of insurance plan (Preferred Provider Organization [PPO], Point of Service [POS] MCO or HMO); the specific carrier(s); the total number going on the health plan; or the geographic location.

Take note that each area of employee overhead has within it far more detailed procedures and management requirements than the outline may suggest. (See Table 20.1). The listing is arranged so that one can see the activities that are the responsibility of the practice without the Professional Employer Organization (PEO) and which of these same activities are assumed or shared by the PEO once the practice becomes a PEO client.

Federal Regulatory Cost Portion

Based upon an updated study for 2000, the average cost per employee to comply with federal regulations was $6,975 for businesses with fewer than 20 employees (see Fig. 20.3). With new legislation and regulatory requirements being added each year, the cost burden will continue to rise.

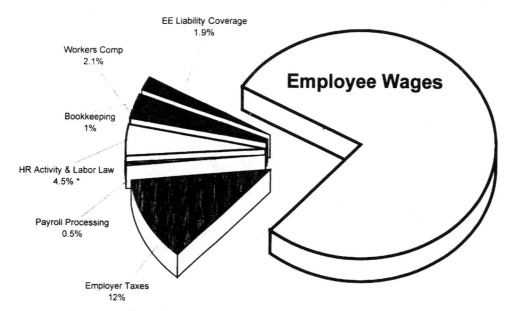

Employee Related Overhead Costs
(National Average as a Percentage of Gross Wages - 22%)

FIGURE 20.2 **For every $100 in employee wages, each employee costs an additional $24 to $26 (24%–26%), not including health insurance costs.**

Source: Small Business Administration, Department of Labor and Staffing Industry estimates.

Employee Turnover Costs

A less obvious but more significant soft dollar cost that is not fully understood and rarely tracked is employee turnover (see Fig. 20.4). This is a huge time bomb of cost to the practice. After spending valuable time seeking, hiring, and then training the employee, for whatever reason, the employee decides to leave for what he or she deems to be a better opportunity elsewhere. The practice then has to start all over and hope for the best. Other employees are disrupted because of a need to cover the increased workload, and morale goes down. It's a continuous cycle of negativity and is very costly in view of all the areas in the business that are affected (see Table 20.2).

A more detailed breakdown of the areas that are affected by turnover can be obtained at no charge by sending an email to Medical Management Consultants (MMC) at Info@mmchr.com (web site www.mmchr.com).

QUESTION

Does it make sense for the practitioner to take on the HR responsibilities and the related liabilities of being the employer and hope for the best, or should the focus be on building the practice and delegate (i.e., outsource) most of these activities (which are headaches to most business owners) to a PEO?

TABLE 20.1   HR Administration Components—Detailed Breakdown

	WITH PEO		WITHOUT PEO
	PEO	Client	Client
Human Resources Management			
Personnel Records Administration/Audits	•		•
Unemployment Claims Administration	•		•
Government Regulations and Compliance	•		•
Department of Labor and other Agencies	•		•
involved in Employment Issues	•		•
and Workplace Safety (60+ Laws)	•		•
Personnel Policies and Protocol	•		•
Hiring, Qualification, Selection Consultation	•		•
Candidate Social Security Verification	•		•
Proper Disciplinary and Termination Procedures	•		•
Employee Administration Consultation	•		•
Wage/hour Law Consultation	•		•
Complaint Procedures and Employee Counseling	•	•	•
Wrongful Termination Consultation	•		•
Sexual Harassment Consultation	•		•
Legal Consultation	•		•
Employee Handbook	•		•
Workers' Comp • Safety Program • Claims Mgmt • Loss Control			
Workers' Compensation Insurance	•		•
Claims Processing and Filing	•	•	•
Claims Management	•		•
Loss Control Program with Video Library	•	•	•
Fraud Prevention Program	•		•
Legal Responsibility for Audits and Defenses	•		•
Communication With Injured Employees	•		•
ADA Americans With Disabilities Compliance	•		•
SB198 Senate Bill 198 Compliance	•	•	•
Safety Management Program	•	•	•
CAL/OSHA Records Administration	•	•	•
Payroll Administration • Employer Tax Filings and Reporting			
Payroll Processing and Delivery	•		•
Direct Deposit	•		•
Employer Tax Routing to all Agencies	•		•
Tax Reporting, Agency Filings, quarterlies etc.	•		•
Payroll Deductions and Garnishments	•		•
W-2, W-4 Preparation	•		•
Reconciliation of Payroll Accounts/Mgmt Reports	•		•
Legal Responsibility for Audits	•		•
Magmedia reporting	•		•
Flexible Employee Benefits Program			
Rate Negotiations With Health Care Providers	•		•
Administration of Benefit Program	•		•
Health Plan Options for Employee and Dependents	•		•
Dental Care and Vision Plan	•		•
Cancer Plan	•		•

TABLE 20.1 *(continued)*

| | WITH PEO | | WITHOUT PEO |
	PEO	Client	Client
Group Term Life Insurance and Disability	•		•
Employee Hot Line	•		•
Credit Union	•		•
Group Membership Discount Programs	•		•
Family Entertainment and Movie Discount Programs	•		•
Section 125 Cafeteria Tax Benefits Program	•		•
Dependent Care Tax Savings Plan (child/elderly)	•		•
Tuition Assistance Program	•		•
Car Rental Discounts	•		•
Health Club Discount	•		•
401(k) Retirement Savings Plan	•		•
Optional Services Available			
Recruiting and Hiring Consultation	•	•	•
Management and Supervisor Training Programs	•	•	•
Forklift Training	•		•
Predictive Index Testing for Key Hiring Decisions	•		•
Candidate Assessment and Qualification Criteria	•		•
Background and Reference Checks	•		•
Drug Testing Program	•		•
Employee Turnover Reduction Program	•		•
Job Descriptions, Salary Surveys	•		•
Worksite Human Resource Manager	•		•

Following is a review of how the typical small to midsize practice may handle their HR responsibilities. We will also assess the benefits to these practices should they choose to utilize the added value provided by the PEO and be relieved of most of the hassle and administrative burden as well as much of the liability.

Alternative 1: The Practice Performs the HR Responsibilities

The typical practice will hire a sharp office manager or administrator who has experience with personnel issues, has lots of common sense. This person will consult with the practitioner and will be backed by a labor attorney on retainer and a bookkeeper and/or CPA. The practice may also purchase Employment Practices Liability Insurance (EPLI) at added cost.

The practice then deals with possibly 7 or more service providers. These would include brokers, consultants for payroll; employer tax administration; filings and reporting; Workers' Compensation insurance; safety, health, and benefit programs; credit unions; tax benefit and retirement plans; employee labor law issues; and so on.

These vendors all have their own agendas, with no connection or vested interest in any of the others' activities. Vendors bill the practice in accordance with their own billing periods, which means perhaps hundreds of phone calls, invoices to reconcile, and many checks to write throughout the year.

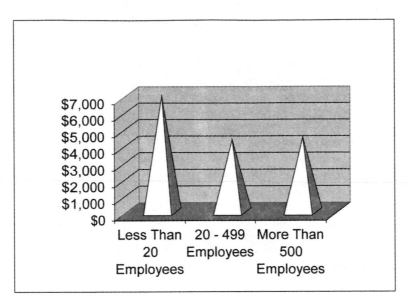

FIGURE 20.3   Federal regulatory costs per employee by business size.

Source: Report for the Office of Advocacy, US Small Business Administration RFP No. SBAHQ-00-R-0027 by:
W. Mark Crain and Thomas D. Hopkins
www.sba.gov/advo/research/rs207tot.pdf

This same office manager or administrator (or, as often is the case, maybe even the practitioner) may also take on the tasks of researching, developing, and distributing an employee handbook; office hiring and selection procedures; compensation policies; job descriptions; and implementing and maintaining compliance with existing and newly issued legislative updates—including HIPAA privacy rules, for example.

Finally, this individual will also be expected to contribute time to enhance caregiving, help ensure a smooth operation at the practice, increase and maintain employee productivity, and assist in the physicians' long-term plan to grow the practice.

This approach to handle HR responsibilities has, for the most part, been the most widely used in the past; however, it has become overwhelming and an enormous distraction and interferes with the focus on the priorities of the practice, the ones that increase the bottom line.

In recent years, the explosion of new employment legislation and a highly litigious society has created an environment in which the physician must continue to seek alternatives to best manage HR including the employee related overhead costs as well as the liabilities.

Liabilities of Being the Employer Doctor

Woven into the employee related overhead costs are the liabilities, risks, and exposures of being the employer. While employees can be one of the practice's greatest assets in today's litigious business climate, these same employees can, on the hand, be the practice's greatest potential liability.

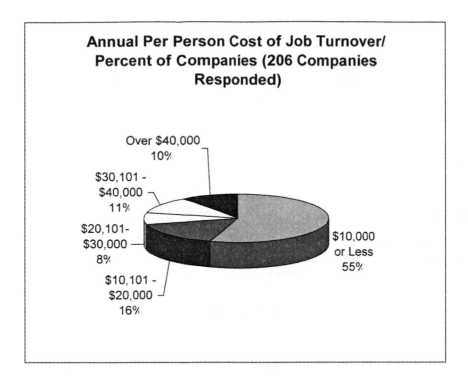

FIGURE 20.4 Annual per person cost of job turnover.

Factor in lost productivity from a vacancy, search fees, management time used to interview and training costs for a new hire.
Source: Data—William M. Mercer, Inc. Business Week Magazine, April 20, 2002 Issue

Figure 20.5 illustrates the impact of the increasing number of employment laws in the form of claims filed for fiscal year 2001. Figure 20.6 provides the median jury award by discrimination type for the period of 1994 to 2000. It also should be noted that the award amount increased consistently every year during this period, and there is no doubt that this trend will continue.

New Employment Legislation

In addition to the existing government regulations, Congress, at any given time, has several hundred employment legislative bills pending. How many will eventually become law is anyone's guess, but the workplace can expect a continuum of new employment laws and regulations as a reflection of today's highly litigious society.

Alternative 2: The Medical Practitioner Outsources the HR Responsibilities to an Experienced PEO, Utilizing Professionals Who Specialize in the Healthcare Industry

In the past, out sourcing of functions that traditionally fall within the human resources domain has already been utilized on a very large scale by more than 62% of all

TABLE 20.2   Turnover—Business Areas Affected

Outline Guide for Analyzing Cost of Turnover

1. Loss in Production Volume
   a. Loss in production volume from lost staff-hours
   b. Estimated loss in overall production volume

2. Increased Operating Expenses
   a. Increase in unemployment compensation premium
   b. Increase in accident insurance rate (new employees are more likely to have work-place injuries in new position)
   c. Additional operating cost in overhead due to low production

3. Production Expenses
   a. Cost of training
   b. Extra labor cost
   c. Cost of vacancy and low production period
   d. Loss of material (spoilage by new employees)

4. Administrative Cost (Service)
   a. Personnel office expense
   b. Medical examination expense
   c. Advertising expense
   d. Pre-job training
   e. Cost of induction and payroll administration
   f. Accounting cost

5. Other miscellaneous costs such as:
   a. Separation (severance) costs for departing employee
   b. Travel/moving expenses for new employee
   c. Potential legal expenses in event of employee litigation
   d. Lower morale, reduced synergy of workforce
   e. Ongoing administration costs such as COBRA or workplace injury follow up

Source: Employment Development Department of California

employers. Payroll processing is just one example (Source: 1997 SHRM-BNA Survey #62). In recent years, with more focus on productivity and the clearly demonstrated benefits of outsourcing, the estimate is over 90%.

Today, physicians must build a foundation to concentrate on caring for their patients, being highly productive, and growing their practices. Practices must also attract and keep in place highly motivated professional staffs of employees that are dedicated to these same principles. This becomes an ongoing challenge in today's highly competitive and often unpredictable healthcare environment.

Enter the PEO Industry, which has come to be recognized as a viable HR services alternative for virtually all small to midsize companies, including medical practices. In prior years, the terms *employee leasing* or *staff leasing* were common references for an alternate approach used by a business to provide for an additional pension plan option for owners/key management that differed from the plan offered to their regular employees. Subsequent tax legislation disallowed this practice and the leasing company's focus moved to reducing Workers' Compensation costs and payroll with very minimal HR support. Any comparison to earlier approaches can leave one with

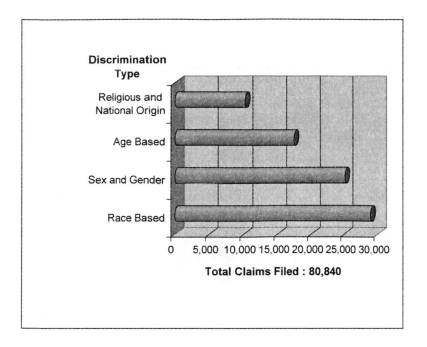

FIGURE 20.5 EEOC claims filed—fiscal year 2001.

Source: Equal Employment Opportunity Commission—February, 2002 Report as cited in Career Journal Publication. www.careerjournal.com/myc/legal/20020226-chen.html

a misconception of the depth of services a highly credible PEO can bring to an organization. Specialization and tailored services and benefits, along with the transfer of employer liabilities, are more accurately conveyed by the contemporary term PEO outsourcing or coemployment. Therefore, these references have been used throughout this chapter.

PEOs became fully recognized as a growing force in the staffing industry in the early 1980s. In 1983 for example, there were approximately 20 PEOs. This grew to over 2,000 nationwide; however, in recent years, consolidations, mergers, and acquisitions have reduced the number of PEOs. In the absence of a specific tracking mechanism, it is believed that there are now less that 1,000 nationwide. Most important is that in terms of revenues, this industry has grown consistently and dramatically year after year with a current average annual growth of 20% to 30%. In fact, PEOs now account for 30% of the entire staffing industry in revenues (see Figure 20.7).

These major industry activities have created several very large PEOs, some being publicly traded. However, bigger isn't necessarily better when you consider that the primary benefactor of the PEO services program is the small to midsize practice or business. Often, large PEOs cannot provide the specialized services, flexibility, personalized attention, or quick response these practices need and expect.

Among the more experienced PEOs are some that have chosen to specialize in specific market segments such as health care, which is the MMC's specialty. Others may deal with such industries as heavy manufacturing, transportation, and contractor/building. These PEOs come to know the unique aspects of their respective

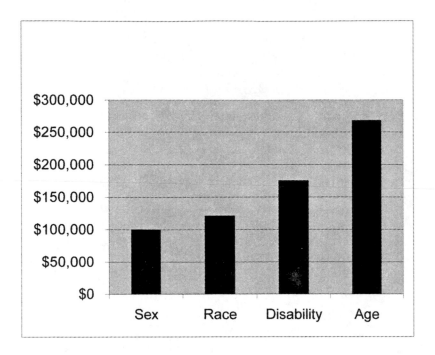

FIGURE 20.6 Jury award median by type of discrimination case (1994–2000).

marketplaces and use their experience and expertise most effectively. This can be critical in an environment where employers face so many exposures, not only in running their practice or business but also in coping with the escalation in employment laws and related litigation.

WHAT ARE THE ADVANTAGES OF OUTSOURCING?

How can the PEO's integrated services benefit all parties in the relationship?

For the Medical Executive and Medical Practice

Outsourcing allows for more focus on patient needs, reducing costs, and growing the practice.

- *It controls and reduces hard and soft dollar costs.* Outsourcing consolidates the activities and costs of a multitude of service providers and vendors into a single and highly specialized PEO. Only one check per pay period need be issued to the PEO for these HR Services.
- *It reduces the liabilities of being the employer.* In most states, liability falls on the employer (employers' insurance carrier) who has the injured employee on

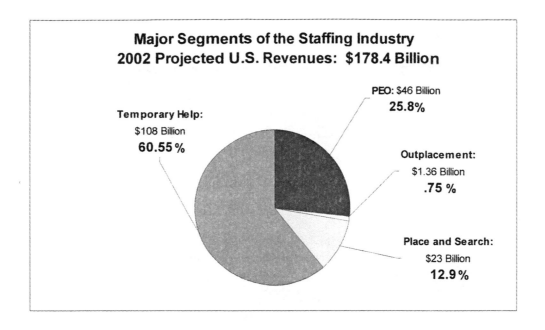

FIGURE 20.7 Major segments of the staffing industry.

The PEO industry has now grown to over one fourth of the entire staffing industry with in excess of 3 million employees nationwide and growing 20–30% annually.

the payroll and who is providing the Workers' Compensation insurance coverage. In both cases, this is usually the PEO, although the workplace employer may have some liability if "gross negligence" contributed to or caused the workplace injury.

Another area in which some liability is transferred to the PEO has to do with OSHA compliance. For example, in California, one of the toughest states for workplace safety compliance, the Division of Occupational Safety and Health issued a policy that applied to dual-employer situations (coemployment, temporary help, employee leasing, PEOs, etc.), which said, in part, "The company supplying the employee is referred to as the *primary* employer [PEO] and the company supervising the employee at the workplace is referred to as the *secondary employer* [the business]." Of course, the workplace employer is generally responsible for maintaining a safe workplace.

A third area of transferred liability relates to *payroll administration and management.* The PEO takes responsibility for proper compliance with all federal and state agency requirements for payroll taxes, filings, reporting, and records management of the employees. This is because it is the PEO's federal and state IDs that are used in the filings. State requirements however, do require that the workplace employers maintain copies of their timekeeping records for a specified minimum period of time.

- *It provides more cost-effective and better employee benefits options.* This allows the practice to attract and retain the best employee candidates and maintain higher morale, and it helps reduce the huge costs, loss of productivity, and disruption associated with employee turnover as discussed previously.

- *It reduces the time spent on employee and government compliance issues for both the practice and its key staff members.* This enables them to focus on adding new patients, increasing satisfaction, and handling their own specific priorities.
- *It promotes synergy of HR components.* By integrating all services into one stream-lined program, each component has a vested interest and interdepends on the shared goals of quality service, value, cost control, and loss prevention of all parties, including the specific needs of the practice and the employees.
- *It provides peace of mind.* Outsourcing ensures that stringent requirements and government regulations are handled by experienced professionals with exper-tise and a vested interest in ongoing compliance.

For the Employee

Outsourcing increases morale, productivity, and job fulfillment.

- *It protects their rights.* Helps foster an environment where the employee's as well as the practitioner's rights in the workplace are respected.
- *It offers better benefits.* Provides employees with greater access to more affordable (big company) health and other benefits options, more selectivity, and a means to participate in self funded/nonmatching, or employer matched retirement plans and tax savings opportunities. Family fun benefits, including theme park and movie discount programs, as well as credit unions, add more value to the benefits program offered by full service PEOs.
- *It addresses and resolves problems.* Puts in place a means to help identify and resolve employee issues and concerns that may otherwise escalate.
- *It results in increased job stability.* Provides for a potentially more stable employ-ment relationship, career growth, and self-betterment opportunities by taking advantage of specialized employee programs offered by the PEO, such as training.

For the Government

Outsourcing offers more assurance of compliance and enhanced communication.

- *It consolidates requirements.* Tax filings and collection of employer payroll taxes from many practices through a single PEO entity reduces administration costs.
- *It brings health care to more workers.* Outsourcing provides more options to the practice to extend medical benefits to more workers.
- *It improves compliance.* Outsourcing provides a more receptive and noninvasive option for practices to comply with the increasing volumes of employment related laws, regulations, and legislative requirements in the workplace.
- *It reduces unemployment.* Outsourcing promotes higher productivity at the prac-tice, which in turn leads to growth and more employment opportunities for those in the labor force.

HOW DOES THE PEO RELATIONSHIP COMMENCE AND WHAT HAPPENS NEXT?

1. The medical practitioner becomes aware of the PEO alternative in the following ways:

    *   Word of mouth from trusted advisors, accountants, attorneys, financial planners, business consultants, or another colleague who is a PEO client.
    *   Membership in a particular medical or fraternal organization.
    *   A special education course in which he or she is participating.
    *   Recommendation of a governmental agency, such as the Employment Development Department (EDD) or Small Business Administration (SBA).
    *   Endorsement by an industry association such as the National Association of Professional Employer Organizations (NAPEO), the local chamber of commerce, networking organization, or similar business support group.
    *   Enduring the pain and anguish of a major employer/employee related problem.

2. *PEO selected and initial meeting.* The practice seeks out a PEO utilizing the selection procedure suggested in the latter part of this chapter ("How Should You Select a PEO for Your Practice?"). During the initial meeting, it is important to achieve open communication. The practitioner should be *forthright* with all concerns regarding employees in the workplace, whether these are for the future or actual events that are happening now. Examples may include sexual harassment issues, a complex termination, unresolved employee issues, suspected fraudulent Workers' Compensation claims for difficult-to-prove cases such as "stress," hostility in the workplace, gaps in or the total absence of government compliance, and so on.

3. Data provided to PEO. The PEO will need copies of various information relating to Workers' Compensation, payroll, and administration costs and must know whether employee health benefits are desired and what, if anything, the practice may have in place in the area of an employee handbook, OSHA Program, and other HR related procedures.

4. *Needs analysis and Proposal Development.* When the practice and the PEO are satisfied that the needs profile has been completed, the resultant analysis is used to develop a proposal tailored to the practice.

5. *Proposal presented.* The proposal is presented to the practice and should not only address the needs of the practice itself, but also the benefits available to the workplace employees. Take note that even though some practices choose not to sponsor health benefits for their employees, there are other employee benefits made available by most PEOs at no cost (retirement plan availability, tax savings programs, credit union, discount memberships and movie tickets, family entertainment, and more).

6. *Proceed or wait.* Any remaining issues are clarified, and the practitioner decides to proceed or wait. Hopefully, after this process, it will be clear that the PEO benefits outweigh other considerations, and the practice should proceed and begin enjoying these benefits. A timetable is reviewed and agreed on. The PEO can then be up and running in as short a period as 1 week for urgent

situations but it is best to allow about 3 to 4 weeks from the time that the decision is made for a smooth transition.

7. *Conclude service agreement.* A standard service agreement (with amendment for any optional services such as a specialized training curriculum) summarizing the terms of the arrangement is reviewed and signed by the practitioner and PEO. The PEO becomes the employer of record for the employees, and the practitioner remains the workplace employer, retaining functional control of the employees. What results is referred to as a *coemployment* or *dual-employment* relationship, extending the benefits of the arrangement to all parties (see Figure 20.8).

8. *Employee orientation.* The employees are given an orientation by the PEO on the services and benefits available to them as a result of the program. In addition, the employees have the opportunity to ask questions and have the PEO address any concerns, and then the paperwork is completed.

9. *Program Benefits Begin.* The HR Services presented in the proposal are initiated in accordance with the agreed timetable. This includes the payroll services and administration. Prior to each payday, the practice reports hours worked to the PEO. Since the PEO already has all employee and wage data in their automated system, an invoice is generated quickly. The invoice includes wages, employer taxes, Workers' Compensation insurance, health benefits costs if applicable, HR services and the preagreed service fees for the pay period.

The invoice is paid by the practice, and the PEO has the payroll checks printed and delivered to the workplace and/or performs direct deposits if this feature is included in the services arrangement. Take note that the payroll checks are *issued from the PEO's own accounts.* This is an important distinction

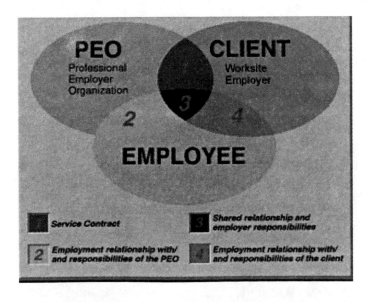

FIGURE 20.8   Illustrating the co-employment relationship.

©NAPEO 2003—reproduced with permission of the National Association of Professional Employer Organizations

as viewed by government authorities, and the IRS and provides an added measure of liability protection for the practice.

Sounds simple, and it can be. A well-established and highly reputable PEO will take a much deeper and will have a vested interest in the specific needs and requirements of the practice from the beginning. Once in place, the PEO will assume most of the responsibility of the HR elements, and this becomes a cooperative effort with the practice.

ADDED VALUE DERIVED FROM THE PEO RELATIONSHIP

What the practice will receive is the full compliment of services discussed above, but with a great deal of added value, depending on the PEO you choose and, of course, their ability to deliver the added value that would be meaningful to your medical practice.

Real-Life Examples of Added Value at the Workplace

Although the basic HR elements are the same, each client has a particular workplace atmosphere, along with specific needs, requirements and priorities that are meaningful to that client. Perhaps it is a brand-new practice with no HR policies whatsoever in place. It may need access to salary and benefits surveys so it can attract the best employee candidates and remain competitive with other practices in the area.

Some practices may be having problems with a high rate of employee turnover—a very costly situation to deal with and one that requires a concerted and directed effort to overcome. In either of these situations, the program of services offered by an experienced PEO can include procedures to help correct the problem and/or put in place the required support.

The following actual cases demonstrate how the experience and professional expertise of a full service PEO can make a substantial difference in the workplace and bring relief to the practitioner.

Case 1

In a recent program developed for a Medical Management Corporation (MMC) client, there was a need for a PC based time-clock system that would also be used for tracking the accrual of vacation and sick-leave hours. This would save much time for the person in charge, who had been performing these tasks as well as preparing the relevant reports manually.

MMC researched candidate vendors and alternative software packages to do the job. After reviewing the operational aspects with MMC, the client company made the selection, and MMC integrated the software program within their own payroll management system. The client company was delighted to not only gain the benefits of the expanded payroll function, but also greatly reduced the hours spent on the manual time-keeping error-prone system they had been using.

The more obvious concern to the business owner is the area of employer liability. The following cases are actual examples that have occurred at MMC clients in recent years. They convey the importance of a *swift and appropriate* response to workplace issues that can literally close a practice if not handled properly.

Case 2

An Administrator recently determined that one of their billers was incapable of handling the duties she was performing and, so as not to look bad, was burying paperwork instead of giving it to a supervisor who offered to help. The administrator decided to terminate the employee, and she told MMC she had a paper trail of memos to the employee, referring to poor performance.

Reviewing the paperwork, MMC found that, in fact, the employee had been told that she was doing a "great job." Termination would have resulted in an immediate claim. The employee's manager really felt like this individual was a nice employee and, thus, MMC helped compose a letter of warning so that the employee was reassigned to do necessary but less vital work. The employee was given a chance to improve, litigation was been avoided, a considerable amount of time was saved, and the practitioner, manager, and employee were happy with the arrangement.

Case 3

This particular example focuses on one of the more vulnerable aspects of a small medical practice and conveys another major advantage of selecting a PEO that specializes in this field. A doctor discovered that one of his staff members had been embezzling money over the course of a number of months. The doctor did not have any insurance coverage for embezzlement, but fortunately for him, MMC's Comprehensive Services Program automatically included this important benefit.

MMC assisted in the investigation and prosecution of the employee. MMC's insurance carrier made payment to the doctor on the claim, and the employee was arrested. The doctor is very happy about the protection he received. Without MMC, he would not have been able to recover any of the stolen money.

These examples clearly illustrate just how powerful and meaningful the element of added value can be when the practice forms a trusting relationship with a well-established and highly specialized PEO.

Without the experience and close working relationship MMC had formed with their clients, these practitioners would have spent much time, effort, and mental anguish trying to resolve these issues alone and/or with the assistance of costly legal counsel, who would have had to reconstruct a complete history with a time consuming and lengthy investigation.

The key element in these examples was that PEO's services personnel had already formed a close working relationship with the practitioner clients. But just as important, when a PEO incorporates a friendly staff of field representatives, they gain a critical familiarity with the work force from the employee's perspective and, collectively, they hold a vested interest in the resolution of any employee related issues, exposures, and liabilities.

Workers' Compensation—Average Cost per Claim

Workers' compensation costs vary by state, but California is a good indicator. In spite of being one of the toughest states in terms of OSHA requirements and enforcement, the average cost for workplace injury claims is continuing to rise (see Fig. 20.9).

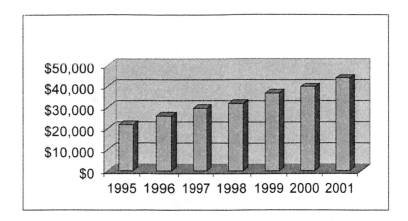

FIGURE 20.9 Worker's compensation average cost per claim in California.

Source: California Workers' Compensation Insurance Rating Bureau as reported in the Los Angeles Business Journal April 22–28, 2002

WHAT ARE THE DISADVANTAGES OR CONCERNS OF OUTSOURCING?

In reviewing the many advantages presented above, one would think there are no disadvantages or reasons why the practitioner would not move forward. After all, the proposal presented by the PEO conveyed the specific advantages and the corresponding added value that can be gained from the PEO relationship.

If there is any hesitation, it is usually because of one or more of the following general reasons, often referred to as the 4 Cs: cost, control, culture, and commitment. Let's explore each.

Considerations for the Practitioner

Cost

Perception: "With a full HR professional staff at my disposal, transfer of liability, labor law and government compliance assistance, Fortune 500 benefits, and employee administration support, aren't the services very expensive for a small practice?"

Reality: The PEO is cost-effective and brings added value. As part of the proposal development process, experienced PEO's perform a careful analysis taking into consideration the various costs (in both hard and soft dollars) of the practice. This analysis also includes important feedback on other areas of added value that the PEO program can bring.

Control

Perception. "If the practice becomes a coemployer with the PEO, and the PEO becomes the employer of record, wouldn't the practice have less control of all employee- and compliance-related matters?"

Reality: The PEO brings greater control to the practice and employee issues. Creating an alliance with a PEO that can provide your practice with the HR expertise you do not presently have actually increases your effectiveness in handling the important priorities of your practice. The PEO enhances the level of confidence and assuredness at the practice by dealing with the daily employee-related administration, giving the practitioner greater control in this important area.

Culture

Perception. If the PEO becomes the coemployer and employer of record, the employees may feel that they no longer work for the same organization, that the relationship will not benefit them, and this may affect their morale.

Reality: The PEO Relationship benefits the employees. Long-standing PEOs are very sensitive to this perception and for this reason make it a point to meet and come to know all employees at the practice both as a group and individually, during the employee orientation procedure. The PEO representative will also be pleased to meet with employees individually to address any specific concerns.

The workplace employees are soon reassured, once they understand that they will continue to perform the same daily workplace duties, with the same individuals, with virtually no change—and the relationship further protects their own rights. The employees also recognize the benefits to the practice, which can serve to form a more stable workplace for them and enhance their own well being, and view the relationship positively.

In addition, when the employees can gain access to a wider variety of benefits—an employee assistance hot line, a retirement plan, a tax savings plan, credit union, discount movies, self betterment opportunities, and more—they can only view this as beneficial to them. And they have the practitioner to thank for bringing these added benefits to them as part of the PEO relationship.

Commitment

Perception. "With so many administrative and liability responsibilities delegated to the PEO, doesn't the service agreement with the PEO require a long-term commitment in which I must be bound by strict terms and conditions?"

Reality: An experienced and reputable PEO will include a termination clause with no penalty as part of the service agreement. Many PEOs require a 1-year service commitment. However, PEOs that have gained credibility over the years, with a loyal following of clients, will include a termination clause or similar arrangement to allow for an easy transition out of the agreement with a minimal notification period.

How Will My Current Office Costs Compare With Those of a PEO?

As in most service businesses, there are a variety of approaches used by PEOs to establish their costs for servicing their clients' needs and to calculate their fees. For simplicity, PEOs generally express their fees as an overall percentage of the average gross wages of a stable work force, stating what is included in this comprehensive fee.

Many cost factors enter into each practice. Remember, there are both *hard* and *soft* dollar costs. *The hard dollar costs* are straightforward and easily determinable.

These may include actual costs for existing Workers' Compensation insurance coverage, payroll processing and employer taxes, health programs, and so on.

In reviewing the comprehensive listing of HR services areas broken down by function (see Table 20.1, shown earlier), you can readily see that the vast majority of the costs are *soft*. This means that they are time consuming in nature and involve interpretative analysis; thus, they pose some difficulty in arriving at an actual dollar cost. The more HR activities performed by the practitioner or key staff members, the more costly they become to the practice.

All things being equal, and based on national averages that incorporate both hard and soft dollar costs, PEOs are highly beneficial. PEOs can reduce the overall employee-related overhead costs of the practice when you consider both hard and soft dollars and, of course, turnover costs if this is an issue.

But What about the Savings in Your Time Spent on These Nonproductive Issues and Your Concerns about Liability?

Even when there is a small cost involved, virtually all practices/businesses stand to benefit in the areas noted previously. This is particularly true when the practitioner and/or key staff members are burdened with these time-consuming responsibilities and problems themselves and are held accountable to perform them in compliance with the applicable regulations. With the transfer and sharing of liabilities, the PEO brings real value and a cost effective and meaningful alternative for the practice and the employees.

How Should You Select a PEO for Your Practice?

We'll assume that you have reviewed the benefits available to your practice as well as to the employees and found that this alternative is worth your consideration. Now you are ready to take the next step and seek a PEO worthy of your trust and confidence.

1. Check the length of time the PEO has been in business, its credibility, and its reputation.
2. Make sure that the PEO can deliver the scope of services that can meet your requirements.
3. Be sure that the PEO has adequate financial resources and professional staff.
4. Seek a PEO that documents the service relationship with its clients and employees.
5. Confirm payment of taxes and insurance.
6. Require a termination clause
7. Select a PEO that has experience in healthcare and in your specific concerns, such as the following:

   - Interviewing, selection, and hiring techniques.
   - Employee performance, assessment, and reviews.
   - Sexual Harassment issues and protocol.
   - Proper disciplinary and documentation procedures.

- Safety in the workplace and office violence.
- Reducing employee turnover.

8. Verify Licensing Requirements.
9. Association Membership in NAPEO or (www.napeo.org)

EMERGING MEDICAL HUMAN RESOURCE ALTERNATIVES

As the business community continues to seek ways to minimize the distraction of nonproductive but necessary workplace activities, other innovative HR service approaches are starting to take form.

Administrative Service Organization (ASO) (Fee Based)

These providers offer complete and centralized administrative servicing of the HR functions including Workers' Compensation, benefits, payroll, HR administration, government compliance, and safety. However, unlike a PEO relationship, the practice/business itself still retains full responsibility as the employer of record and, as such, uses its own federal and state identification numbers on all employer/employee related documentation. Some PEOs however, may also offer an ASO alternative should this be the preference of the client.

ASP—Application Service Provider (Fee Based)

These providers are more leading edge, in that they extend the power and efficiencies of today's web-based technology into the HR function, providing on-line service capabilities. These may include employee self service processes from simple address changes to monitoring their 401(K) plan, checking credit union balances or making health plan changes. In so doing, ASPs incorporate a variety of Internet tools, software, specialized applications and processes along with consultative services to maximize cost effectiveness and streamline their offering.

Expanded Insurance Brokerage Services (No Added Costs or Fees)

For larger practices/businesses (in the range of 50 or more employees), a few select insurance brokerages have expanded their service portfolios to include a variety of cost-free services that bring substantial value and savings to their clients' practice/business. The actual services they provide are paid for by the reinvestment of a substantial portion of the commission dollars they receive, which are already included in the insurance premiums paid by the practice/business. With this alternative, there is no extra cost to the practice/business for these services, which may include HR and benefits administration, professional consultation, employee handbook, risk management services, OSHA and Labor Law compliance, comprehensive seminars, management/supervisory training workshops, and many other valuable services. A pioneer in this innovative approach is a California company named *Employer Benefits.* (*www.employerbenefits.com*).

Neither ASOs, ASPs, or expanded brokerages provide the full scope of services of a PEO. For this reason, the fees would typically be lower than a PEO (and perhaps nonexistent as is the case with expanded insurance brokerage services). Nevertheless, they are certainly worth a mention in the context of HR outsourcing. Following are the primary differences:

1. Unlike a PEO, there is no coemployment relationship, in that the client company of an ASO or ASP still remains the employer of record for the worksite employees.
2. There is ordinarily no liability transfer from the business owner as would exist in the PEO relationship, a major consideration for many entrepreneurs. However, in some instances, liability may be transferred by contract for certain services provided such as COBRA administration.
3. Although the ASO and ASP can provide meaningful HR support, their program orientation is to deliver quality HR products and services as opposed to the PEO whose program orientation is to deliver a full scope of quality HR products, services, value and liability protection.
4. With regard to the so called soft dollar employee administration costs, it is too early to tell whether an ASO or ASP versus a PEO addresses these as effectively. The PEO has a clearly defined vested interest and the synergy of HR components in working with the client, and this translates to more accountability.
5. There is no national accreditation or quality standard for the ASO or ASP, although each can certainly provide verifiable evidence of their credentials and experience, as well as client testimonials.

Business Process Outsourcing (BPO) (or Outsourcer, Fee Based)

The BPO is also a very new arrival on the HR scene and appears to be an all things to all people approach. Essentially, in its broad definition, a well-established BPO can present itself as being able to deliver an ASO, ASP, or even a PEO type of program to the client company. Conversely, many HR consultants with no specific focus are also using the BPO marquee for the coattail benefit. There are a few large BPOs that are integrating their offerings to Fortune 500 companies and who may also consider expanding their target market to include the medium size business community—and perhaps even small businesses as well.

Assessment of Emerging HR Alternatives

The ASO, ASP, and BPO have a relatively short history and their HR offering is spread among varied approaches with a current focus on a larger client base. Thus, it will take some time before a specific and consistent definition is developed for them. In addition, one will need to understand and then consider the cost versus value equation in the selection process, as opposed to other HR alternatives such as a PEO. The expanded brokerage services option is certainly worth consideration for those larger organizations in view of the many no-cost features and benefits.

CHAPTER 21

Medical Practice Noncompete Agreements

Frederick William LaCava

> My stepfather, a heart surgeon, was correct. Advances in medicine
> have never taken place in courtrooms or lawyers' offices.
>
> —James M. Kramon, Esq.
> Kramon & Graham, PA

The angriest individuals I have ever met in my life are parties to litigation over contractual covenants not to compete. Not medical malpractice cases, not even divorces, produce the fury, the expense, the feelings of betrayal and fraud that infect doctors fighting over whether, if, and how a paragraph in what was once a friendly business deal should be interpreted. The anger and grief probably spring from a failure of the parties to achieve mutual understanding at the time that the agreement is negotiated. These covenants are necessary, but over-reaching by one side or the other leads to terrible legal conflicts.

DEFINITION

The covenants in question are agreements that in certain circumstances one of the parties is committing himself or herself not to practice his or her profession for a period of time within a geographical area or with members of a defined population. The covenants arise in two sets of circumstances: sale of a practice or as a term of an employment agreement. The law treats the two types quite differently, favoring agreements as part of the sale of a practice and entertaining challenges to covenants in employment contracts.

A covenant not to compete is legally based on preservation of a protectable interest in goodwill. Though goodwill is an intangible property right, it is very much a real one. Accountants and the IRS have recognized methods of quantifying it. The federal government's fraud-and-abuse enforcement arm is very interested in the goodwill factor to make sure that it is not in fact a disguised kickback (divorce lawyers love it when divorce prompts an evaluation of marital property). Goodwill is the value attributed to an ongoing practice's name recognition, location, telephone numbers, business names, and all those things which would make a potential patient come to one doctor's office rather to than another's. The law recognizes that a practitioner has the right to protect that value from a competitor who unfairly tries to appropriate it.

COVENANTS IN THE SALE OF A PRACTICE

Goodwill should be protected in a sale of a practice because much of the value of such a practice is encompassed by the element of goodwill. A practice may include a building or suite of offices, either owned or leased; the equipment, furniture, and supplies on hand, records of patients; and other financial interests. But the biggest value of a practice is the propensity of existing patients to come to that location for medical services. The goodwill has been created by the practitioners who have provided those services in the past. To the extent that patients have liked Dr. Washington and have been satisfied with his medical treatment, they will tend to come to his office after Dr. Adams has acquired the practice. A large part of what Dr. Adams has paid for is the likelihood of transfer of that patient loyalty from Dr. Washington to him. A necessary part of the sale of the practice, then, is a commitment from Dr. Washington not to compete with Dr. Adams in that location or nearby for some reasonable amount of time. If Dr. Adams were not to require such a commitment from Dr. Washington, Dr. Washington would be free to open a new office across the street from the old one and attract the patients who were loyal to him in the old office to come to the new office. Unless Dr. Adams only bargained for some secondhand equipment and shop-worn office space, he would not have gotten the goodwill he paid for.

Covenants not to compete which are incident to the sale of a practice are favored by the law, almost universally enforced, and play a logical and necessary part of the sale or transfer of goodwill. Disputes and litigation over these covenants arise when the seller tries to find a way to get around the commitment.

As an example, an imaginary scenario follows: "Yes, I signed the covenant not to compete with Dr. Adams, but my wife, Dr. Martha Washington, did not. She can start up a competing practice across the street from the old office. She doesn't use the business name Washington Internal Medicine Associates that I sold to Dr. Adams; she uses Dr. M. Washington Internal Medicine, P.C. I don't practice medicine in any way at her office; I just sit out in the waiting room and drink coffee and chat with the patients."

Sellers who try such tactics usually lose. In negotiating the sale of a practice, either as seller or buyer, use an attorney who is expert in the area of covenants not to compete. Don't use a real estate lawyer, your tax attorney, or your divorce attorney! Don't use your brother's former college roommate just because he would do it cheap! You would never have a psychiatrist set your broken leg; so pay for the appropriate specialist. Make sure that the terms of the covenant are reasonable. A covenant whose terms are draconian may be voided by a court, leaving the purchaser with no protection at all.

COVENANT AS PART OF EMPLOYMENT CONTRACT

A covenant not to compete that is part of a contract of employment (or part of a stockholder's agreement) is far more likely to result in litigation, because these covenants are far more likely to be used or avoided unfairly. Many an employer would like the covenant to function to punish an employee who would dare to leave a job with an ongoing practice and compete with it in any conceivable fashion. Many an employee has signed an employment contract without ever giving thought to the possibility that the covenant would not be enforced against him or her, or worse, thinking that the covenant could not be enforced. If the covenant is drafted to be reasonable, it will be enforced, and it should be enforced. The reasons are easy to see.

A young associate, Dr. Johnson, joins an elder practitioner, Dr. Lincoln, in an ongoing practice with goodwill created by Dr. Lincoln. Dr. Johnson gets to know Dr. Lincoln's patients and impresses them with his own abilities. Dr. Johnson and Dr. Lincoln do not agree on an extension of the employment contract, and Dr. Johnson is notified that he may not practice medicine within the terms of the covenant not to compete contained in his employment contract. Dr. Lincoln has a protectable interest in the goodwill of his practice, which Dr. Johnson should not be allowed to appropriate and use against his former employer as a competitor. If the covenant is reasonably drafted, it will do no more than protect that defined interest belonging to Dr. Lincoln. The problem is defining what interest may be reasonably protected.

"REASONABLE" TERMS OF THE COVENANT

A covenant not to compete will not be upheld by a court if its effect is to go beyond the interest that Dr. Lincoln has in his goodwill. Current patients who have a current relationship of trust with Dr. Lincoln should be recognized as a legitimate interest. But, what about persons who have never been patients of Dr. Lincoln's, patients who may never have heard of Dr. Lincoln? What about patients who have not seen Dr. Lincoln in years and who may no longer have any tendency to consult with him on a new problem? The courts have struggled with this concept, and decisions can be found that both enforce and strike down covenants that cover future or possible patients. The covenant must be for a reasonable amount of time. How long is there a reasonable expectation that a patient would come back to a doctor who treated him or her earlier? Covenants up to 2 years have been almost uniformly upheld, while covenants longer than that have had varying fates.

The covenant must extend over no more than a reasonably necessary geographic area to effectuate protection of the legitimate interest. That geographic area may be far wider in a rural area than within a metropolis. The size of the geographic area may also vary with the kind of business interest being protected. In some cases, an area of a whole county is too big, while in others an area of 12 states is deemed reasonable. The definition of the geographical area is many times given little review by a court, and instead, another covenant with protection of one county or a 50 mile radius is cited, with a conclusion that a similar-sized area is also reasonable. A more particular examination of the facts of the particular case may distinguish it from that other case.

An alternative to a geographic limitation is a specification of certain persons whose business may not be solicited by the former employee, usually a designation of "current" patients or customers who have been served by the employer within the time of the associate's employment. In these cases, there is no geographic area of coverage, and the patient or customer may reside anywhere. Courts approve of these current customer limits.

A covenant may be declared unenforcable if one of its terms is unreasonable and cannot be separated from the remainder of the covenant. The law will not apply a blue pencil to rewrite the terms of a covenant to bring it within the scope of reasonability, but it will strike down a term that is unreasonable which can be isolated from the other terms of the covenant. However, a covenant may contain a *cy pres* clause (medieval French for "as close"), which directs the court to enforce the covenant within the limits of the law as closely to the meaning of the parties as possible.

REMEDIES (THE LEGAL RX)

No, a remedy in legal matters is not a medical prescription but the things that courts can do to protect or compensate a person who has been harmed by violation of a covenant not to compete. The possible remedies are (1) an award of actual damages proven after the fact, that is, how much monetary loss can be attributed directly to the unfair competition of the former employee; (2) liquidated damages calculated in advance at the time the covenant was drafted; and (3) injunction, that is, a court order that the former employee stop violating the covenant immediately. The first remedy is almost never used and is included in this analysis to show why the other two remedies are used instead. Actual damages after the fact requires that the whole period of the covenant run before any remedy can be considered. Employers argue that they could be put out of business before they ever got to be heard in court. Employers also argue that it would be so difficult as to be impossible to calculate. I have my doubts about how impossible it would be, but it is not very practical. I will come back to liquidated damages and why they a far more appropriate for physicians later.

An injunction is an order by the court, that is, the government, that a doctor not practice his or her area of medicine within the area and time limits of the covenant. In order for a court to issue an injunction, the court must find that the damages that may be done to the former employer are irreparable, that is, that no amount of money that can be reasonably calculated can compensate the former employer for the harm done by the former employee's competition. Further, the court must determine that it is in the public interest to issue the injunction. Very, very frequently, an employment agreement with a noncompete covenant in it will have recitations in it that the parties agree that damages to the employer would be irreparable and that it would be in the public interest that an injunction issue to enforce the covenant; that is, that the covenant should try to supply these necessary areas of proof by incorporating them into the language of the covenant. No court is bound by such recitations. It is only the court that determines the public interest, not the parties, and it is only the court that can determine that an alleged damage is or is not irreparable.

There are a million arguments and counter arguments between medical practitioners over whether the financial damages that may be done between them can or cannot be calculated. Once a court turns, however, to damages that may be done to patients, arguments tend to be more one-sided. Courts are beginning to pay serious attention to the public interest, which may be affected by the issuance of an injunction in circumstances in which it may be shown that an injunction would endanger members of the public who may need a particular specialty of medicine or even the ability to perform a specific procedure within that area of specialty; for example, by having physicians available to make full use of a particular facility in a community hospital that would otherwise suffer damages. Arguments have also been made that a covenant between doctors is or should be against public policy, because the enforcement of such an agreement forbids a patient from seeing the physician that he or she prefers without allowing the patient any say in the matter. Sec. 9.02 of the Opinions of the Council on Ethical and Judicial Affairs of the American Medical Association (1986), provides for agreements restricting medical practice.

AGREEMENTS RESTRICTING THE PRACTICE OF MEDICINE

> The counsel on Ethical and Judicial Affairs discourages any agreement between physicians which restricts the right of a physician to practice medicine for a specified period of time or in a specified area upon termination of employment or a partnership or a corporate agreement. Such restrictive agreements are not in the public interest. (Counsel on Ethical and Judicial Affairs)

I am unaware of the AMA giving any practical support against covenants not to compete. Courts in some states have taken the position that the covenants are void because they are against public policy. You must consult with an attorney to find out the legal handling of covenants not to compete between physicians involving injunctions.

Liquidated damages are specifications within a contract, in advance of any breach, which reasonably determine what monetary damages are likely to result from a breach of the covenant not to compete. The liquidated damages may set a specific figure or provide a certain formula for calculating the damages based on specified elements such as collections at a particular office, and so on. If the covenant is for longer than a year, the contract may provide that liquidated damages for breach during the first year will be this amount, and a breach after one year would be that amount. The law highly favors liquidated damages because the two parties have calculated the amount in advance and relieve the court of having to determine damages from the many different ways by which they can be calculated.

It is my own position that a specification of liquidated damages in a contract eliminates the claim for injunctive relief as well. The basic argument for injunctive relief is that a monetary award cannot compensate for the injuries done. Liquidated damages specify that amount and eliminate that claim. Some courts have, however, granted both damages and injunctive relief, perhaps because the parties did not raise the logical conflict before the court. I personally advise my clients to seek or offer provisions for liquidated damages because I find it repugnant to use the power of the state to tell a patient that he or she may not seek medical treatment from Dr. Kennedy or Dr. Nixon. The patient's choice is not to be sacrificed for a business concern, while the monetary damages will protect the loss of any goodwill that may be suffered.

Liquidated damages, however, have their own set of abuses. The amount of the damages may not bear a logical relationship to any reasonable way to calculate damages. An amount that is obviously in excess of such an estimation is legally a penalty on the person violating the covenant rather than compensation of injuries sustained by the complaining party. The law will not enforce a penalty or private punishment. An employer who overreaches may find himself or herself with no protection at all.

CONCLUSION

When faced with the prospect of drafting or of signing a covenant not to compete, consult a lawyer experienced in that specific area of law. Such a covenant is a reasonable and appropriate protection for the legitimate property right of goodwill, but such covenants will lead to bitter conflict if they attempt to restrict competition beyond what is legitimately protectable.

CHAPTER 22

Physician Recruitment

Allison McCarthy

> Medical career identity is that part of your life related to occupational and health care organizational activities. It is the unique way in which you believe that you fit into the health care industrial complex.
>
> —Eugene Schmuckler, PhD, MBA, CTS
> Institute, of Medical Business Advisors, Inc.

Improving financial performance in medical organizations today—be they group practices large or small—is a skillful balance between cinching the belt and investing in the right growth strategies. Whether that strategy calls for expanding a practice, moving into a key market, improving overall market share, or adding a new clinical program, recruiting the right physicians becomes all-important in achieving the organization's strategic goals. Without physicians, there are no patients. Indeed, doctors are key drivers in any medical organization's growth strategy. Simply put, finding and hiring the right physician is a surefire prescription for success.

An effective recruiting strategy is a process-driven long-term approach that requires

- planning and preparation,
- organizational (team-building) commitment,
- persuasive sales and marketing skills, and
- good retention practices.

Recruitment has become a refined art in recent years, as practices and physicians themselves grow increasingly savvy about the finer points of marketing positions and securing employment. It's more competitive than ever, too. Many organizations are going after the same physicians. Add to that a shortage of doctors in key specialties and certain geographic areas and the pressure becomes that much more intense. In addition, the aging of the physician workforce, their increased dissatisfaction with managed care, and changes in doctors' work expectations (they want more free time) have affected the demand and supply.

Also, both practicing physicians and residents fresh out of training have become more discerning and skillful in managing the search process. Candidates have learned to be selective based on how they're treated on the phone, how they're treated in person during site visits, or how smoothly the negotiations go. One small bump in the road and they could choose to go elsewhere. In truth, they look to rule organizations out, not in.

Even the smallest of practices must have an effective recruitment plan because they compete directly with the big guys—larger practices and hospitals that have polished their efforts and perfected their processes.

Centralized Effort

Physician recruiting is most effective when centralized by an individual within the group. The best approach is to assign one internal person to lead the effort, with support staff or assistance as necessary.

Appointing one person to oversee and coordinate the process—managing candidates, CVs, site visits, and contract negotiations—gives prospects a personal contact for any questions or concerns they might have.

Some practices and organizations choose to augment internal recruiting staff with seasoned outside consultants. Outsiders can be effective at taking a segmented piece of the recruiting effort, such as generating a first initial prospect list or creating a medical staff development plan. Outside agencies can also help with a politically charged or an unusually complex search, such as locating a physician with special language skills or ethnic background.

In addition, recruiting agencies can give the organization a better sense of how attractive its competitive package is in the marketplace because they know what others are offering.

However, totally outsourcing the recruiting effort may not be organizationally sound or cost effective in the long run. Successful physician recruiting really requires at least one knowledgeable and diplomatic individual on the inside who understands the medical community and practice dynamics, who can persuasively sell the opportunity to the right candidate and who can handle, with confidence, the fine print in contract negotiations. Would-be hires will value the recruitment process even more when it's driven from the inside.

Winning Traits

The in-house recruiter needs a myriad of skills to manage the recruiting process and land the right candidate: *diplomacy, discretion,* and *determination.*

- Diplomacy is essential because not everyone within the group or medical community always agrees that a position needs to be filled in the first place. A successful recruiter must be adroit enough to defuse any differences of opinion.
- Determination is important to see the project through to completion.
- Finally, discretion is vital in matters pertaining to personal and professional background and salary negotiations.

Not surprisingly, top-notch recruiters enjoy being with people, going out to dinner, talking on the phone. First-rate interpersonal skills are a must-have. Equally important are sound business practices—a key asset when it comes to managing budgets wisely. It helps to be organized, too, as there are numerous balls to keep in the air as the process moves along.

A final consideration is accessibility to decision makers in the top of the organization, most notably, the group practice leadership. An effective in-house recruiter has the executive director or medical director's ear in order to share differing opinions and perspectives gleaned from the medical staff, and to solicit input on conflict resolution.

With a centralized effort and the right internal person in charge, how do organizations small and large build and sustain a top-notch physician recruitment operation?

Determine Need

The physician recruiting process begins with the group's strategic plan. Physician leadership and key administrators need to pinpoint niche services and outline strategic goals. Where does the practice see itself in 5 to 10 years?

The in-house recruiter gathers this information into a medical staff development plan that outlines the number of physicians and specialists the practice should hire to accomplish the goals. Each position needs a plan, timeline, and budget. And the group must be patient: the process can take up to 9 months before a recruit is completed. While it is hard to anticipate sudden departures, it is possible to forecast long-term requirements and implement an overall long-range recruiting strategy to do as much preplanning and preparation as possible. Once in place, it is important to follow the process and hire right. The worst thing any practice or organization can do is to take just anyone.

Part of determining need is to decide how to get the work done. What resources are necessary to do the job? Will the in-house recruiter need staff, external resources, or a combination of both?

A contact management software program is especially helpful to manage the process and flag key details on prospects. People can choose among several off-the-shelf products, such as ACT or Goldmine, which can help capture and keep track of conversations and candidate information. The software programs can

- segment the database by specialty or practice opportunity,
- create tickler lists of "to do" items to manage candidates through the process, and
- maintain notes on activities and conversations with prospects/candidates.

Software programs also make it easy to generate reports to demonstrate activity and the numbers of candidates in various stages of the recruitment funnel (to help benchmark against standards), and to demonstrate within the organization where there is room for improvement in the recruitment process.

Getting Ready: Set the Parameters

The practice must establish its search criteria before prospecting can start. This means having the group leadership determine the following:

- Who is the ideal candidate?
- What does the practice want in education and professional experience?

- What about personality?
- What personal style blends most harmoniously with existing colleagues?
- Does the candidate need to be proficient in any specific languages or have a particular ethnic background to cater to key groups of patients?

This information, and additional details about how and where the candidate will be contracted, whether locum support is needed, how the reporting relationship will work, and defined roles and responsibilities, become part of the selection criteria. The in-house recruiter should put it all down on paper in a one-page detailed description about the practice opportunity. This information becomes a guide for people to follow when they are screening and evaluating candidates, and it is sent to prospective candidates who want to learn more about the position.

Compensation and Contracts

Each position needs a compensation package and contract. Putting the financial pieces together begins by researching and reviewing all available data about market opportunities. Recruiters use the American Board of Medical Specialties, the AMA database, and other resources to learn about numbers and locations of physicians in key specialty areas.

It is important to gather statistics about the target market nationally and regionally. This will help determine the competitive nature of the search and how challenging it will be to recruit each position.

For example, what is the local market bearing in terms of compensation levels and benefit packages for the recruited specialty? How can the organization structure or "sell" the position as the most attractive employment opportunity in the marketplace? (See Fig. 22.1.)

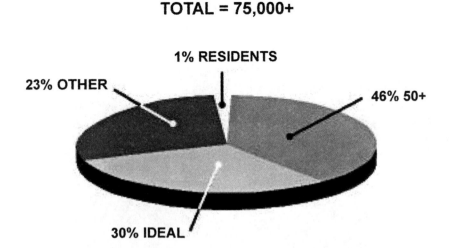

FIGURE 22.1   Median physician compensation per physician work relative value unit (RVU) by specialty.

Practices should make sure all financial pro formas and contracts are in place before the first would-be hire arrives on the doorstep (see Appendix 1).

Assemble Internal Team

Teamwork is the name of the game in the recruiting business. One of the in-house leader's first steps is to establish an internal recruitment team made up of physicians and administrators who are asked to be part of the search process. Group involvement, specifically leadership from key physicians, is essential to the success of the overall recruiting effort. Physicians on the committee can help troubleshoot any problems that arise, such as responding to doctors on the staff who grumble about adding a new specialist. These leadership physicians can also act as initial mentors and support systems when the new doctor arrives on board. Other team responsibilities include making screening phone calls, completing on-site interviews, assessing candidates' strengths and weaknesses, and assisting with social events.

Team members must have dedicated time available to receive calls, faxes, or e-mails from interested physicians who might have questions about the opening. The team must be well versed in the practice arrangement and the compensation plan in order to field the calls. Team members should be able to address community and lifestyle questions knowledgeably and comfortably.

The team leader needs to coach the group to sell not only the organization and the opportunity, but to carefully evaluate candidates to be sure they are the right fit for the job. Training sessions are very helpful for ensuring that people understand how to conduct effective telephone screening interviews, how to host informative site visits, and how to mentor new doctors coming aboard.

A recruitment effort is only as successful as its buy-in from physician and hospital leadership. Management must be committed to the effort in terms of time and dollars.

Fill the Funnel

The best-kept secret about physician recruiting is to keep the funnel filled with a pool of candidates. Organizations can't afford to wait for doctors to beat a path to their door; they have to go after the physicians they want. That means generating a sizeable list of prospects on the front end to narrow it down to the 100 or so doctors who will be called for an initial conversation. From there, the team may do some 50 telephone-screening interviews to generate 5 site visits in order to select the one perfectly matched prospect who will sign on the dotted line.

Depending upon the opportunity, there are a number of ways to generate a list of prospects:

- Direct mail, using a purchased list of physicians culled from criteria such as medical specialty and current geographic location. The American Board of Medical Specialties, the AMA, and licensure boards can supply these lists. The organization sends direct mail announcing the opportunity and then has a team member follow-up with outbound calling. If the physician is not interested, the caller should ask if he or she knows someone who is.
- Personal calls following recruitment fairs and specialty meetings.

- Advertising in medical and specialty journals and on the Web.
- Resident campaign using posted flyers and announcements.
- Physician networking based on group member recommendations.

From the initial pool of candidates, the internal recruiter must call prospects and conduct preliminary screenings to verify licensure status and board certification, gather professional and personal details about the candidate, and answer his or her questions about the opportunity. Whenever possible, research should be done to secure the prospect's home telephone number. Calling prospects in the evening at home gives them more time and privacy to talk freely.

This screening step generates a smaller list of credible prospects that meet the search criteria that was generated at the beginning of the recruitment process.

Recruitment Materials

Another early step in the recruitment process is to gather, or produce as necessary, promotional materials to describe the geographic area, local hospital and/or group practice, surrounding communities, and schools. Resources may include brochures from the chamber of commerce, Web site linkages to other sites, group/hospital-general brochures, and, of course, the one-page description about the practice opportunity. All of this information can be mailed to key prospects upon request. A sample direct mail piece is provided in Figure 22.2.

Interviews, Reference Checks, and Site Visits

It is best to have two separate people on phone detail: one team member can follow up briefly on the first direct mailing and another can conduct screening interviews. The first person is present to "sell" the organization and employment opportunity; the second is not selling the position as much as weeding out candidates who just don't fit.

The physician's CV should be available to the person doing the screening interview so that he or she can confirm professional information as well as ask questions about unclear time periods.

Following the telephone conversation, the team recruiter should verify the physician's credentials by contacting licensure boards to confirm that the candidate has an active license to practice medicine in the states he or she has indicated and that there are no liabilities associated with those licenses. It is also worthwhile to double check physician credentialing information with the American Board of Medicine Specialties, using annual publications, which are available in most hospital libraries, or going online at www.abms.org. Checking online requires registration to access information.

Provided the credentials verification returns positive information, a screening interview report should be given to the internal team, along with a copy of the candidate's CV and credentials verification. A sample telephone interview report is follows.

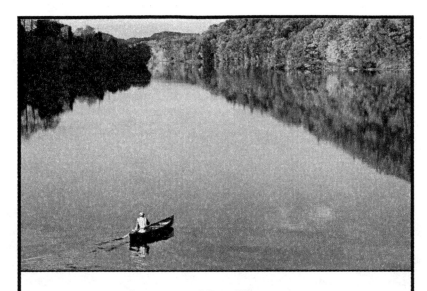

FIGURE 22.2 Sample physician recruitment advertisement.

Telephone Interview Report
Internal Medicine Physician
Sample: Dr. Joe Miller, MD/DO
Home: 1234 Bank Street
Office: 301-828-3270
Cell Phone: 310-445-2312

Dr. Joe conveyed his interest in practicing in New England through the PracticeLink database.

Personal History

Dr. Joe grew up in New Jersey and has lived in many locations throughout his medical school and training. He and his wife currently reside in San Diego, CA, where he is completing his residency training. They would like to settle in the northeast; they have with a strong preference for Massachusetts. His wife is from that area, and they spend most of their vacations in the northeast. They enjoy outdoor activities such as hiking, camping, and fishing. He indicated that they prefer a suburban area with easy access to urban offerings.

Education/Training

See CV. Dr. Joe is licensed in California and is completing his residency training in June 2004.

Professional Goals

Dr. Joe is seeking a general internal medicine position. He would like an office-based practice, with the opportunity for office, hospital, and nursing home management of his patients. He could be interested in a hospitalist position as well. He has special interest in diabetes care. He also has extensive critical-care experience that he feels is necessary because some hospitals do not have depth in that area or even have an intensivist on staff.

When choosing a practice, he indicated some preferences. He stated that he is not particular about the size of practice, but feels that a call schedule of 1 in 4 would be acceptable. He also mentioned that he would consider a multispecialty group, but would not want to be on call for pediatrics since he is not trained in that area. He stated that he realizes some opportunities are employed positions, but he would like the opportunity for partnership.

Dr. Joe chose internal medicine because of the variety it offers. He considered various subspecialties but never found one area of emphasis that seemed to fit. He has greatly enjoyed the camaraderie he has experienced through his residency training. His training has emphasized being close to the patients. They even do house calls, which is part of their ambulatory training. This aspect has been very rewarding and enriching for him.

Personal Goals

Dr. Joe seeks a practice in the northeast, since he and his wife love that area of the country. Access to the city is important, as well as the opportunity to practice in a suburban community where the cost of living and real estate is affordable.

First Impressions/Summary

The conversation with Dr. was open, honest, conversational, and relaxed, even though he had been up all night on-call! He was eager to share his ideas and goals for his first practice. Location is an important factor for him and his wife, and he was very interested in Massachusetts. We discussed his interests and desires first, and then the opportunity was described to him. He was agreeable and open to a variety of practice structures, with concerns around support, coverage, and how well he would be able to connect with the physicians he would work with on a regular basis.

If the internal team is in agreement, a second screening between the physician candidate and organizational leadership and team members takes place. This conversation can happen in person, if the candidate is within driving distance, or over the telephone if not. Team members typically ask the physician candidate questions such as the following:

- What do you like about your current practice?
- What factors do you think make up a satisfying practice?
- What type of practice arrangement are you looking for?
- Why do you wish to join a practice affiliated with (name of hospital or organization)?
- What do you expect to receive from the (name of hospital or organization) in return?
- What are your current and future professional goals?

Site Visit Basics

When the phone calls and reference checks are complete and everyone involved in the process has had an opportunity to reflect on the candidates' strengths and weaknesses, it is time to decide on the short list of star prospects and issue an invitation to these prospects to visit.

Generally, candidates spend one to two days on site, during which time they

- meet with administrators to discuss organizational philosophy and budgets,
- take orientation tours of the office location(s) and hospital,
- mingle with potential colleagues,
- connect with a realtor for a community tour, and
- have dinner with the internal recruiting team, medical staff, and spouses

All the while that the candidate is on campus, the recruiting team should evaluate him or her on the following criteria:

- communication skills
- work ethic
- interpersonal skills
- maturity
- judgment and common sense
- long-term interest
- education and experience
- ability to mange a practice
- cultural fit within the community
- ability to work with the medical staff

It is helpful to have an interview report form listing the criteria so that team members can easily rate each candidate and register their assessment and opinions.

Recruitment as a Sales Process

Successful recruiting is not unlike sales—it takes a persuasive personality and a winning attitude to position the opportunity to outside prospects and internal staff alike. A positive get-to-the-other-side determination is essential to go after, and secure, the best candidate for the organization.

Through the entire process, the recruiting team must put its best foot forward, representing the practice with quality and class. The recruitment team is the prospect's first introduction to the organization and first impressions can be lasting.

Selling Over the Phone

The telephone is an indispensable part of the recruiting process and is a pivotal selling tool in the recruitment strategy. Excellent telephone skills are critical at the prospecting stage, when team members are soliciting interest in the opportunity, and during the screening interviews, when team members must deftly and simultaneously evaluate the candidate and weed out those who don't fit.

The trick in telephone interviewing, is to build rapport quickly. Suggestions for effective phone screening and for building instant rapport include the following:

- Eliminate distractions; turn off beeper and ask the office assistant to screen calls.
- Have a planned opener to start the conversation.

- Prepare questions that call for open responses, not merely "yes" or "no" answers. Address clinical, philosophical, and lifestyle issues.
- Determine what motivates the candidates; if they are entrepreneurial in spirit, they won't fit neatly into a salaried position.
- Create a dialogue. Look for common ground.
- Control the discussion.
- Keep the conversation short—no more than 20 minutes.

Features vs. Benefits

Another way the recruitment process is sales oriented is that during the telephone interview, team members must do a good job of assessing features versus benefits. Over the telephone, team members must solicit the candidate's needs by asking the right questions and listening carefully to understand their idea of an ideal position. In this way, team members can assess if the practice opportunity is a good fit for the candidate. Once the team member knows the prospect's needs, he or she can more effectively describe or "sell" the practice opportunity by defining benefits versus features. Benefits are those aspects of the opportunity that will directly meet the needs of the physician candidate. Features are the specific aspects of the practice opportunity that may or may not fit the needs of the physician candidate but are worthy of his or her consideration.

Accept the Positive

Part of the selling game is to play up all that is good about the opportunity and control the objections as much as possible. There isn't any position open today that doesn't have a share of potential weaknesses, be they organizational politics, too little or too much HMO penetration, skyrocketing malpractice rates, the geographic location, or the cost of practicing or living in the area. Staff must first recognize the challenges and then demonstrate to prospective candidates that leadership is willing to work with them to manage the issues. For example, if high malpractice rates are a deal breaker with the perfect candidate, then leadership must build insurance coverage into the compensation package.

The recruitment team also has to sell the candidate on the location of the opportunity. Team members should consider what the local market has to offer of value to physician prospects, such as lifestyle (family, cultural, recreational, housing costs, and spiritual), professional development, specialty competition, and type of practice. The team can emphasize these points when marketing a recruitment opportunity for the region.

Every region has its pros and cons. Don't be discouraged if the market seems to have less appeal—either because of geography or other features that can't be changed. Hard-to-recruit markets take more effort in the way of mailings, personal calls, working with residency programs, networking, and following-up with every candidate who seems the least bit interested. Statistics prove that a large percentage of physicians choose to practice where they have ties, either because they grew up in an area, went to school there, or have family ties. Team members should network to find physicians with a geographic kinship. Review the backgrounds of the current medical staff, and if they come from the same geographic area or training program, use that information to target that regional group. Sometimes the existing staff can work connections they might have with medical schools or professional organizations. Don't exclude physicians already settled in the area as potential candidates. Consider internationally based physicians, particularly Canadians, many of whom already speak English. And in especially challenging markets, take advantage of U.S. Public Health Service, National Health Service, and Indian Health Service opportunities for loan repayment to physicians who practice in underserved areas.

While "choice communities" and practices may be able to run an advertisement or just talk with the local residents, in hard-to-recruit markets dedicated time must be spent on the phone. Mailings, working with the residency programs, networking are a part of any process. Every position has physicians that will eventually come to the location. The team's role is to find these qualified candidates and attract them to the organization.

Clinch the Deal

Once the team and decision leaders have found the perfect match, the practice may need to offer relocation assistance, volunteer to help the spouse find new employment, or gather information on special needs and school issues for children in order to ink the deal. It is money and time well spent to be sure the organization gets the candidate it needs and wants to further its strategic goals and growth strategies.

Once hired, the internal team needs to continue to be attentive to the new physician through an effective retention strategy.

Retention Planning

The final step in the recruiting process is a strong mentoring program. In fact, retaining a new physician takes just as much energy and time as recruiting one. New people require attention early on to be sure all is well. While many people play a supporting role—from various department members and office staff to medical colleagues and partners—there needs to be one person assigned specifically to help the new hire settle into the job and community. The responsible person can be a physician, administrative leader, or a member of the physician relations staff. It isn't necessary for the mentor to take on all of the orientation items and responsibilities, but,, rather, to make sure someone is following through with each task.

Selecting a mentor is the best way a practice or organization can nurture its long-term investment in human resources.

The most successful retention efforts follow a planned timetable of activities to address all aspects of fitting into the work and community environment. Activities include clinical aspects, the business side of practice development, and the socialization needs of the doctor and his or her family. It is important to have an orientation plan that builds in the hospital and clinic. And listing orientation activities by category—for example, clinical, financial, office routine, social—ensures that all areas are covered.

Scheduled Chats

The mentor should schedule weekly, monthly, and, finally, quarterly conversations to address and resolve any issues that might arise. Mentors should also host and introduce the new hires at key meetings and activities. The mentor should get others from the practice and hospital involved in the orientation process so that the new physician can begin to place names and faces with responsibilities.

It is important to spread out the learning because even the brightest and best human brains can get overwhelmed. The new physician also needs time to explore on his or her own. If the physician approves, the mentor should also check in with his or her spouse to see how things are progressing on the family and home front.

At the end of three months, the mentor should schedule a lunch or office meeting to check in about professional and personal satisfaction. The mentor should ask the doctor candid questions about his or her experience to date: Have orientation activities met the new hire's expectations? and Where does the new hire need additional insights?

After the new hire has passed the 3-month mark and the honeymoon is over, there is still an ongoing need for support and validation. The frequency and nature of the interactions will change—moving from introductory to more integration activities, such as getting the new person involved on hospital committees, or in presenting at continuing medical education (CME) seminars or grand rounds. It is a great show of support if the mentor can attend when the new hire is presenting at any courses.

Customized Program

There is no one perfect format for creating a physician retention plan. The key elements involve developing a budget, timetable, planning tactics, accountability, and a desired outcome. Sound retention practices will safeguard the investment the organization has made to bring the new hire on board. Taking a proactive approach to retention planning ensures that the new hire's needs are addressed before issues become too hot to handle.

Key Elements of Success

Finally, when it is all said and done, there are a few key points to keep in mind to ensure a top-notch and successful recruitment effort:

- Success depends on persuasive selling, an understanding of features versus benefits and a firm hold on all that the opportunity encompasses—from job responsibilities and compensation to community living.
- Community and lifestyle are key to a new hire's happiness and longevity on the job.
- Candidates can slip away when organizations are slow to respond. Moving quickly separates the winners from the losers.
- Everything and anything that pertains to recruiting should revolve as much as possible around the candidate's convenience.
- Be prepared! Written plans, timetables, and budgets for each position are essential.

A sound recruiting strategy requires a full funnel of candidates and a solid approach for internal positioning. The internal team must be persuasive and have a knack for selling. The practice or organization can hire consultants as needed and rely on physicians already on staff to help position the organization for success. An effective physician recruiting effort demands a good opportunity, a market-competitive compensation package, strong internal support, solid organization, and the drive and determination to hire the candidates the practice wants.

SAMPLE: SITE VISIT ITINERARY

8:00–9:30	Medical director meeting

- group mission, vision, values
- practice philosophy and expectations
- desired candidate qualifications

9:30–11:00	Executive director meeting

- group strategic plans, financial position, and organizational structure
- review of sample practice budget
- call coverage schedule
- review of administrative support structure
- review sample contract

11:00–12:00	Practice manager meeting

- scheduling parameters
- medical record systems
- staff organization
- testing procedures
- tour of facility, office site, and staff introductions

12:00–2:00	Lunch with group members
2:00–3:00	Q&A session with medical director and executive director
3:00–5:00	Community tour with realtor
6:00–9:00	Dinner meeting with group leadership and spouses

SAMPLE: PHYSICIAN CANDIDATE EVALUATION

Physician's Name: _____

Interviewed by: _____ Date: _____

Substantiate your comments or impressions in writing, and where possible, include a quotation to support your view.

Please rate from 1–5 (1 being lowest and 5 highest)

Professional Qualifications

_____
_____
_____

Education/Experience

_____
_____
_____

Communication Skills

_____
_____
_____

Ability To Lead a New Group Practice

_____
_____

Ability to Fit into SJH Medical Community

_____
_____

COMMENTS: (Please note any additional impressions about the candidate's qualifications, background and suitability.)

_____
_____

Hiring recommendations:

_____ Would hire.
_____ Would not hire.

Please fax completed form to Allison McCarthy at 508-760-6911.

Thank you for your cooperation and assistance

APPENDIX

List of Physician Recruitment Agencies

- Action Medical Search. Recruitment firm offering physician placement throughout the United States. Includes job-searching strategies.
- Advent Associates, Inc. Provides physician recruitment services across the United States in all medical specialties, with particular expertise in oncology, cardiology, and radiology.
- Agent.MD. Recruiting, consulting, and representation of physicians on all compensation and contract negotiation issues for new health care practice opportunities at hospitals or groups.
- Alliance Physician and Associates. A physician recruiting firm specializing in opportunities in Washington, Oregon, Idaho, and Alaska.

- American Medical Consultants, Inc. Physician recruitment company offering practice opportunities, listed at the site, throughout the United States.
- APC Medical Resources. A recruitment firm offering both locum and permanent placement of physicians. Searchable database of jobs, with call ratio and some details of practice opportunity.
- ApolloMD. A physician staffing firm that focuses on providing quality services to all components of the emergency room—hospitals, physicians, and patients.
- Cornerstone Physician Consulting. A recruitment firm specializing in physician employment and search nationwide.
- Daniel Stern & Associates. A physician recruitment firm specializing in the field of emergency medicine. Conducts and makes available an annual national salary survey for emergency medicine physicians.
- EHL Ecare Health Ltd. A consulting firm offering recruitment, retention, and training for health care facilities.
- Emergency Staffing Solutions. Provides emergency department and emergency physician staffing.
- Enterprise Medical Services. A physician recruiter placing Canadian doctors in the United States. New positions are listed regularly.
- Eva Page and Associates. A recruitment firm that specializes in employment for physicians in the Pacific Northwest and Alaska.
- Farr Health care. Recruiting physicians for jobs nationwide. Searchable database of opportunities at site.
- Geneva Health International. A recruitment and staffing consultancy catering exclusively for the nursing and medical sectors internationally.
- Global Medical Search, Inc. A national physician search firm with its jobs listed in text-based directory.
- Gutermuth Medical Services. A contingency-based physician recruiter for clients who have multiple recruiting needs and a guaranteed-retainer program for need-to-fill searches.
- Hayman Daugherty Associates. Successful permanent placements of physicians with clients all across the United States.
- Health Search USA. A nationwide physician recruitment agency. Search hundreds of employment opportunities in an on-line searchable database. Services include developing plans for retention programs, compensation, and succession.
- Health care Transitions. Physician recruitment firm with searchable database of opportunities and a FAQ section for physicians interviewing for employment.
- The HealthField Alliance, Inc. "We work on both a contingency and a retainer basis, depending upon our clients' needs." Provides assistance and input in critical areas including: compensation, contract interpretation, contract negotiations, income guarantees, and visit/interview plans.
- HealthMatch Services. Physician recruitment firm with listings of current openings.
- J and C Nationwide. A recruitment firm placing physicians in temporary locum tenens jobs and permanent practice.
- Jackson and Harris. Offering permanent search, placement services, and salary survey for physicians.

- K Group Online.com. A physician recruiter showing its list of nationwide job opportunities and applicants.
- Kay Martin Associates. A contingency placement firm exclusively recruiting physicians. Site includes references from clients.
- LAM Associates. Employer-paid physician recruiting agency placing full-time and locum tenens positions in Hawaii and the U.S. mainland.
- Latter Associates. A physician recruiting company with a regional focus. Job search of database allows for customization of results for each applicant.
- Locumotion. Medical recruitment and education services company. Education and career planning service for health professionals for the UK, Australia, New Zealand, and South Africa.
- Marsh Group. Provides physician recruitment services for health care profession opportunities throughout the United States.
- MDR Associates. A national permanent placement physician search firm. Member of The National Association of Physician Recruiters.
- Med2020. Multispecialty physicians' jobs and resources site. Contains positions searchable by specialty and location.
- Medical Placement and Search. A contingency radiology search firm offering references and a searchable database of jobs for applicants.
- Medical Search Consultants. A recruitment firm specializing in the placement of orthopedic surgeons and physicians nationwide. Offering either contingency or retained fees searches.
- Medicorp, Inc. A recruitment firm offering physician recruitment and retention services. A physician compensation survey is available at site.
- Medipro. An American company with offices in Central Europe which provides English-speaking, trained medical staff to hospitals in the United States.
- Medstaff National Medical Staffing, Inc. A physician locum tenens that focuses on physicians who specialize in emergency medicine, pediatrics, obstetrics and gynecology, and primary care.
- MedSuccess. Physician placement services with individual attention given to physicians seeking new employment opportunities. CVs presented, with permission, to client base after complete job opportunity discussion.
- National Physician Associates. Physician recruitment firm based in Arizona specializing in full-time and permanent part-time Physician placement and the sale of medical practices.
- Nephrology Resource Group. Physician recruitment and placement agency focusing on renal physicians.
- NephrologyRecruiters.com. Dedicated nephrology physician placement service. Offers qualified candidates a convenient and confidential job placement resource.
- Office of Celeste Tabriz. A physician consulting firm specializing in helping J-1 and H-1 physicians obtain the waiver positions that they are seeking.
- The O'Kane Group. Physician recruitment and placement specialists for Northwest USA. Includes company background, list of services, and contact information.
- Olesky Associates, Inc. Physician employment recruiters for both permanent and locum positions for all specialties nationwide.

- Physician Employment Advocacy Services. A physician and health care executive recruitment firm.
- Physician Finders. Employment agency for physicians. Directory of job openings at site.
- Physician Recruitment Solutions. Otolaryngology recruiting and placement services on a nationwide basis.
- Physician Solutions, Inc. National locum tenens, permanent placement of physicians and health care professionals.
- Physicianfit.com. Recruitment firm for physician practice opportunities, employment and recruitment.
- PhysicianRecruiting. Physician recruitment firm offering information and opportunity descriptions for employment in numerous fields of medicine.
- Physicians Search. A recruitment firm offering practice opportunities of hospitals, medical groups, and health care systems, plus job search information and tips.
- Pinnacle Health Group. Hundreds of physician opportunities throughout the country. Resources include employment articles at the site and e-mail newsletters for clients and physicians.
- Placement USA. Physician placement and medical staffing. Jobs for medical professionals.
- Radiologix, Inc. Recruiting for radiology, magnetic resonance imaging, computed axial tomography, and positron emission tomography opportunities.
- RDS Medical Recruiting. Specializing in the recruitment of physicians of all medical specialties for permanent placement.
- Rock Medical, Ltd. A physician placement that provides customized employment arrangements between health care facilities and qualified physicians.
- Southeast Physician Search. A physician recruiting service working to build bridges between opportunities and physicians—whether you are a resident, a seasoned practitioner, or a medical facility.
- Southeastern Physician Placement. Provides physicians with position placement opportunities.
- St. John Associates. A national physician placement firm, representing practice opportunities in all specialties, including psychiatry, neurology, orthopedic surgery, urology, neurosurgery, cardiology, and internal medicine subspecialties.
- Team Health. A firm providing hospitalists for physician management and staffing in emergency medicine, radiology, anesthesia, critical care, hospitalist programs, and pediatrics.
- United Search Associates. Physician recruitment firm with searchable database of opportunities.
- Ursula Thomas and Associates. Professional physician search firm offering quality placement services to physicians nation wide. Free service to physician candidate.
- U.S. Physician Resources International Inc. Includes description of the recruiting process, job opportunities listed by specialty, and blind curriculum vitae.

Source: www.pohly.com

APPENDIX 1   Median physician compensation per physician work relative value unit (RVU) by specialty.

Physician Compensation

Specialty	Average	Lowest	Highest
Primary Care			
Family Practice	$147,516	111,894	197,025
Internal Medicine	160,318	117,984	205,096
Pediatrics	149,754	111,113	201,086
Primary Care Surgical			
OB-GYN	238,224	184,045	350,455
Ophthalmology	246,823	161,763	417,000
Otolaryngology	254,978	180,084	392,890
Internal Medicine Specialties			
Endocrinology	160,085	123,984	221,633
Neurology	196,563	130,872	252,765
Hematology/Oncology	269,298	155,475	473,000
Pulmonary	198,956	143,229	280,278
Rheumatology	165,218	119,076	218,113
Nephrology	233,824	161,039	405,142
Gastroenterology	282,133	179,000	381,340
Cardiology	300,500	186,667	434,607
Surgical Specialties			
General Surgery	261,276	175,314	364,279
Cardiovascular Surgery	558,719	351,108	852,717
Colon/Rectal Surgery	291,199	186,000	420,175
Neuro Surgery	438,426	279,655	713,961
Oral & Maxillofacial	208,340	157,404	352,879
Orthopedic Surgery	346,224	237,731	540,524
Plastic Surgery	306,047	196,711	411,500
Urology			
Vascular Surgery			
Miscellaneous Specialties			
Dermatology	232,000	168,988	407,000
Psychiatry	150,610	121,000	189,499
Hospital Based			
Anesthesiology	265,753	219,850	392,960
Radiology	309,361	225,181	429,716
Emergency Medicine	210,830	160,000	250,000

Source: Physician's Search: 2003

CHAPTER 23

The Case for Concierge Medicine

Allison McCarthy

> Concierge medicine just gives the rich the illusion of comfort and good care. Not only do you not necessarily get better outcomes—you can, in fact, get worse outcomes.
>
> —Meri Kolbrener, MD

Steep cuts in Medicare reimbursement rates, skyrocketing premiums for medical liability insurance, and mountains of managed care paperwork have squeezed physicians into a corner. Frustrated because they spend less time with patients and more time with bureaucracy, and exasperated because they work longer hours for less income, some physicians are contemplating leaving the profession altogether. Others are opting for early retirement. And many are considering concierge or premium-service medicine as a new practice model because they believe it allows for improved care coordination, enhanced services, and better prevention strategies.

Concierge medicine (retainer medicine) first emerged in the mid-1990s in Seattle, Washington. For an annual fee, primary care physicians offer patients top-drawer treatment that includes amenities such as same-day and extended appointments, house calls when necessary, enhanced referral coordination that can include accompanying patients who need to see a specialist, and 24-hour access via pager and cell phone. Patients pay annual out-of-pocket fees for the white-glove service, but use traditional health insurance to cover allowable expenses, such as inpatient hospital stays, outpatient diagnostics and care, and basic tests and physician exams. Typical annual fees can range from $875 to $4,000 per patient, to family fees that top $20,000 a year.

Stress and Strain

According to data from the American Association of Medical Colleges, the average physician graduates from medical school $95,000 in debt. Add that pressure to the stark reality that reimbursement rates are shriveling, from managed care organizations to Medicare, which adjusted for inflation in medical practice costs, was 6%

lower in 2001 than it was in 1991. Even as state and federal reimbursement rates plummet, physicians are expected to ratchet up productivity while staying ahead of mounting paperwork that, according to some studies, can count for as much as 36 minutes of nonreimbursable pencil pushing for every hour of care. Increasingly pricey overhead, staff support, and malpractice insurance add to the stress and strain of everyday business. The result is a groundswell of disillusioned physicians, eager to invent a better model of care.

Good-bye Gatekeeper?

There are growing numbers of doctors who are fast losing faith in the notion of physician as gatekeeper, a key tenet of the managed care movement. An internal medicine physician in the Northeast, writing in a letter to the editor, decried the gatekeeper role as having taken over the offices of the nation's primary care doctors, increasing their costs, decreasing their income, and forcing them to spend less time with patients. Drug formulary choices and referral paperwork, not coordination of patient care, said he, have become the major focus in doctor offices today with preventive medicine relegated to an even lesser role.[1]

Principled physicians are discouraged by the pace at which they need to practice medicine in a managed-care environment, agrees a prominent attorney in a large metropolitan area who specializes in health care and in setting up premium-service practice models.

His clients say it is not about the money; but, rather, a desire to provide a more personalized level of care with better patient outcomes. Incentives that require these physicians to see as many people as possible in as short a period of time as possible just do not allow for quality interaction. They want more time with their patients.

It's a common refrain. A national tracking study released recently by the Center for Studying Health System Change found that although doctors spent about two additional hours a week on patient care in 2001 than they did in 1997, a growing number felt they just didn't have enough time with each individual. Physicians are frustrated because, as medical care and treatment become more complex, they feel they have too much to discuss with patients in too little time.[2]

Scarcity of time impacts physicians' satisfaction with their own lifestyle and quality of life issues. Is it any surprise that, like so many others today, they want more leisure and free time to enjoy families and friends?

An Answer for Many

There are those—consumer advocates, insurance regulators and even fellow practitioners—who have voiced concern about premium-service practices, citing issues such as discrimination and exclusivity. But for many doctors, frustrated with their inability to practice medicine as they see fit, this type of practice arrangement is the

---

[1]Pamela Moore, PhD, *Physicians Practice,* January/February 2003.
[2]Sally Trude, "So Much to Do, So Little Time: Physician Capacity Constraints, 1997–2001," tracking report published by the Center for Studying Health System Change.

ticket to improved physician and patient satisfaction. Physicians who have converted to premium-service medicine say they have more time to provide personalized, dedicated care and more time to focus on prevention strategies tailored to meet individual needs.

Which Approach?

Physicians interested in setting up premium-service practice models have several options: franchise, affiliation, or independent ownership. Several national firms specializing in concierge medicine offer franchise arrangements or affiliated relationships. The plus in hooking up with a national firm is a turnkey operation, with guidelines to follow in everything from office set up to marketing initiatives. Physicians benefit from the experience and expertise but incur long-term financial and revenue sharing obligations to the parent organization.

Physicians who go it alone retain their independence and ownership. Outside expertise from experienced attorneys and healthcare consultants can help with practice development, legal and transition issues, office set up, and positioning. These professionals can help physicians make very individualized choices for their premium service practice, based on personal philosophy, local market, and the kind of patient base they currently have.

Seek Legal Counsel

Any physician contemplating a new practice arrangement would be well advised to seek legal counsel. It is imperative that physicians who are setting up their own independent premium-service practices get counsel to minimize or eliminate their risks. It helps to work with an attorney who has had experience in setting up these types of practices because there are a number of legal steps to consider.

Background survey. The first step is to investigate the legal environment. The lawyer needs to review the legal and regulatory lay of the land in the state where the physician wishes to practice to make sure there are no unique impediments to setting up a premium service practice.

Corporate formation. The new practice needs an organizational structure that complies with legal requirements and applicable payer contracts. Generally, this structure is a two-entity model, including both a business and a professional practice entity that, together, have a relationship.

Contract agreements. Next, the attorney must put contracts into place between the practice entity and the business entity to define the relationship from a service and financial perspective. What will one entity pay the other for services, and how will the two organizations allocate costs between them?

In addition, the attorney needs to write a membership agreement for patients who join the business corporation, stipulating that the annual fees paid to that corporation cover a range of amenities, the key features of which are the premium-services the practice offers.

Taxes and accounting. An accountant or tax attorney needs to examine the practice's tax structure to make sure that funds flow within the new corporate system in such a way as to minimize tax to the owners. In addition, the practice must be set up so that cost allocations that are made within the system are supportable.

Payer relations. Ideally, the physician's attorney has experience in negotiating wrap-around agreements with payers, so patients can use their existing health insurance, including Medicare and Medicare managed care, to cover allowable services. The amenities the practice provides as part of its premium-service offerings must wrap-around, in a complementary way, patients' existing health-insurance plans.

As physicians structure premium-service practices, there are a number of additional legal issues they should discuss with their attorneys. Among these are the following:

- Ban on balanced billing, which is the law that prohibits physicians from charging for covered services in excess of the payer's allowable amount for those services. Attorneys must structure agreements to stipulate that physician fees for amenities are distinct and apart from covered services.
- Nondiscrimination provisions, both in law and contract, stipulating that the physicians cannot discriminate against payers' insured members. All members of the practice must be treated the same way in matters pertaining to access, style of practice, substantive medical advice, and payment.
- Corporate practice of medicine issues, which allow that only a professional corporation or physician can engage in the practice of medicine. There must be a clean separation between the professional corporation that provides insurance-covered services and the separate business entity of the practice that provides the range of amenities that are not covered by insurance.

When physicians seek legal counsel they should search for attorneys who are experienced in a variety of subject matters so as to include the health care regulatory environment, the health insurance regulatory environment, and issues pertaining to corporate and tax structuring and accounting.

Setting Annual Fees

Panel size and patient annual fee structure depend on the services offered, the target population served, and the physician's desired revenue projections. Physicians must take into consideration the going rate for other concierge-type practices in the market and position fees and services accordingly. If a competitor's annual patient fees are less, the physician should be sure his or her palate of services offers more.

Generally speaking, patients who are interested in what premium-service practices have to offer are willing to pay for access, personal care, and attention. While many presume that it is only the affluent population that becomes practice members, they are a minority of the patient base, with the majority joining for the added convenience, attention to medical complexities, and preventative focus.

Surveys among the physician's patient population can help test the service complement against the pricing. What services are patients willing to pay for? Then, armed with information, physicians can tailor their service smorgasbord to meet patient expectations.

Many service components, such as same-day appointments and 24-hour access, are standard fare, while others—like visits to specialists or making house calls—are variable luxuries. Physicians should choose services for their particular patient population.

Catering to Patients

Physicians and office staff transitioning to premium-service practices need to place significant emphasis on customer service and patient relations. Patients expect, and are paying for, a higher level of customer service and a real personal relationship from doctor and staff. Often, staff will benefit from special programming in customer service training and orientation. Some physicians may consider paying top-notch staff two to three times above the going market rate because retaining quality staff is a critical component for practice success. Patients appreciate staff continuity and the opportunity to form long-lasting attachments, which enhance patient happiness and overall satisfaction.

While the entire support staff needs to be oriented to the new practice model, only a few office staff—those skilled in managing telephone sales—should talk with interested callers and handle follow-up conversations. This transition period is often confusing; it will be best for office staff to be well coached, even scripted, to make sure these telephone conversations provide clarity and offer sensitivity.

Investing in Technology

Along with staff training, there are a host of operational issues involved when transitioning to a premium-service practice model. Technology is an especially valuable tool. The practice may need to purchase new telephone and computer systems and arrange for Internet access if it is not already available. Initially, the office will need a preliminary tracking system to follow who is staying with the practice, which patients are moving, when and where to forward their medical record, and which patients have paid the membership fee. As the practice grows, contact management software is a key investment to keep track of everyday patient activity, with reminder prompts for physicians and staff to call before and after specialty appointments or tests in order to talk to patients about their results and any care needs.

The office may also want to consider an Internet-based billing and bookkeeping system and an electronic medical record (EMR). Patients can view the EMR online, as can physicians in other parts of the country, if the patient is traveling and needs care.

Many of these premium-service practices promote email communication for quick and easy access to physicians and staff. Patients can email their physician and schedule appointments and prescription refills on-line. Providing easy and expanded access is one of the hallmarks for these types of practices. Patients will need to feel the difference between old and new practices and be well satisfied with the service enhancements.

Physicians may choose to invest in office renovations of an existing practice site or relocate to a new office setting. It all depends on the target market for the practice, the image it is cultivating, and how eager physicians are to reach out to the upwardly mobile young professional, successful baby boomer, the affluent retiree, or those who live more modestly but are willing to make an investment in a premium-care arrangement. If the physician chooses to retain the current practice site, it will be important to communicate a definitive start for the new practice and the service and environment differences must be easily recognized by the patient—the sense of added value must be conveyed.

Access and Communication

The service elements considered most critical to patients in premium-service practices are increased access and communication with physicians and how thoroughly doctors and staff manage their medical care. Same-day or next-day extended appointments are the rule, not the exception. Annual physical exams are more comprehensive than in traditional medical practices. In addition to the general examination, physicians typically spend one full hour with the patient and conduct tests and procedures during the annual exam that are not routinely offered by traditional practices such as chest x rays, EKGs, and lab workups.

Further, follow-up appointments for specific problems are available within 24 hours of the patient's request, and the physician will spend a good 30 minutes with that patient. It is crucial to reinforce the service elements of the practice: The patient is paying a premium for access and time.

Other perks that premium-service practices may offer include the following:

- Helping patients research the best facility for tertiary care, nationally and internationally, and then making all necessary appointment arrangements.
- Offering patients special after-hours access via telephone, cell phone, or pager number to easily reach a personal medical assistant or physician.
- Making Web site, e-mail, and dedicated fax line available to patients.
- Providing medical information and advice via Web site and telephone and creating on-line access to medical records, tests, and appointment scheduling.
- Escorting patients immediately upon arrival into consult or exam rooms, without having to wait.
- Scheduling appointments with specialists and providing patients with reminder calls for those specialist appointments.
- Generating more in-depth letters to provide information to specialists prior to the patient's specialty consult appointment.
- Arranging for physicians to accompany patients to their specialty appointments if desired.
- Making house calls as needed.
- Closely following patients to guide them through their specialty care or to monitor inpatient treatment and plan of care.
- Calling the patient to explain test results and treatment options following the specialty visit.
- Calling new prescriptions into the patient's pharmacy during the office visit.
- Handling prescription refills and arranging delivery via mail or directly home.
- Safeguarding confidentiality and security by granting office access only to those patients who are practice members.

- Offering yearly consultations with a physician-recommended physical fitness trainer, chiropractor and/or nutritionist.
- Developing personalized preventive care plans to help patients minimize their risk for certain chronic diseases by using innovative diagnostic techniques, when appropriate, such as DNA/gene testing, and offering antiaging programs and herbal remedies

Premium-service practices are all about providing personalized, attentive service. With this level of detail, physicians really get to know their patients. They are available to see them more often and more quickly, which helps cut down on trips to the emergency room. And they go out of their way to make a connection.

In an office hallway in Florida, a physician in a premium-service practice happened to bump into one of his patients outside an exam room. They stood in the hall and talked for 10 minutes; the physician asked about the patient's health and inquired after her husband and his health. Afterwards, he confided that he never would have been able to converse with her like that in his old practice setting because of time constraints. "I would have avoided patients in the hallway so they wouldn't stop me," he admitted.

There is no evidence yet, but physicians practicing in these new arrangements often admit they believe medical outcomes will be improved. Others, like Meri Kolbrener, MD, of Washington, DC, strongly disagree. The more traditional practice places an emphasis on episodic treatment while there is time and a strong relationship to focus on prevention and care for the whole person in the new practice model.

Spread the Word

Success won't happen without a marketing plan. Physicians must develop a marketing strategy using the existing patient population as the first target. Not surprisingly, the majority of premium service practices are built from the preexisting patient panel.

When it comes to transitioning, the most successful physicians are those with a full panel made up of a cadre of patients who have, through the years, formed lasting attachments to office physicians and staff.

And while the new practice needs to count on old loyalties, it is important to create a new image for the practice, including name and logo identity, to demonstrate the high customer service orientation the new practice will feature.

Once the practice identity is in place, a letter to patients needs to go out explaining the basics of the new service. It helps to develop collateral materials to describe the service offerings in greater detail for those patients who express serious interest. Other marketing ideas include an informational night, where interested patients can come and meet the physician and tour the office. Radio and cable television spots, advertisements in local newspapers and direct mail campaigns can inform the public. Some physicians are comfortable doing community lectures. Others feel word of mouth is the most effective marketing vehicle to steer new patients into the practice.

Marketing is an important and ongoing effort. The concept of paying a premium for greater service and access to one's physician is still in the early stages. Many patients will not be familiar with will have some resistance to change. How the new practice description is made and processed can really make a difference for that patient. Some patients will only be testing in the first year seeking proof that there is value in the new practice that is equal to their additional expenditure. And because 10% of the patients, on average, fall out every year due to personal relocations, transitions to long-term care settings, finances, or because they feel they don't have enough health issues to warrant this specialized treatment, physicians must continually market to retain and replenish their patient panel.

As a courtesy, it is important for physicians to write an explanatory letter to colleagues and to the hospital where they admit patients. Physicians can also hold meetings with medical colleagues and hospital leaders to educate them about the practice model and work with them to develop effective access points for their patients. Hospitals tend to accommodate these patients, as they can typically become their donors. Some hospitals even refer large donors to premium-service practices for extra-special coddling and care. Also, during the practice's transition, physicians should consider sending a letter expressing their expectations and a description of their new practice model to local specialists.

Timetable for Launch

It generally takes from 3 to 6 months to launch the new practice arrangement. Physicians need to be financially prepared for a decline in one patient base while the new patient base is slowly increasing. A full panel could take as long as 12 months to 2 years. In the meantime, because of upfront start-up expenses, it may take several years before the practice realizes a solid return on investment.

The financial investment and length of time needed to transition into these practices depends on the degree of change made from the traditional medical practice. Change factors include accepting third-party reimbursement, redesign of the office structure, and redesign of the pricing structure of the program.

Obviously, physicians would do well to invest significant thought and planning into the transition phase. The practice must do everything it can to diminish any fear and anger that people might have over this transition. As a local, and more often than not, longstanding fixture in the community, practices cannot leave patients who decline or are financially unable to join hanging in the wind. Physicians and staff must work together to find a care arrangement for each individual.

Outside consultants can help manage patient placement and other transition and start-up issues. Sometimes, consultants are called in to help the physician decide if a premium-service practice will be successful in his or her particular market area. Here is where surveys can be extremely valuable. Following a carefully scripted questionnaire, experienced market researchers can call patients in the practice to test pricing and "trigger" service points. Questions explore the kinds of services that are important to patients and ask them directly whether they would be willing to pay out of pocket for personalized care and, if so, how much and for what type of services.

Key Decisions

The key decisions physicians need to make when proceeding into a premium service practice include the following:

- Target population—based on age, gender, clinical focus, and target geographic areas
- Service offerings—while many service components are standard, others like house calls, specialty visit participation, and office ambience, are variable.
- Fee structure and panel size—depends on the physicians' target income level, the number of patients to be served, and the services the practice offers.
- Legal considerations—take steps to minimize and eliminate risks and draw up contractual agreements.
- Health plan participation—will the practice continue to be a preferred provider or disenroll provider participation in health plans?
- Approach to take—franchise/affiliate with a current premium-service plan, or remain independent? While membership in a current practice offers the advantage of experience and expertise, it does require a long-term sharing of revenues. If physicians choose independence, then they must also decide on whether to use outside consultants for transition assistance.
- Annual fees—determine pricing based on the desired number of patients in the panel. That patient number can range from 100 individuals to upwards of 600 people.
- Operational issues—review the need for operational changes, from staffing and informational systems to billing procedures.
- Marketing—promote services with launch information and ongoing public relations.

CONCLUSION

Physicians who have made the transition to premium service practices find the experience extremely rewarding. This model of care not only enhances physicians' lifestyles by reducing time commitments within the practice, but it also improves their professional satisfaction with more focused time and attention on fewer patients. Proponents argue that it is a viable system that allows for effective coordination of care by caring and conscientious physicians. For these physicians, the opportunity to practice unhurried medicine as they see fit is priceless.

CHAPTER 24

Customer (Patient) Relations Management for Health Care Organizations and Physicians

DeeVee Devarakonda

> When people call upon health issues, it's not the same thing as ordering a shirt from Lands End, or putting money in an account at Morgan Stanley. It's their health, or the health of somebody dear to them. So there's an emotional aspect to this industry that most industries don't have.
>
> —Jeff Wilson
> Deloitte Consulting

Sophistication, competition, scrutiny, Internet-age companies, and technologies have all raised the bar on patient expectations. Patients that have tasted the level of information and customer service from Amazon.com, or webmd.com, now demand and expect similar services and information from their health care organizations. However, traditional brick- and-mortar health systems have vastly different marketing and technology infrastructure.

WHAT IS CUSTOMER (PATIENT) RELATIONSHIP MANAGEMENT (CRM)?

In the health care industry context, a patient's (the patient is often referred to as a "customer") relationship with physicians (referred to as business or practice) has increased in complexity. Today, health care organizations are expected to reach out to patients, wherever they are, with the right personalized offers, whenever the patients want them and however they want them. Despite this dynamic economic environment, health care providers—both established and young—are expected to be conducting their transactions and providing service in the Internet age while continuously building loyalty by providing impeccable experiences for the patient.

Building these impeccable patient experiences requires listening to patients closely and understanding their needs so as to provide products and services tailored to these needs. This requires patient data collection and building and executing programs around the patient insights.

Health care organizations are being challenged more than ever. The reasons stem from

- *Dynamic economic climate.* Economic downturn, rising health care costs, and fierce competition are forcing health care organizations to look closely at their patient assets and forcing both consumers and care providers to look at technologies such as internet. According to HCFA (Health Care Financing Administration), U.S. health expenditures will rise from $1.2 trillion in 1999 to $2.1 trillion in 2004–2005 (estimated).
- *Role of technology.* eBusiness, CRM, remote sensing, and related health care technologies are propelling health care organizations to reengineer the entire value chain for more efficient and profitable operations. According to Forrester, a leading research and advisory group, the health care industry will reach $370 billion in online transactions in 2004. Consumer adoption will drive online sales to $22 billion, but business trade will quickly outstrip consumer spending, reaching $348 billion. By 2005, consumers, providers, insurers, and medical suppliers will come together to form a health care eBusiness network (Figure 24.1).
- *More regulatory scrutiny.* Consumers are very concerned about privacy of the data that resides with health care organizations, and regulatory bodies are watching marketing practices closely. There are more than 35 privacy bills pending on the floor to protect consumer privacy.
- *Health Insurance Portability and Accountability Act of 1996 (HIPAA).* HIPAA mandates regulations that govern privacy, security, and electronic transactions standards for health care information. HIPAA compliance enables health care

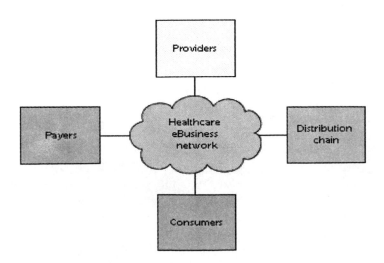

FIGURE 24.1   Health care eBusiness network.

Source: Forrester Research, Inc.

organizations to better manage the way they collect, process, and use patient data to strategize and execute their marketing programs. HIPAA gives patients greater access to their medical records and more control over how their personal health information is used.

- *Lack of know-how.* Lack of know-how, breadth of technical and domain expertise to implement viable technology-enabled patient programs at price points that work for health care organization is yet another concern.
- *Expensive upfront investments.* Investing in enterprise-level patient relationship infrastructure upfront without adequate visibility into the returns is even more challenging today given the economic climate and perception of marketing within corporations as cost centers rather than investments.

CRM can help health care organizations achieve their business objectives while addressing the above-mentioned challenges. In the last few years, CRM came to mean different things to different people. CRM has become a general buzzword, which often came to mean an expensive initiative that costs millions with not so great to nonexistent results. Not true. Due to various reasons including lack of clarity around business, consumer vision, inadequate requirements gathering, inappropriate software, vendor selections, and messy and expensive implementations, CRM acquired the negative image, which need not have been the case.

CRM is a business philosophy; a mind set that health care organizations need to cultivate to design, develop, and operate health care organizations around patients in away that is mutually beneficial. This is the mindset needed for health care organizations today. This is true for a two-employee privately held health care practice or a mega corporation spanning several continents with multiple product lines. CRM allows you to

- develop a single and consistent view of your patient,
- find and keep your best patients,
- improve patient satisfaction and retention,
- gain competitive advantage,
- develop long lasting and profitable relationships with your patients,
- improve sales and marketing effectiveness, and
- improve your downstream business operations.

CRM efficiently helps health care organizations differentiate themselves from their competitors through superior patient relationships and streamlined business operations with all stakeholders—patients, suppliers, and partners.

The twenty-first century began with an uncertain economic environment and an uncertain geopolitical climate in which new political ideologies and destinies are being shaped. Bioterrorism scares and emerging sociopolitical equations are impacting health care organizations and consumers worldwide and the way people choose to communicate with each other. In general, the environment is one of distrust and suspicion. Governments across the globe are debating security versus privacy issues, which are affecting both businesses and consumers and the way they transact and communicate with each other. Scares similar to the Anthrax contaminations of October 2001, SARS in 2002, and the energy grid meltdown of August 2003 are not only disrupting normal communications and the way of life that people were accustomed to but will have implications for health care organizations and how they communicate with their patients. This opens up new avenues for electronic communications such as e-mail and the Internet (Figure 24.2).

In this environment, it is imperative for businesses, especially young health care organizations and physicians who are not yet established brands, to develop patient trust systematically. CRM helps health care organizations do exactly that. Remember, your best patients are also the ideal constituents for your competitors. To survive and flourish, health care organizations need to provide not only an impeccable product and service but also need to lock patients into their business, making it difficult for them to switch over to competitors. Impeccable brand experience and CRM are the keys to achieving this goal.

CRM elevates the patient relationship away from the one transaction mode and makes health care organizations realize the lifetime value of a patient. Small and medium health care organizations are very well positioned to implement CRM philosophy and concepts. Young health care organizations already practice these concepts in their daily business to some extent in one form or the other, and these organizations have less corporate bureaucracy and less complexity in delivering cross-functional, cross-team CRM.

What kind of company, practice or industry needs CRM the most? Simple: any company that has customers and aims to provide products and services at a profit needs a CRM vision, strategy, and roadmap. CRM is the way health care organizations should bring people, processes, and technology to develop long-lasting and profitable relationships with their patients and other stakeholders. No more, no less. In order to achieve these objectives, health care organizations need:

- a team that is committed to the same business and patient vision,
- simple business processes that are responsive to changing patient needs,

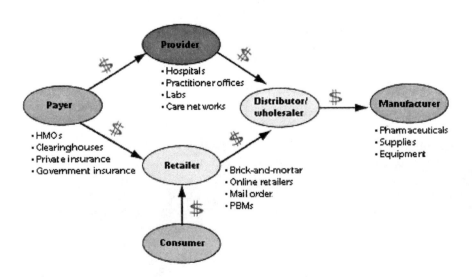

FIGURE 24.2   How health dollars flow online.

Source: Forrester Research, Inc.

- patient 360-degree view or at least a "good enough" patient view,
- real time patient information and insights, and
- a consistent communications strategy and execution across multiple channels.

While implementing CRM, it is essential to remember CRM is more than technology. CRM is a philosophy that needs to be embraced by the health care employees who are committed to deliver the organization's promises to the patient while being guided by clear business objectives, with supporting processes and technology. CRM possesses technical, organizational and strategic challenges for businesses.

Technological needs. As for CRM technology, there is no perfect silver bullet. In addition, young health care organizations and physicians often do not have the resources—money, professional talent, infrastructure, domain expertise or the process maturity—to make heavy upfront technology investments or implement them at the pace that business needs dictate.

Organizational needs. CRM initiative is cross-functional in nature. It involves employees from various groups and departments and is often fertile ground for corporate dynamics and turf battles. One of the great advantages young health care organizations have is relatively less hierarchical organizational structure, with several degrees of freedom and ability to implement ideas at fast pace. CRM demands processes with clearly defined roles that various constituents can play to serve patients. The phrase "processes clear roles" may sound at odds with young-company culture. However, that need not be the case. CRM can help streamline business processes, greatly reduce the drudgery of work for employees, and help employees take up value-added and more stimulating tasks. In any case, CRM is no longer an option but is the cost of doing business.

Strategic needs. Young health care organizations often need to change their directions to go with the flow, be flexible to sustain and survive and grow their business. Small health care organizations are proficient at quickly and nimbly reacting to the business needs or their most valuable patient needs. Therefore having a rigid CRM roadmap that takes years to complete and implement does not work for them. Hence CRM strategy needs to be in accordance with business strategy and has to have room for mid course corrections, to allow 180-degree change in business directions as business realities dictate.

Circle of CRM—Key Phases

There are three phases at the core of a CRM infrastructure to facilitate meaningful, personalized, and profitable patient relationships and help the company to be a closed-loop of learning within a medical organization.

1. Data to Information:
The Foundation for Personalized Patient Relationships

Clean, correct and intelligent data is the lifeblood of any CRM initiative. Success of a patient insight-driven organization depends on how data can be converted to information, information into insight, insight to action, and action into closed-loop marketing. The first critical step for any CRM initiative is to build an effective and robust patient data mart. You want to build initial data marts to house the clean data on your most profitable or valuable patients.

Unless health care organizations have a clean-data infrastructure that this campaign management software can use, it will not be possible for them to personalize communications with patients in a meaningful and profitable way. If communications are not personalized, they risk not only massive missed-opportunity costs, but also wastage and time-to-value—not to mention faulty patient experiences. A personalized data warehouse that converts data into information is required for health care organizations to make better-informed decisions and effectively manage patient relationships. The goal of your decision support system and data warehouse is to provide an easy, quick look at historical patient data. On this journey to convert data into information, ask yourself the following questions:

- *How far back do I want to look into the practice?* You may want to look at weeks of data for your patients or years of data for a handful of high-net-worth patients
- *Who owns the data?* Many health care organizations today are grouped around products. Chances are that patient data is duplicated across the business, which can create territorial divisions within the company. An advantage of young health care organizations is that you don't have the historical baggage and you can start from a clean slate.
- *What is our privacy policy and strategy?* It is imperative for health care organizations to be proactive and self-regulate with a coherent privacy policy and design their systems to comply with this strategy. This will affect the way you manage your HIPAA compliance.
- *Do I need a 360-degree patient view or a "good enough view"?* A patient 360-degree view is a marketing mantra today, but how doable is this? It's more challenging than you think! Health care organizations must wade through technical, organizational, and business challenges before they can accomplish this.
- *How can I get my groups to share data so my enterprise can speak with a single voice?* While CRM is the Holy Grail at a 50,000 ft level, when it is time to discuss the grassroot-level details, territorial conflicts invariably surface and hinder groups from sharing data. Executive sponsorship and reinforcement of a common vision from senior management becomes a critical ingredient. While young health care organizations may face this issue on a smaller scale than large business conglomerates, it is still critical to enforce a common CRM vision across rank and file.

The complexity of building a data warehouse depends on how many data sources you have, on what kind of systems your data resides, and so on. For building effective and successful patient data marts, an incremental approach works much better than a big-bang approach, wherein a company divides the project into ambitious multimillion dollar, multiyear phases. An incremental approach helps health care organizations to build data marts, mine them, and then execute programs based on the insights. Organizations can then analyze the successes, gain internal support, get additional resources, slowly expand the scope, and build on the previous successes in an iterative manner.

Steps Involved in Building a Data Warehouse

According to a Standish Group survey, more than 70% of IT applications go over budget and time—data warehouse applications are no exception; however, if you adopt a process, an oriented development approach, and implement a rigorous project management discipline, you increase the likelihood that your CRM data warehouse will be effective. The following is a simplified list, but it reveals some of the key steps needed to build a data warehouse:

1. Extracting data from the data sources. This can be very challenging, as data might reside on different systems, and this forces you to prioritize what data you want and what role that plays in your CRM decision-making. This step involves moving data from the source (e.g., to your Web site) to a central location (e.g., to your marketing data mart).
2. Transforming the data. This is the key activity after data extraction. It is critical to have clean data and involves modification, enhancement, or elimination of data based on the job instructions.
3. Loading the transformed data into a dimensional database.
4. Building reports for decision makers. This could consist of a report for your marketing management outlining the analysis of your latest patient acquisition campaign.

The first three steps: Effective data processes that (1) extract, (2) transform, and (3) load (ETL) represent the number one success factor for your data warehouse project and can absorb up to 70% of the time spent on a typical warehousing project.

Add data incrementally. Even in a small practice with few employees, you will be amazed to know how fragmented data can be and in how many data islands it resides—medical charts, op reports, patient brochures, e-mail contact lists, address books, spreadsheets, and so on. It can be an overwhelming task to gather all this information in a central electronic repository. It is best if you take an incremental approach to integrate the patient data available in electronic format and then proceed to more manual and laborious components such as business cards and paper lists. Health care organizations may house patient data in central repositories, thereby providing the enterprise with a memory, but it is data mining that adds intelligence to the enterprise. To convert information into insight through data mining, ask yourself the following questions:

- *How good is my data?* A health care provider who sends the company brochure to its long-standing patients asking them to sign up for its services certainly needs to ask itself this question.
- *Is the application of models to new data appropriate?* When you "model" data using data-mining techniques to obtain patient insights, beware that the data you model could be different from the data you are going to apply this model to.
- *How long can you use your model?* The ability of a model to classify, estimate, and predict diminishes over time. Therefore, your models need to be maintained and enhanced, which requires ongoing maintenance.
- *How long does the prediction stemming from data mining remain viable?*

- *How do I interpret the results?* This can be a source of unexpected challenges. It is a that task requires experts who not only understand and interpret the results for you and what they mean to you but who can be objective and consistent
- *What is our privacy policy and strategy?* It is imperative for health care organizations to be proactive and self-regulate with a coherent privacy policy and design their systems to comply with this strategy. This will affect the way you manage, mine, and communicate data.
- *What tools should I use?* There are several data mining techniques available today, decision trees, on-line analytical processing (OLAP) queries, neural networks, and so on, but no one technique solves all business problems. Commercial software may be linked to particular data-mining technique(s). So you need to decide: what works best for your technical/business environment. Is an integration effort required? If the answer is "Yes," how much will it cost? How user friendly are the tools? How much should you invest in training?

Where Do You Begin?

There are several decisions that you need to make while mining the data. You can do this in-house and control the complete process if you have the expertise, or you can outsource the activities that are not to your strategic advantage. Both options have pros and cons. In today's economic climate, health care organizations are also increasingly looking at outsourcing options to minimize upfront technology investments and also for leveraging quick ramp-up and ramp-down of operations. If you decide to do this in-house, ensure the software you select is scalable, supports your current IT investments, and is likely to be compatible with emerging technologies. Also, make sure you understand the product you are purchasing and how it mines the data.

2. Insight to Action: Building Meaningful Campaigns

Success of a knowledge-driven organization depends on not only how data can be converted into information and then how this information can be converted into insight. Those insights have to be put into action by building meaningful campaigns.

Campaign Management. This is the process of designing, executing, and measuring marketing campaigns through the use of applications that help you to

a. select and segment patients,
b. design campaigns and execute the campaigns to contact patients,
c. track the contacts made with patients,
d. measure the results of those contacts, and
e. learn from these results to more efficiently target patients in the future.

Some key questions to ask while you build campaigns:

- Do you have a CRM roadmap that fits in with your overall patient vision and strategies, and does it outline the course of action for campaign management?
- What is your privacy policy and strategy? It is imperative for health care organizations to be proactive and self-regulate with a coherent privacy policy; they must

design their systems to comply with this strategy. This may affect the way you design and execute campaigns.

- What tools should you use? There are several campaign management tools available today, but no one tool can solve all business problems. You need to decide, What works best for you technical/business environment? Is any integration effort required? If the answer is "Yes," Then you need to ask, How much will it cost? How user-friendly are the tools? How much should you invest in training?

Critical components of campaign management include the following activities:

- *Patient Segmentation.* The process of identifying groups of patients for better targeting marketing and communications efforts.

  Segmentation is critical for effective and intelligent one on one communications with your patient. Some issues around segmentation are the following:

  1. Ensure your data quality is excellent, which can give you meaningful segmentation.
  2. Consistency of treatments and processes are of paramount importance.
  3. Buying a software tool is not enough for effective segmentation. You also need to understand what the software tool does in the back end. Watch out for anomalies, and take steps to make reparations.
  4. Make sure you administer the initiative to a small sample and that the business rules are in place before you roll out your campaign to the larger group.

- *Personalization.* Ability to customize your product/service to each patient:

  1. Good personalization is possible, especially when you have a good patient history.
  2. You also need to have all business rules in place for effective personalization.
  3. Ensure your patient data is of high quality (e.g., addressing a female patient as Mr. or sending mail asking a patient to sign up for your service to a person who is already your patient can defeat the purpose of personalization).
  4. If you model data before personalization, you can target more effectively and personalize it.
  5. It pays to have a clear privacy policy and to ensure that your personalization philosophies are in tune with that policy.

- *Execution.* Actual implementation of your marketing programs and messages.

  1. Before you execute, ensure that you are equipped to fulfill promises you are making in the campaigns (e.g., If you are printing a toll-free phone number in your direct-mail piece for your patients to use, that toll free telephone number should work)
  2. Make sure your sales and service channels are aware of the campaigns, and publish a general calendar for the whole company
  3. Develop business rules and strategies for follow-up campaigns

What Campaign-Management Software Is Not?

Campaign-management tools are comprised of any software that attempts to address the complete automation of marketing-campaign processes. Excluded from this definition are project-management and workflow-management applications that do not actually automate campaign management; sales force automation; patient service and call center support tools; data mining and modeling; content management; and basic e-mail delivery tools that are not fully integrated into a campaign-management solution.

3. Close Loop Marketing: Building a Learning Organization

In order to reap the true benefits of CRM, it is imperative for health care organizations to collect, measure, analyze, report, and learn from the results of various patient acquisition and patient retention campaigns they undertake so that they can continuously improve their CRM effectiveness and success rates.

- *Response measurement.* Ability to track a patient's response to the message delivered to him/her—measures the return on investment (ROI).

    1. Consistent reporting is key to gauge effectiveness of your campaign.
    2. Compare how your campaign is faring with past promotions to continuously improve.
    3. Develop new ways to capture data, actionable recommendations.
    4. Encrypt patient ID to parse the data and analyze.

- *Reporting.* Ability to report the campaigns and the results to various constituents within the organization in customized way. This is an excellent way to continuously improve CRM effectiveness, gain champions. and boost the morale to continue to embrace CRM.

    1. Establish the goals and continuously monitor the effectiveness of campaigns so you can improve.
    2. You may also want to have clear vision of the campaign expectations from all stakeholders from the outset. This can help develop your reports.

- *Promotion history.* Ability to view the components and results of past campaigns so critical for patient 360-degree view. This is often an overlooked area in most businesses. It is important to document the results of all the campaigns and programs a business conducts to continuously refine patient insights.

    - Central repository of data is extremely useful.
    - Match inbound/outbound communication by patient IDs.
    - Too many people tracking/people leaving the organization can be detrimental to maintaining the patient history. Make sure you have processes in place to protect you against that business reality.

Measure the responses and calculate the cost per contact/ROI over a period, collect data points to monitor how the patients are responding and how it is adding to the bottom line and communicate across the company to continue to build support for CRM. If you execute a campaign that does not yield expected results, it is more important to analyze and learn from the campaign than sweep the results of the campaign under the proverbial carpet. In order for CRM champions to do this, the organization culture has to be one that is supportive rather than one that indulges in blame games and corporate politics.

TO CRM OR NOT TO CRM?

Young health care organizations are often strapped for lack of resources, and do not have established brand equity enjoyed by large health care organizations. Physicians who set up their practice often work with unstructured processes, fledgling infrastructure, and immature processes. They do not have the luxury of time to achieve success by trial and error. Today they also stand in danger of an uncertain future, as the economic vagaries don't spare even large health care organizations from going bankrupt. Therefore, CRM is critical for young health care organizations to help them build and cultivate a loyal patient base that contributes to a steady and increasing revenue stream and helps them survive and thrive even in adverse business climates.

Some small or medium size health care organizations are family owned or controlled by a limited number of stockholders. Some entrepreneurs may be interested in limited growth objectives, while others may be interested in growing business at a different pace. For entrepreneurs with very limited growth objectives, patient retention could be more important than patient acquisition, while for some, patient acquisition may be as critical as patient retention.

CRM is a powerful tool to enrich patient retention and patient acquisition for new products and new services. To develop appropriate patient retention programs, it is critical to understand the patient data and the context of patients' interactions with the company and then develop personalized programs for each patient and communicate that the company values them. CRM can help young health care organizations use their resources productively. CRM is no longer an enterprise-only product or concept. Small- and medium-sized health care organizations are ready to adopt CRM concepts and technology that delivers—not the type of technology that requires armies of consultants and years to implement. Small health care organizations need CRM without bells or whistles and a CRM solution that is suited to their needs.

CRM can help young health care organizations acquire and keep the patients as they grow their business in a profitable manner. You can start CRM with very little investment. It can be suited to your needs and easy on your resources.

- *Find your best and most valuable patients.* Use the data you have of your patients and find out who your most valuable and profitable patients are. You must try to keep your best patients with you at all times—remember they are also the patients your competitors may covet.

- *Profile your best patients/understand them.* Understand what makes your very best patients different from your other patients. Then acquire other patients who look like your top patients by using messages/offers that worked for your best patients. Armed with this insight, start the dialog with them and learn with every interaction. Personalize and continue to build on your CRM successes. Amazon.com effectively uses well thought out personalization strategies and supporting technologies to provide Amazon browsers with a wealth of information and recommendations based on similar behavior of other buyers.
- *A two way street.* Any relationship is built on two-way conversations. Building relationship with your patients is no exception. The first step is to listen to your patient. Do you remember what they bought and returned at the Web site, in person, with your sales team, or on the phone? Are you aware of their behavior on the Web site? Do you listen to their complaints in the call center and read their responses to e-mails, then link them all so that when they contact the company next, you can communicate with them meaningfully? Do you ask them questions and remember the answers? Personalization is all about using this information to position your next conversation with the patient. Plan how you will use this to make the experience more relevant to your patients; cross sell, up sell—make your patients so satisfied and happy that they will come back to you again and spend more.

Internet has taught patients to expect the information, products, and services you put in front of them to be relevant and, in general, the Internet has raised the bar on patient expectations. Small health care organizations cannot afford to be forgotten/neglected by the patients, prospects, or suppliers. To constantly remind them and meaningfully interact with them, health care organizations need organizational memory and the ability to deliver personalized services.

1) Interacting and transacting with you should be a low risk for patients.
2) You cannot afford to slip up on your promises. If you have a privacy policy, never ever break it.
3) What differentiates your service or product from others? Patient interaction and service can be a big difference.
4) Don't get carried away by the great technology you bought and implemented or the cool product or service you have. Always ask yourself, Why should patients bother with my messages? What is in it for them?
5) Electronic media are very valuable and cost effective for you. Focus on them. Make your Web site easy to navigate and personalize. Provide valuable content, and have features to obtain patients' permission for future communications.

Young health care organizations have relatively less bureaucracy and less history. They have few hierarchies. This gives young health care organizations quite an advantage to sculpt the company processes and mind set around patients at an early stage to let the company grow along these lines. CRM concepts and technology can support health care organizations in this endeavor.

CRM benefits for health care organizations are as follows:

- CRM helps you understand patients and enables you to offer them the right products at the right time through the right channels. This improves the patient response rates, which directly translates into top-line revenue.

- CRM helps you build great brand experiences with your patients and helps develop long lasting relationships—this is critical for growing health care organizations.
- CRM helps you target your resources more effectively, thereby improving your revenue and employee productivity.
- CRM helps cut costs and improve profit margins by minimizing waste.

Chances are that health care organizations are already implementing CRM at some level. To fully reap the benefits of CRM and have a multiplier effect on your patient profitability, it is critical to adopt a ROI approach of CRM initiatives.

RETURN ON INVESTMENT FOR CRM INITIATIVES

Gone are the days when marketing could go to the board and ask for millions to "build the brand" and for related warm fuzzy reasons. Health care organizations today cannot afford to spend money on programs that do not show returns on investment. Today's business climate is especially harsh for functions and programs in a company that cannot present a clear ROI for their existence. Marketing as a function and patient retention and acquisition programs are especially vulnerable in this climate unless the marketing and especially CRM initiatives are supported with a sound ROI argument.

A very basic challenge for young business is not only pooling the resources but also allocating resources wisely, and ROI arguments help young health care organizations make those choices. Typically marketing budget and outlay decisions focus on operating expenses like public relations, advertising, trades shows, and direct mailing. However, CRM can involve capital investment decisions. To be successful, marketing/CRM practitioners should learn to speak the language of business and build ROI analysis to support CRM initiatives.

How Do You Calculate the ROI for Your CRM Initiatives?

1. Detail the CRM costs:

   - hardware—computers, servers, accessories
   - software—database, campaign management software
   - implementation costs of hardware and/or software
   - internal resource costs associated with the deployment of the capital improvement
   - upfront investments in call centers, staff, equipment, and so on

2. Estimate the revenue impacts:

   - increase in patient response rates
   - increase in patient conversion rates
   - increase cross-sell ratio
   - decreased account attrition rates
   - increase in fees
   - increase in average spend per account
   - increase in average number of transactions

Health care organizations can use past experiences to guesstimate the revenue impact. Firms with limited CRM experience can use public information and expert's knowledge to estimate the revenue impacts.

Once you calculate the revenue and cost impacts, you need to calculate the net present value (NPV) of your CRM initiative. For a CRM initiative (or any other project), if the NPV is greater than zero, that means your project/CRM initiative will make money for you; if it is less than zero, that means it will not (you typically need a compelling business reason to implement a project with an NPV less than zero).

NPV calculations include:

1. Investment—money you expend for the initiative at the beginning.
2. Revenues that you accrue as a result of the initiative over a period—can be one time or a recurring revenue.
3. Costs that you accrue as a result of the initiative over a period—can be one time or a recurring item
4. Discount rate—your accountant or Finance department can give this rate.
5. Time Period—define the time period for which you would like to compute the NPV.

NPV is the cumulative differential between the revenue and cost stream discounted at the discounted rate minus the investment.

$$\text{NPV} = \frac{\Sigma \ (R_t - C_t)}{(1 + r)^t) - I} \qquad T = 1$$

where t represents time, n represents the number of time periods, R is revenue impacts, C is cost impacts, r is the discount rate, and I is the Investment.

Again, NPV > zero means the project will pay for itself, < zero means the project does not pay for itself, and an NPV of zero will give you a break even.

Remember, NPV is simply a guideline to help you quantify the CRM results to make informed investment decisions. Note NPV calculations include assumptions and guesstimates, so allow room for error. Microsoft Excel or Lotus 123 can help you calculate the NPV for a CRM initiative. This simple software can also help you develop "what if" scenarios with various values for NPV components and CRM options.

WHERE DO YOU BEGIN?

Practice and Business Objectives

Through 2005–2006, more than 50% of all CRM implementations will be viewed as failures from a customer's point of view, according to Gartner, Inc. (NYSE: IT and ITB). Gartner continues to say these failures will be due to a combination of inability to link channels, lack of process redesign, or failure to provide any real patient benefits. Clarity of where your industry, consumer and company are going in the short term and long term helps you define your business objectives and the patient benefits that are essential to clarify before you chart out your CRM map. Involve all stake holders from various function—sales, service, production—take their inputs to arrive at your business objectives. Communicate the business objectives to all constituencies. CRM affects not just marketing but functions across the company. Establish your company vision, role for CRM, and CRM metrics. CRM metrics-driven business objectives will help you derive the requirements for technology, people, and process and will also help you with capacity planning and strategies right down to execution. In small health care organizations, it is not unusual to make midcourse corrections to strategies and modify business objectives. Nevertheless, the process we are detailing out in this section will help you minimize chaos and implement CRM as seamlessly as possible.

Requirements Gathering

The success of any project depends on clear and detailed definition of the specific requirements of the initiative and of course a systematic implementation. A recent survey of IT executives revealed that less than 20% of business technology projects are completed on time, on budget, and according to original specifications. According to the Standish group survey, more than 70% of projects fail to be completed on time/ on budget. Main contributors to project failure are inadequate user input and incomplete, unclear, or changing requirements and project specifications. If the business pays attention to the process of gathering and documenting requirements, it can pave the way to a successful CRM initiative. Gathering requirements and including them in the project management process enables

- users to participate in the process, to build a working solution, to learn the system early on and to build a working relationship with other functions,
- the technical team to build a solution that can work in a way that reflects the user needs and helps bridge the gap between the user and the IT community, and
- managers to measure project success, to feel assured of project adaptation.

Technology Selection

CRM technology evolved rapidly and the plethora of options today at your disposal can be baffling. You as a CRM champion and user need to pay utmost attention to the process of selecting CRM technology that is appropriate for your needs. CRM deployments for a 360-degree patient view and real time patient interactions are great, but not if they take several million dollars and drag over several years, which could be kiss of death for young businesses.

Therefore, when you examine the CRM toolscape, note that most vendors are improving their footprint and chances are they can offer you a "cutting edge toolkit" at bargain prices—applications that you may need, not today, but in the near future. Ask yourself this question: Do I need it—the capacity, the price, and the scale? Do you know with absolute clarity how your business needs are going to change in the near future? Even if you buy more than what you need, can you handle it and implement this in the timeframes and with the resources and constraints you have? It is very critical to be clear about your objectives, gather requirements, and then prioritize what you need the most and what you can take up based on your resources.

In addition, the rapid pace of technology consolidation is creating a market in which specific technologies are more dependent on other technology decisions and affect larger parts of an organization. This change is forcing more business and IT personnel to be cross functional over a wider breadth of technologies:

- deliver as much as possible electronically
- asynchronous
- automate

Small- to medium-size health care organizations don't need costly and extensive CRM suites. On the other hand, they need solutions that can give them quick returns on investment and prove their worth within a short period of time. For example, for a patient data mart, spreadsheets are very handy. You can conduct preliminary data functions using spreadsheets and use e-mail software to conduct campaigns. You may be better off with simple Excel software or MS Access, which costs a few hundred dollars, than industrial strength databases that cost more to implement and maintain with multimillion dollar and multiyear implementation efforts. The CRM Spotlights in following sections of the chapter will outline how health care organizations are leveraging CRM technologies.

Today's software vendors, both those who started out with call centers and those who began in campaign management or sales force automation, are racing to provide a suite of solutions that enable practices to address small business needs.

A Partial List of Activities That Will Go a Long Way While You Choose Your Technologies

- Before selecting a package or best-of-breed solution based on sales presentations, develop a business case for your CRM initiative and calculate ROI models on your investments (some sample guidelines are included in the chapter under ROI on CRM).
- Ensure that the software solution is simple and amenable to scaling up or down as per your business needs.
- The CRM infrastructure does not stand alone. To provide intelligent patient service through multiple touch points, it is imperative to have a clear view of the patient. This requires CRM to be integrated with the front office, back office, and workgroup infrastructure—enterprise resource planning (ERP) and supply chain software to facilitate the flow of transactions and patient data.
- While you are evaluating CRM technologies, look for software that allows you to integrate your CRM with other enterprise applications and existing technologies. Even if you do not need this integration today, make sure your new CRM technology can integrate well with your existing technology infrastructure in the future.
- Software is not the only expense you will incur. You will also incur implementation expenses and opportunity costs if technology is not chosen and implemented well.

It is essential for you to have a clear CRM strategy and approach the implementation in an incremental way while digesting CRM in realistic modules. Therefore you need to critically evaluate your needs and accordingly choose appropriate CRM solution. Today, software vendors are realizing the potential of CRM for health care organizations and are offering software or hosted solutions to address CRM needs of young companies that are within their budgets.

Criteria for Technology Selection

- What tools are available?
- How do they compare?
- Which live up to expectations?

Both research and experience reveal an often confusing, complicated world of claims, features, and upgrades, a wide array of technical architectures, and an even wider array of pricing structures when it comes to choosing CRM software. Critical Criteria for selection include:

Scalability. As a young practice, a scalable marketing program and CRM infrastructure should be flexible enough to accommodate industry/company trends and realities effortlessly and seamlessly without crushing your marketing infrastructure of people/processes. A scalable CRM infrastructure should allow you to add a new channel, a new patient segment, a product, or a service line seamlessly with minimum incremental effort. Make sure you have a CRM technology that is scalable.

Interoperability. You may need an authoring tool today to develop your collateral; for this purpose, you might select MS Word. Later you may want to conduct campaigns to introduce your company or gauge satisfaction among current patients through an online survey. The software you build or purchase for all these individual activities should be able to coexist and talk to each other. The software you purchase does not have to be monolithic software, but, rather, needs to be modular so that it can work with your other programs. For example, your e-mail software should work with your authoring tool. In today's complex and fast paced evolution of technologies that need to coexist with legacy technologies, interoperability is one of the important criteria for CRM technology selection.

Ease of Use. As a young company pulled in different directions, it is important to have a CRM solution that is easy to use and does not necessitate extensive user training.

Cost structure. CRM software comes with obvious costs as well as hidden costs. Ask the right questions and find out the hidden costs for systems implementation, integration, and user training.

CRM TOOLSCAPE

According to a Gartner release, worldwide CRM software revenue is projected to reach $4 billion in 2005. Today, there are a wide array of options available in various CRM areas—be it sales, customer service or marketing—to buy stand-alone products or complete suites. Software product health care organizations even offer hosted solutions that work for small company budgets. Here is a partial list of vendors offering CRM products, services, and hosted solutions spanning marketing, sales, call center, customer service, Web-based self-service functions. Functionalities range from simple contact management to complete set of CRM capabilities, including patient analytics, personalization, and multichannel execution

Vendor Selection

There are several small as well as large CRM companies that offer software and services. Young health care organizations need flexible and prompt personalized service. Today even large software and service providers are going after the small-business segment and are offering very attractive options. Some suggested steps in vendor selection:

1. Develop your criteria for selection and shortlist.
2. Invite CRM companies for demos, proofs of concept, and in-depth discussions—see if they understand your business. For example, when a company invited a software vendor to present their CRM solution, the vendor focused exclusively on how well they support e-mail campaigns, though the client mentioned several times that their target audience relies on direct mail and they wanted to see how the software can help them with that. Needless to say, the software vendor lost the deal. Therefore, it is critical to figure out if the vendor understands your business need and can provide a solution that works for you.
3. Talk to references and also visit reference sites; talk to industry analysts like Gartner, IDC, META, or Forrester—these can be good sources of information.
4. Explore to see if payment to the CRM organization can be tied to performance.
5. Ensure that you get the support—especially if you are going with a small vendor. Find out how stable and solvent they are. Your finding may impact how well you will be supported if you purchase their product/software/solution (this may be true even for large businesses).

CRM SUCCESS FACTORS THAT NEED SPECIAL ATTENTION

Successful CRM implementation also depends on the top management's ability to develop clear vision, strategy, and people and processes that are interwoven to effectively utilize the technology and execute the tasks.

People

A well thought out and implemented CRM involves all groups. The team dynamics can make or break CRM success in a company. Today, different functions within an organization are required to work together as health care organizations are rallying to be more patient-centric than ever before. Though cross-functional and departmental collaboration sounds idyllic, it is often a playground for organizational politics that make building scalable marketing programs more complex.

COLLABORATION AND COMMUNICATION

As you roll CRM out—at a 50,000-foot level, of course—all groups pledge to work together for common good; at the grassroots level, this could very well translate into giving up your resources or sharing your rewards with your colleagues from other functions or even giving up control and ownership of assets including patient information. This is tailor made for turf politics and disruptive patient service. All this requires a strong commitment and continuous communication and reinforcement of clear vision from the senior management across the organization and teamwork.

REQUIREMENTS GATHERING AND PROJECT MANAGEMENT

Requirements gathering. As technological advances open up more communication channels between the company and the patients, patients are taking advantage of them. This forces health care organizations to incorporate multiple access channels (including fax, e-mail, Web, and video) and address patient inquiries in any format. These trends have created enterprise-level changes for patient service, which includes stakeholders from other divisions and functions. More than 70% of technology projects fail (go over time and over budget or simply flop) due to inadequate requirement gathering process, according to a Standish Group Survey. What this means is that health care organizations will be have to carefully identify all the users and stakeholders in the initiative, identify their business needs, then mesh this with the company's overall vision and strategies to establish a rigorous requirements-gathering process that takes all necessary user inputs into account to shape a viable CRM initiative.

Project Management. Project management can be one step that stands between the success and failure of a CRM initiative. Large organizations can spend between $30 million and $90 million over a 3-year period investing in technology, labor, consulting services, and training related to CRM initiatives. With organizations investing substantially in CRM initiatives, Gartner analysts say project management is becoming crucial to contain costs and increase successful CRM projects. Many organizations are implementing CRM strategies, but a majority of them will underestimate the costs of CRM projects by as much as 40%–75%. It is critical for health care organizations to develop a robust project plan that contains the right estimates of deliverables; the right people, with clear roles for them; the right responsibilities; the right project costs; and the right processes to track the progress of CRM initiative with timely phase reviews.

THE CRM TEAM

It is sufficient to say that with changing CRM technologies, changing business dynamics, changing objectives, and high consumer expectations, health care organizations need to reevaluate the role of patient facing as well as other "back office" patient-servicing skill sets, performance measurements, and compensation requirements.

Why Do We Need Processes?

Processes help improve the quality of your operations and also help improve the productivity of your resources. CRM requires teams to cross sell/up-sell or coordinate seamlessly with other internal groups to provide a consistent patient experience at all the patient touch points. This cannot be accomplished seamlessly without right processes, which need the following:

Executive Sponsorship

For profitable CRM, it is imperative for your contact centers, sales force teams, and other patient touch points within the practice to collaborate and deliver a consistently excellent and seamless patient experience. This means coordination between various groups within the practice, sharing resources, responsibilities, successes, and challenges without territorial conflicts. This requires a strong commitment and reinforcement of clear vision from the senior management across the organization to facilitate teamwork and minimize territorial conflicts. Executive sponsorship is essential so that appropriate processes can be formulated and implemented.

Cross-Functional Teams

As technological advances open up more communication channels, health care organizations are required to incorporate multiple access channels (including fax, e-mail, Web, and video) and address patient inquiries in any format. These trends have created enterprise-level changes that include stakeholders from other divisions and functions. Therefore, health care organizations should have cross-functional teams that involve frontliners and other stakeholders to actively engage in formulating the processes and have the requisite buy-in from their peers and senior medical executives.

Build Vs. Buy Vs. Outsource

There are options to build, buy, or outsource your CRM infrastructure. There are advantages and disadvantages to all three options.

Build. Rapid technology advances are transforming the business landscape. This makes it very challenging for health care organizations to keep abreast of the technologies, to train and manage resources on tools, to grapple with cross-functional, cross-departmental dynamics, and build the CRM application. In addition, mergers/acquisitions and other market realities can make CRM operations complex and distract health care organizations from delivering excellent patient experience.

It is very tempting for small health care organizations to think they can develop what they need in-house themselves. Maybe—maybe not. It is very essential to stay focused on your main business and see if the solution is available elsewhere. Figure out if you are in the business of whatever you are doing or, let us say, in the business to develop a patient survey tool or a low-end database. It is best to get outside help wherever you are dealing with an initiative/task that is not your core competence or where it is to your strategic advantage—be it time-to-value or cost savings.

Buy. Depending on your business needs you can either buy CRM package solution and implement or build best of breed solutions that are suited to your business needs. You need to pay very close attention to what the software vendors are promising. Naturally, they will be more interested in making the sale, than advising on whether it integrates well with your existing technologies, so the onus is on you as a buyer to ask the right questions and make appropriate purchases.

Outsource. Especially for very young health care organizations today, outsourcing can be an option worth exploring to de-risk technology decisions. Outsourcing de-risks marketing program—avoids unnecessary upfront massive capital investment and will also equip the marketers with the flexibility to ramp up or down as the situation demands. Outsourcing does not mean health care organizations can wash their hands of the CRM function. Still, it is the business that will have to provide the strategic direction and control the CRM process and outcome. There are also application service provider (ASP) solutions that de-risk technology decisions.

One of the attractions of going the hosted route becomes very clear when you have a two-doctor practice marketing medical services that require 24-7 availability of information, transaction, and service. They have attractive pricing that encourage the pay-as-you-go paradigm, which is of enormous help to young businesses. However, the disadvantages of ASP are (1) you can't integrate with your other enterprise systems for patient 360-degree view, (2) you can't customize to reflect your exact needs, and (3) you can't work offline, which can be a disadvantage if you are mobile.

Privacy and Security of Patient Data

An Accenture Consulting/Vanderbilt study found that 95% of people who go online have significant concerns about the loss of their personal information. Pew Charitable Trusts funded another recent study that indicates that two thirds of the online population feel that businesses should not be allowed to track people.

As health care organizations have started opening up more channels so that consumers can communicate and do transactions with them, the number of channels that are available for health care organizations to collect patient data—including social-security numbers and financial information—is going up. E-mail spamming has turned up the heat on the aspects of consumer privacy, and spamming on other channels, such as the telephone, is also under scrutiny. In fact, telespamming is so acutely felt, businesses are coming up with products such as Telezapper to help consumers avoid telespamming. As Internet technologies continue to mature, cyber crime incidents are going up and have come to be considered as a class of their own in cyber terrorism, which is not going to be discussed in this chapter.

In a post 9-11, Patriot Act (PA) or West Nile Virus world, there is an increasing regulatory and government scrutiny on corporate practices affecting consumer interests. Even prior to 9-11, the government moved to make health care organizations' patient data more secure through the Health Insurance Portability and Accountability Act of 1996 (HIPAA), which allows patients better access to and more control over their data.

As privacy legislation (online or otherwise) moves forward at the federal and state levels, there is a growing awareness in the business world of the need to protect patient privacy. With increasingly sophisticated and aware patients, the failure to respect their privacy could result in eventual patient attrition. Increasingly, health care organizations are devising their own privacy policies and deploying tools to better manage patient information stored in sales-prospecting files, transaction histories, and other databases.

Health care organizations also need to tailor their services/products to suit individual patient needs by collecting and understanding patient data better and thereby reducing the clutter in the consumer's life. This ambition entails collecting better patient data, but does this mean more consumer monitoring thereby invading their privacy? If privacy is protected, does that mean health care organizations cannot collect and track the data well enough to provide personalized offers? What can the health care organizations do in this situation to have an approach that helps them help their patients? There is a way out.

The 3C Privacy Mantra for Businesses

The patient privacy issue is one of trust management. Your patients need to trust you with their confidential and sensitive information and need to feel that they can control how you, as their data custodians, treat their data. It does not matter whether you have a two-employee company or a 1,000 employee company, you still have to be careful about how you collect the data, what you do with it, how you store it, and how you use (always with the patient's permission). It does not help that patients may have low tolerance for privacy snafus by young businesses. Patients are known to cut less slack for young health care organizations, so follow the 3C Mantra:

Collaborate among cross-functional teams.

Comply with your privacy policy and regulations.

Communicate with your patients continuously.

Collaborative Medical Marketing Trends

Given the economic environment and competitive pressures, health care organizations are focused on patient acquisition and patient retention. Health care organizations are teaming together to offer comprehensive and end-to-end solutions. If you are partnering with other health care organizations to pool in your expertise, offer joint solutions, and take up joint marketing and patient communications programs, be careful how you execute these functions and about what principles you are in agreement with your partners on in regard to sharing patient databases. It is advisable to formulate a simple and clear privacy policy and adhere to that in the partnership agreements. Comply with the policy at all patient touch points. Communicate this very clearly with your business partners and patients in all your channels of communication. Inventory your data collection processes and gateways. Select appropriate projects to add security to your data across extended networks and partners. Note that there is no silver bullet to protect the privacy. Privacy compliance is as much a business issue as it is a technical issue, sometimes more so.

Implications for Patient Strategies

While you are formulating and implementing privacy policies; you need to address the following questions:

- Do your patients *respond* to your company's privacy strategy?

  It is not enough to have a privacy policy that is so confidential no one is aware of it. It is imperative for businesses, once they implement their privacy strategies, to understand how consumers are responding and loop the feedback to fine-tune your policies accordingly.

- How do *you* consider the impact on the patient from every privacy decision you make?

  Every privacy decision you make will impact the patient and your business, but to what extent? How do you determine this impact? Some of them will be patient facing and some will be in back end office operations. This step is essential so that you can make appropriate decisions and make optimum usage of your resources.

- Will your medical business operations support the privacy initiative?

  Privacy enablement requires resources and training with perhaps no immediate, or apparent short-term value-added to the top line or bottom line. Health care organizations that take a proactive view of privacy enablement as the cost of doing business in the twenty-first century will benefit. Health care organizations still need to adopt critical processes and technology that agree with their resources and gradually enable privacy in an incremental way.

Role of Technology

There is no technological silver bullet. Privacy-enabling a business is composed of elements of company loyalty toward patients, commitment to build long-lasting and profitable patient management by building trust, and engaging cross-functional teams that can pick and deploy suitable data security across the network. Here are some salient steps for secure data management that affect technology choices of the business:

- *Privacy-compliant database development.* Health care organizations have to listen and record what patients are saying. Organizations need to know how patients prefer to be contacted (they may prefer not to be contacted at all). All these details will have to be stored in a secure database, which is regularly refreshed with the outcome of the company's communications with the patient. This will be the central repository that the company will draw upon to design and execute consistent and privacy-enabled patient communications.

- *Enterprise data management.* Protect the data across the organization, from group to group, from network to network. It is not enough for health care organizations to protect data from external intruders—they must protect it from internal data abusers as well. It is not enough that patient data is secure during transmission at the patient touch point. It also needs to be safe where it is stored. It is not unusual to have patient data stored or lying around where it is accessible by internal intruders. Therefore, it is imperative for health care organizations to go beyond traditional firewalls to have multilayered security at the data level.

CONCLUSION

Privacy issues are here to stay for health care organizations at any given stage in CRM implementation. The discussion around security and privacy can only be expected to become more prominent. Health care organizations should keep privacy on their laundry list of action items while devising their CRM plans.

CHAPTER 25

Ethical Issues in Modern Medical Practice

Render S. Davis

> The dogmas of the quiet past are inadequate to the stormy present. The case is piled high with difficulty, and we must rise with the occasion. As our case is new, so we must think anew and act anew.
>
> —Abraham Lincoln, 1862

> The times, they are a-changing.
>
> —Bob Dylan, 1962

A century separates the eloquence of Lincoln and Dylan, yet both were witnesses to trying, turbulent times that left our society profoundly changed. There are few who would doubt that the practice of medicine today is both dramatically changing and piled high with difficulty. The standards that stood vanguard a generation ago appear to no longer drive the rapidly evolving relationship between physicians and patients. Others entities, most notably payers and regulators, have interposed themselves into the relationship, and the result is a radically different approach to health care.

Yet, the ethical principles of beneficence, respect for autonomy, and justice that served as a foundation for the healing professions since the age of Hippocrates, remain as important today as two millennia ago. Ethical dilemmas arise, not from clear choices between good and evil, but when there are no clear choices between competing goods. Often, these issues surface when ethical principles themselves are weighed in relationship to each other. Questions such as, when does a physician's obligation to treat conflict with a patient's right to self determination? and, When does an individual's demand for autonomous choice offend our society's sense of justice and fairness? are but a couple of examples of ethical principles in conflict.

EVOLUTIONARY SHIFTS IN THE PRIMACY OF ETHICAL PRINCIPLES

For nearly 2000 years, the principle of beneficence, the profession's obligation to be of service to others, was the foundation of the practice of medicine. In taking the Hippocratic Oath, physicians swore that they would "perform their art solely for the cure of patients," and patients viewed their doctors as wise, caring, and paternalistic healers unwaveringly committed to their welfare. Until the era of modern medicine dawned in the early twentieth century, sincere, caring, and compassionate service probably were the most effective instruments in the physician's meager armamentarium.

World War II and the decades that followed saw an unprecedented explosion in medical knowledge and technology. As a direct consequence, physicians were called upon to become increasingly sophisticated technicians and specialists, demands that pulled them farther from the bedside and diminished the close, personal relationship with patients they once enjoyed. This increasingly impersonal relationship, combined with the starkness and technically intimidating nature of hospitals, led to a dramatic shift in the traditional patient-physician relationship. No longer did the patient see the family doctor as the caring, paternalistic figure who held his or her interests foremost. Instead, an overwhelming array of specialists appeared before the patient to explore illness etiology or examine a particular body part—too often appearing more interested in the malady than in the person afflicted with it.

The covenant of trust that once bonded the physician and patient was rapidly eroding and, amid the social turmoil of the 1960s, patients began to demand that physicians treat them as equal partners, both informing them of the nature of their disease and seeking their permission to initiate treatment. After all, patients reasoned, they should have the final say regarding what was done to their own bodies.

Consequently, the principle of respect for autonomy, an acknowledgment of an individual's right to self determination, slowly took precedence over, but did not eclipse, beneficence. Physicians still cared for their patients, only now they were obligated to take extra steps to bring patients directly into the decision-making process by explaining treatment options and requesting "informed consent" on the plan of care from the patient

Both principles were supported in the prevailing system of fee-for-service private-practice medicine. There were few constraints on physicians' clinical autonomy, and their professional judgment remained, for the most part, unquestioned. In this climate, physicians reasoned that patients would likely benefit from more tests and procedures; patients, especially the well insured, demanded almost unregulated autonomy over their health care choices. For those with the means to pay, access to nearly all that medicine had to offer was considered an unquestioned right.

This proved to be a formula for potential economic disaster. There was an explosion in new and expanded facilities and unwavering demand for the latest technological innovations, much of it supported by the government as vital to a healthy economy. Nonetheless, a fundamental problem existed because health care was being delivered in a financial vacuum, in which both physicians and patients had only a vague understanding of, or interest in, the economic consequences of the services they felt either obligated to provide or entitled to receive.

Both beneficence and respect for autonomy could be invoked to support this nearly unbridled use of health care resources in the care and treatment of individual patients. Insurers, both private and governmental, paid "reasonable and customary" charges, almost without argument; while as patients' advocates, physicians could garner six-figure incomes from fees generated in providing virtually unlimited care.

The inevitable financial fallout from medicine guided by these laissez-faire rules eventually led to an unsustainable inflationary spiral in medical costs. In the 30 years following the passage of the Medicare Act in 1965, the health care sector of the American economy soared from 4% of gross domestic product (GDP) to over 14%, and there was no clear end in sight to the upward rise. Yet, a growing number of Americans actually saw their access to medical care diminish due to rising costs of employer-paid insurance (when it was offered at all), and restrictions in eligibility requirements for Medicaid and other government safety-net programs tightened. Even as the nation increased overall spending for medical care, many Americans were losing access to the system.

This trend has continued, and even accelerated, during the recessionary period that began in 2000. An especially troubling characteristic of the increasing number of Americans now without health insurance is that, for the first time, it includes expanding segments of the middle class—white collar executives, middle managers, and skilled workers who had, historically, been immune from such cutbacks. Today, lack of access to affordable medical care is no longer just the domain of the working poor.

Alarm over rising health care costs began to spread in the 1970s as both private and government payers sought any means possible to stem the hemorrhaging outflow of dollars. President Richard Nixon tried unsuccessfully to implement wage and price controls to slow it; a few years later, President Jimmy Carter attempted to cap Medicare expenditures. Both efforts failed for two primary reasons. First, there was a fundamental misunderstanding of the nature of health care competition. Health care providers did not compete directly for patients, but, rather, for physicians who held the legal authority to admit patients. As independent contractors, physicians could, for the most part choose to join the staff of institutions that provided the latest technology, the most-up-do-date facilities, and even the most luxurious amenities. Consequently, hospitals competed fiercely for doctors, a process that actually caused prices to rise, not fall. Second, the dominant indemnity-based fee-for-service approach to medical care remained fundamentally intact, continuing to insulate both physicians (the consumer's agent) and patients (consumers of care) from the true costs of the services provided. But economic concerns arising from double-digit inflation and business downturns in the late 1970s assured that fundamental and inevitable changes in the financing and practice of medicine were on the horizon.

The first major initiative to have a significant cost constraining effect occurred in the early 1980s with the implementation of the Medicare Prospective Payment System (PPS) and its health care provider payments pegged to diagnosis related groups (DRGs). This system ushered in a new era of controlled, predetermined prices for health care services. The inflationary spiral of government payments for health care slowed, and soon private payers also were considering adopting alternatives to traditional insurance. Slowly, the concept of prepaid, managed health care provided by health maintenance organizations (HMOs), a concept developed by the Kaiser Foundation and other organizations on the West Coast in the 1940s (and strongly opposed by organized medicine), began to spread nationwide as a possible answer to the country's health care ills.

By the 1990s, HMOs and other types of managed care organizations that provided integrated health care services and financing through insurance or other means had gained a serious foothold and were in positions of dominance in American medical care. The growth in the popularity of managed care signaled the next evolutionary change in the predominance of the key ethical principles.

Just as respect for autonomy superceded beneficence, the principle of justice, representing a new approach of balancing the health needs of an individual with the availability of finite resources for the larger population rose to take its place as the primary principle, becoming the vanguard force driving the movement toward managed care. Physician-ethicist, John LaPuma, MD, in his book, *Managed Care Ethics*, writes that managed care has gone so far as to "sever the link between autonomy and justice that once existed to support the care of individuals."

Embedded within this drive toward a fairer distribution of health care resources was the urgent, but highly controversial, desire to rein in costs. Despite years of active suppression and condemnation by health professionals and providers, the hard economic realities of American society's love-hate (love to have it, hate to pay for it) relationship with health care had finally reached the bedside. The result has been an irrevocable sea change in the landscape of American medicine.

THE PHYSICIAN'S DILEMMA: CARING FOR PATIENTS AND POPULATIONS

In today's health care environment, physicians face a myriad of dilemmas in their daily practice. Time constraints, diminished professional autonomy, declining incomes, explosive growth in technology, and deteriorating public trust combined with increasing public demands are only some of the most obvious problems plaguing practitioners. While some who have been adversely impacted by these changes are quick to lay blame at the foot of managed care organizations (MCOs), this anger may be, to some extent, misdirected.

While there are ample faults in managed care as it is currently practiced, its theory and principles are ethically sound. Health care should be "managed"—for continuity, quality, value, and optimal outcomes—regardless of the mechanisms by which the caregivers are paid. Practicing medicine within managed care still entails obligations to care for patients and to respect their autonomy, but now providers have been placed in a disquieting role as resource managers, requiring a new approach to finding better, more cost-effective ways to meet these obligations, while being held accountable to a larger community to which the individual belongs (e.g., a health plan or employee group) for the costs incurred in delivering care. An article in the *Hastings Center Report* summed up this new approach by noting that managed care is based "on the foundation of a philosophy of care that, however well or poorly articulated, responds to the needs of individual patients in the context of population-based mechanisms to assess needs and distribute resources."

In light of the above-referenced ethical principles, an examination of the current practice of managed care reveals an uneven and troubled landscape that continues to be impacted by declining sources of revenue for nonprofit MCOs and falling profits for the proprietary companies. Across the board, both types of MCOs have been damaged by the precipitous drop in investment income in the wake of the stock market's decline since 2000. Consequently, to maintain adequate services or meet shareholder expectations, managed care organizations have further restricted coverages and/or pushed up premiums to either employers or enrollees.

Although MCOs' emphasis on health promotion and illness prevention is viewed as very good, there remain many highly publicized instances in which the health of individual patients has been jeopardized by apparently arbitrary policies and decisions made by managed care organizations, ostensibly in the name of cost containment. Among especially notable issues have been the following:

- Delayed referral of patients to specialty physicians, or denials of access to specialized services, primarily based on resource allocation and cost considerations.
- Rigidly enforced practice guidelines and programmatic standards that potentially penalize a physician's exercise of his or her clinical judgment.
- Crafting of incentives that encourage physicians to withhold clinically pertinent information from patients and to discourage physicians from serving as advocates for their patients.
- Declining consumer choice of health plans and providers. Increasingly, consumers with health insurance are unwilling to demand improvements for fear of losing the coverage they have.
- Failure of many MCOs, especially those operated as proprietary entities, to acknowledge an obligation to improve community health and broaden access to services to persons such as those with handicapping conditions, the poor, the disenfranchised, undocumented aliens, and others with legitimate, unmet health care needs.
- Apparent subordination of quality considerations in access and treatment to cost containment in delivery of services.

These issues, according to LaPuma, make managed care "morally vulnerable" and fraught with public suspicion regarding its core values. Consequently, physicians practicing medicine today are faced with very real dilemmas in such areas as patient advocacy, access to and scope of care, informed consent, conflict of interest, continuity of care, and patient choice.

In a speech given at Georgetown University, Marcia Angell, MD, executive editor of the *New England Journal of Medicine*, described the physician's primary dilemma within the framework of managed care practice as one of "double agency," whereby physicians are being asked to be "both advocates for individual patients and allocators of finite health care resources to the larger populations of enrollees of health plans." This is a role that seems to impinge on the fundamental tenets of patient advocacy articulated in the Hippocratic Oath. By the terms of many managed care insurance plans, a physician's income is directly related to savings generated in the delivery of care, a tactic criticized by former Surgeon General C. Everett Koop, MD, who wrote, "Something is wrong with a system that spends more and more each year to provide less and less service."

Many of the proprietary (for-profit) MCOs acknowledge their primary business objective is the return of value to shareholders, with obligations to provide expanded access and broader health care coverage to plan enrollees a secondary consideration. While he was Speaker of the Oregon State House, former Governor John Kitzhaber (a physician) addressed this concern when he wrote of the "insidious problem permeating our health care system . . . the perverse set of incentives that leads health care providers to act as isolated economic entities focused on their own well-being, instead of viewing themselves as community resources whose primary role is—or should be—to promote the health of the nation." In light of this troubled environment, let us examine some specific dilemmas confronting physicians in their daily practice.

PATIENT ADVOCACY

Few areas of life are as personal as an individual's health, and people have long relied on a caring and competent physician to be their champion in securing the medical resources needed to retain or restore health and function. For many physicians, the care of their patients was the foundation of their professional calling. However, in the contemporary delivery organization, there may be little opportunity for generalist physician "gatekeepers" or "specialty hospitalists" to form a lasting relationship with patients. It is becoming more difficult for them to utilize the full range of their professional judgment when care is directed through programmatic protocols or algorithm-based practice guidelines; and it is more difficult for their personal values to be unimpeded by substantial bonuses, withholds, and other financial incentives that may directly conflict with their advocacy role—especially if a patient may be in need of expensive services that may not be covered in their insurance plan or offered by the MCO.

CONFLICTS OF INTEREST

Conflicts of interest are not a new phenomenon in medicine. In the fee-for-service system, physicians controlled access to medical facilities and technology, and they benefited financially with every order or prescription they wrote. Consequently, there was an inherent temptation to over-treat patients. Even marginal diagnostic or therapeutic procedures were justified on the grounds of both clinical necessity and legal protection against threats of negligence.

In managed care, the potential conflicts between patients and physicians take on a completely different dimension. By design, in health plans where medical care is financed through prepayment arrangements, the physician's income is enhanced not by doing more for his or her patients, but by doing less. Patients, confronted with the realization that their doctor will be rewarded for the use of fewer resources, could no longer rely with certainty on the motives underlying a physician's treatment plans. One inevitable outcome has been the continuing decline in patients' trust in their physicians.

COMMUNICATIONS

In contemporary medicine, ethical dilemmas in communications are increasingly common and may come in many different forms:

- Physicians are failing to communicate necessary clinical information to patients in terms and language the patients can truly understand.

- Physicians are offering only limited treatment choices to patients because alternatives may not be covered by the patient's insurance plan.
- Physicians are failing to disclose financial incentives and other payment arrangements that may influence the physician's treatment recommendations.
- Physicians are under time constraints that limit opportunities for in-depth discussions with their patients.
- Physicians are finding it difficult to maintain a continuing relationship with their patients that would foster open communications.

While so-called gag clauses implemented by some Managed care organizations to prohibit physicians from informing their patients about noncovered treatment alternatives, have been declared illegal in most states, the duty of physicians to be fully truthful and informative in their communications with patients remains under considerable suspicion.

CONFIDENTIALITY

Whether it is an employer interested in the results of an employee's health screening; an insurer trying to learn more about an enrollee's prior health history; the media in search of a story; or health planners examining the potential value of national health databases, the confidential nature of the traditional doctor-patient relationship is seriously threatened by new demands for clinical information and the increasing reliance on electronic records that may be susceptible to tampering and unauthorized access. Clearly, employers and insurers are interested in the status of an individual's health and ability to work; but does this desire to know, combined with their role as payers for health care, constitute a right to know? The patient's right to privacy remains a volatile and unresolved issue.

The recent implementation of the Health Insurance Portability and Accountability Act (HIPAA) has added a new layer of complexity to the issue of patient confidentiality. When first proposed in the mid-1990s, the legislation was intended to both protect patient information and to provide mechanisms for continuity of health insurance coverage as individuals changed employment, and so on. However, through the regulatory process, the law has become a labyrinth of rules and requirements designed to protect patient privacy in all aspects of medical care, from emergency departments to grocery-store pharmacies. It remains to be determined if the value of the confidentiality benefits will truly outweigh the cost burden hospitals, physicians, pharmacies, and other health care providers have incurred in meeting the letter of the law.

CULTURAL SENSITIVITY

While America has always been called a nation of immigrants, it has never been more true than today. Consequently, the challenge for physicians and other health care providers, in both large cities and small communities, is meeting the health care needs of an increasingly diverse and multicultural population, who speak foreign languages and have social norms, traditions, and values that may substantially differ from their physicians'. Problems arise when clinicians expect, even demand, that patients and their families discard their cultural foundations and adhere to the health care provider's view of the care and decision-making process.

Instead, the health care team should be more aware of and sensitive to the values and beliefs of patients that come from differing cultures; the team should work within that framework to assure that the patient's individual rights are validated and their wishes honored to the fullest extent possible.

Former U.S. Surgeon General David Satcher, MD, PhD, now directs the National Center for Primary Care Medicine at the Morehouse College of Medicine in Atlanta, Georgia. A key component of the center's training program is a special curriculum designed to foster greater cultural competence among physicians and health care providers. Called the "CRASH Course," the program is designed to address these issues:

- *Cultural Awareness.* Acknowledging the diversity and legitimacy of the many cultures that make up the fabric of American society.
- *Respect.* Valuing other cultural norms, even if they differ from or conflict with your own.
- *Assess and affirm.* Understanding the points of both congruence and difference among cultural approaches to decision making; learning how to achieve the best outcomes within the cultural framework of the patient and family unit;
- *Sensitivity and self-awareness.* Being secure in your own values while willing to be flexible in working through cultural differences with others;
- *Humility.* Recognizing that every culture has legitimacy and that no one is an expert in what is best for others; being willing to subordinate your values for those of another to achieve the goals of treatment.

There is little doubt that multicultural sensitivity will continue to grow as an increasingly integral component of medical education and health care practice.

Case Report

An elderly Asian-born patient is diagnosed with fast-growing cancer requiring immediate surgery. The patient is alert and competent. The physician approaches the patient regarding her diagnosis and to seek consent for the operation. In the family's culture, patients are protected from bad news and such health care decisions are delegated to a spouse or child. The eldest son intercedes with the doctor and indicates that he speaks for the patient. The physician counters that "this is the United States" and that the patient has a right to make her own decisions; the doctor demands to talk directly to the patient. As another member of the health care team witnessing this episode, what should you do?

ACCESS TO CARE

In his book Back To Reform, author Charles Dougherty wrote that "cost containment is the goal for the healthy. Access is the goal for the sick." So, for an increasing number of Americans, the concerns described above are almost meaningless because they are, for the most part, outside the structure of the current health care system. Employers are downsizing staff or cutting out health insurance benefits in an effort to be financially successful in a global economy; while demands for greater government accountability in the expenditure of tax dollars have brought about increasingly more stringent eligibility requirements for safety-net programs such as Medicaid. As insurance becomes more expensive or government programs undergo budget cuts, people are being excised from the system.

At the same time, new competitive demands have fostered unprecedented consolidations, mergers, and closures of health care facilities. This shakeout may have served to greatly reduce the overcapacity that plagued the system, but it has been done with greater emphasis on cutting costs than on fostering efficiency and effectiveness in creating a true system of care delivery.

Those who view health care as little different from any other commodity available through the free market see the present access concerns as simply a byproduct of the inevitable restructuring of the system. While they argue that we must adhere to market solutions to solve our health care access problems, others demand a different approach, calling for governmental national health insurance or some form of subsidized care providing at least a basic level of treatment for all citizens. While Americans continue to proudly tout that we do not explicitly ration care as do some other countries (notably Great Britain), we tacitly accept a health care system that implicitly excludes citizens who are unable to overcome financial barriers to access.

Access to care represents the most visible issue at the very foundation of the ethical principle of justice. In their text *Principles of Biomedical Ethics,* authors Thomas Beauchamp, PhD, and James F. Childress, PhD, point out that justice is subject to interpretation and may even be evoked to support the positions of parties in direct opposition. For example, those who support the predominant principle of distributive justice—the fair allocation of resources based on laws or cultural rules—still must decide on what basis these resources will be used. Utilitarians argue for resource distribution based on achieving the "greatest good for the greatest number"; Libertarians believe that recipients of resources should be those who have made the greatest contributions to the production of those resources—a free market approach to distribution—while egalitarians support the distribution of resources based on who is in greatest need, irrespective of contribution or other considerations. Consequently, developing a system of access based on "justice" will be fraught with enormous difficulty.

In the current health care environment, access to medical care is approaching crisis levels as increasing malpractice insurance premiums are driving physicians from high risk specialties such as obstetrics, emergency medicine, and surgery in record numbers. The impact is most dramatic in rural and under-served areas of the country where sole-practitioners and small group practices are discontinuing services, leaving local citizens with no choice but to forego care or travel greater distances to regional medical centers to find necessary treatment. At the same time, significant budget cuts at both the federal and state levels have seriously eroded funding for Medicaid, leaving this especially vulnerable segment of the population with even fewer options than before.

Two areas of the care access dilemma are moving to the forefront. The first is in emergency medicine. A recently completed study by the Federal Centers for Disease Control and Prevention cites statistics showing that in the decade ending in 2001, emergency room visits increased by 20%, while the number of emergency departments shrank by 15%. Increasingly, hospitals have closed emergency departments due to increasing costs, staffing shortages, and declining payments for services. This crisis comes at a time when post 9-11 fears of terrorism and global disease outbreaks like Severe Acute Respiratory Syndrome (SARS) have placed an even greater burden on the delivery of emergency services. Arthur Kellerman, MD, director of emergency services at Atlanta's Grady Memorial Hospital, the city's only level one trauma center, writes that "the situation is alarming and has been for some time. . . . It's unconscionable that we are not coming to terms with the Achilles' heel of our health care system."

The second area that will grow in significance is in the area of genetic testing. As technological capabilities improve, medicine's ability to examine an individual's genetic makeup will open up remarkable opportunities to predict a person's susceptibility to certain diseases or handicapping conditions. From a scientific standpoint, we are on the threshold of an extraordinary new era in medicine, in which identifications of and treatments for potential illnesses may begin before the person is even born.

However, there is a more troubling side to the potential of genetic testing as noted by Johns Hopkins University president, Dr. William R. Brody. He describes genetic testing as "medicine's iceberg," wherein serious dangers for access to care are lurking beneath the surface. According to Brody, heated debate has already begun regarding the value of genetic information to insurance companies who could use the information to determine premium levels, even the overall insurability, for individuals and/or families with a member identified through testing as predisposed to a catastrophic and/or potentially expensive medical condition. In this scenario, infants manifesting a genetic predisposition to certain illnesses or potential behavior disorders may find themselves faced with lifelong uninsurability based on the results of prenatal genetic testing.

Dr. Brody persuasively argues that the potential of this technology, regardless of the incredible scientific potential it offers, could lead to dramatically diminished access to health insurance for tens of thousands of individuals and families and bring about an end to private health insurance as we know it. He suggests that some form of community-rated universal health insurance may be the only reasonable alternative to assure that Americans at all levels, from indigent and working poor to the most affluent, may receive needed, basic medical care. The ethical dimensions of this debate, from questions of beneficence, autonomy, and justice are only beginning to surface and may dominate our deliberations before this decade is over.

Case Report

A young, working-class couple expecting their first child learn through genetic testing that the fetus has a neurological defect that will require lifelong treatment. The insurer sends a letter informing the family that the infant's illness is not covered under the terms of their policy. The family approaches their primary care physician, who is a member of the insurance company's panel of preferred providers, asking what they should do. If you were their doctor, what would you do?

PROFESSIONAL AUTONOMY

Not so long ago, a physician's clinical judgment was virtually unquestioned. Now, with the advent of clinical pathways and case management protocols, many of the aspects of treatment are outlined in algorithm-based plans that allied health professionals may follow with only minimal direct input from a physician. Much about this change has been good. Physicians have been freed from much tedious routine and are better able to watch more closely for unexpected responses to treatments or unusual outcomes and then utilize their knowledge to chart an appropriate response.

What is of special concern, though, is the restrictive nature of protocols in some care plans that may unduly limit a physician's clinical prerogatives to address a patient's specific needs. Such plans may prove to be the ultimate bad examples of "cook book" medicine. While some may find health care and the practice of medicine an increasingly stressful and unrewarding field, others are continuing to search for ways to assure that caring, compassionate, and ethically rewarding medicine remain at the heart of our health care system.

Case Report

Patient is 36 hours post-op from surgery to remove a ruptured appendix. Patient remains febrile, and the attending physician is concerned about a possible abdominal infection. Patient's managed-care provider indicates that, according to treatment guidelines for this surgery, he is covered for only 2 post-op days. The physician's request for an additional day of hospitalization to treat the possible infection is denied, and the MCO representative states that the patient should be discharged with a prescription for antibiotics. What should the attending physician do?

FOSTERING ETHICALLY SOUND MEDICINE WITHIN THE FRAMEWORK OF MANAGED CARE

In Managed Care Ethics, LaPuma notes that, " . . . just as physicians helped society get into an over-spent, over-built, over-utilized health care rut; physicians should help society get out." While the patient-physician relationship has undergone significant erosion, it still remains somewhat tenuously at the center of the medical care universe. There is much that physicians can do within the framework of managed care to both restore their role as patient advocates and as compassionate care givers.

In order to do this successfully, it is important to recognize that irrevocable changes have occurred, but the future evolution of managed care is not yet established. It is much like a pendulum that has swung from one extreme (unregulated fee-for-service medicine) and is now on an arc toward another, as yet undetermined, destination. Will it be a government controlled national health care system? A market driven service bought and sold like any other commodity? Or something in-between? Physicians and other health care providers still have the power to influence the answer.

Managed care may yet prove to be a highly functional and effective system committed to providing cost efficient and clinically effective care as articulated by William Steinman, MD, who teaches his students at Tulane University Medical School to "order only tests and perform screening procedures that will help provide a diagnosis and treatment plan . . . do the right things, at the right time, and for the right reasons." Renowned physician-ethicist Edmund Pelligrino, MD, of the Kennedy Center for Ethics at Georgetown University, goes on to note that "what our health policies do to the individual patient serves as a reality check to what values we hold most dear and the ethical foundation of the policies we develop and impose." So those who truly believe that we can still have a caring and compassionate system of managed care must actively work within that system to bring it about, and not abdicate it. The following sections present some recommended beginning steps in this process.

BEING A PATIENT EDUCATOR, COACH, AND MENTOR

Never has the well-worn adage, "patient heal thyself" been more true. With their emphasis on health promotion and disease prevention and their tightening restrictions on access to expensive acute care, HMOs practically scream at patients to take charge of their own health and well-being.

It is no longer enough for physicians to be healers, intervening when a patient appears at their door with an acute or chronic illness. They must be proactive educators, even coaches, providing patients with the information needed to change poor health habits like smoking, drinking, and obesity, and encouraging them to adopt healthier lifestyles. Unfortunately, this task is more difficult than it appears. Historically, Americans have refused to accept the consequences of their poor health habits, preferring to seek medicine's help in repairing the damage after it has been done. Results from America's Health Report Card, a study completed by the Gallup Organization, showed that while Americans express concern over such things as cholesterol levels, high blood pressure, cancer, and weight reduction, many do little to reduce their risks. George Gallup, Jr. noted in the report's conclusion that

> some of the messages aren't getting through, although people are very much under a constant bombardment of information. It's ironic in a sense that some of the diseases have been conquered, but people have not done their share to stay healthy because they are indulging in habits that are self-destructive. . . .

Even when confronted with the time constraints and discontinuity inherent in frequently changing health insurance plans, it is clear that physicians must be diligent in assessing their patients' health habits and helping them articulate their health goals; assuring that patients understand the terms, limitations, and costs associated with their health plan, and serving as mentors and partners to provide them with the knowledge and self-motivation to change for better long-term health.

Instead of being "gatekeepers" charged with limiting access to the system, physicians should view their roles as that of "navigators"—guiding patients through an increasingly confusing maze of treatment alternatives, and leading them in the direction of informed choices and optimal outcomes. In today's health care environment, the principle of beneficence is inextricably woven into the premise that physicians must do more to help patients help themselves.

BECOMING QUALITY DRIVEN

Whether care should be "managed" is no longer a legitimate question. The fundamental question now is for what purpose is care to be managed? The present moral vulnerability of managed care rests with its apparent overriding concern with cost reduction through limitations on access and service—possibly at the expense of clinical appropriateness, quality, and the health needs of the individual patient.

If physicians are to be credible advocates for their patients, they must unwaveringly stand for quality and against arbitrary and unjustifiable restrictions on access to clinically justified and needed care. This does not imply a return to unregulated fee-for-service medicine, but rather a demand that MCOs be held accountable for both cost effectiveness and quality. The earliest HMOs were established for this purpose, and it has only been in the last decade that managed care has become the de facto tool for driving down cost and squeezing excess capacity out of the system.

Unfortunately, this has not taken place in a coordinated fashion with any clear goal of establishing a cohesive, seamless health care system. Consequently, we have a fragmented, patchwork system, described by Marcia Angell, MD, as a "hodgepodge of temporary alignments, existing independently, often working at cross purposes . . . " that leaves many patients and providers with inadequate tools and information to make truly informed health care choices.

Physicians, other care providers, and managed care organizations should work in concert to develop a system of care that is integrated and coordinated, epidemiologic-data dependent, consumer-driven, sensitive to privacy and confidentiality concerns, and clearly responsive to the legitimate health care needs of enrollees and the general population.

We as a nation can have a health care system that embraces compassionate, clinically appropriate, cost-effective care, with universal access to basic services if we are willing to make difficult, but publicly informed and debated, choices regarding our health care priorities. Physicians must be proactive and central to this process.

DEMANDING HIGH PROFESSIONAL MORAL STANDARDS OF BOTH YOURSELF AND OF MANAGED CARE ORGANIZATIONS

It has been argued that physicians have abdicated the moral high ground in health care by their interest in seeking protection for their high incomes, their highly publicized self-referral arrangements, and their historical opposition toward any reform efforts that jeopardizes their clinical autonomy. In his book *Medicine at the Crossroads,* Emory University Professor Melvin Konnor, MD, notes that "throughout its history, organized medicine has represented, first and foremost, the pecuniary interests of doctors." He goes on to lay significant blame for the present problems in health care at the doorstep of both insurers and doctors, stating that "the system's ills are pervasive and all its participants are responsible."

In order to reclaim their once esteemed moral position, physicians must actively reaffirm their commitment to the highest standards of the medical profession and call on other participants in the health care delivery system also to elevate their values and standards to the highest level. Daniel Callahan, PhD, former executive director of the Hastings Center, articulated this concern when he wrote, "The change cannot only be in our health care system, in its mechanisms, institutions, and practices. It must be no less a change in our values and goals, our ideas of good health and the good life. The change must, moreover, come from inside ourselves."

In the evolutionary shift toward managed care, physicians have been asked to embrace business values of efficiency and cost effectiveness, sometimes at the expense of their professional judgment and personal values. While some of these changes have been inevitable as our society sought to rein in out-of-control costs, it is not unreasonable for physicians to call on payers, regulators, and other parties to the health care delivery system to raise their ethical bar. Harvard University physician-ethicist Linda Emmanuel notes that "health professionals are now accountable to business values (such as efficiency and cost effectiveness), so business persons should be accountable to professional values including kindness and compassion." Within the framework of ethical principles, LaPuma writes that "business's ethical obligations are integrity and honesty. Medicine's are those plus altruism, beneficence, non-maleficence, respect, and fairness."

Physician practice groups should consider proactively developing mission and values statements that clearly articulate the group's collective beliefs and the ethical principles that govern their delivery of care. When they consider joining MCO practitioner panels as either contractors or employees, physicians should carefully examine the organization's mission and values statements, read its access policies and procedures, review for fairness its denial and grievance processes, and inquire about its internal and external ethics forums, evaluating the degree to which they complement the practitioner group's established values. If it is not a good fit, the group may choose to not join the panel. If that is not a reasonable business option, the group's physicians may work from within the organization to strengthen and enhance the MCO's moral position.

A study by the Rand Corporation identified seven key components of a quality managed care plan: financial accessibility, organizational accessibility, continuity of care, comprehensiveness of treatment, coordination of services, interpersonal accountability, and technical accountability. These and every other facet of the health care delivery system should reflect a commitment to honesty and integrity that provides clear assurance to payers, providers, and patients that the system is designed to offer compassionate care, clear communication, explicit fairness in distribution of resources, and a commitment to the highest organizational values and ethical principles.

Incumbent in these activities is the expectation that the forces that control our health care delivery system—the payers, the regulators, and the providers—will reach out to the larger community, working to eliminate the inequities that have left so many Americans with limited or no access to even basic health care. Charles Dougherty clarified this obligation in *Back to Reform* when he noted that "behind the daunting social reality stands a simple moral value that motivates the entire enterprise. Health care is grounded in caring. It arises from a sympathetic response to the suffering of others."

DEVELOPING SKILLS NEEDED FOR THE NEW HEALTH CARE

Medical practice today is vastly different from what it was a generation ago, and physicians need new skills to be successful. In order to balance their obligations to both individual patients and to larger groups of plan enrollees, physicians now must become more than competent clinicians. Traditionally, the physician was viewed as the captain of the ship, in charge of nearly all the medical decisions, but this changed with the new dynamics of managed care. Now, as noted previously, the physician's role may be more akin to the ship's navigator, utilizing his or her clinical skills and knowledge of the health care environment to chart the patient's course through a confusing morass of insurance requirements, care choices, and regulations to achieve the best attainable outcome. Some of these new skills include the following:

- Negotiation—working to optimize the patient's access to services and facilities beneficial to their treatment.
- Team Play—working in concert with other care givers, from generalist and specialist physicians to nurses and therapists, to coordinate the delivery of care within a clinically appropriate and cost-effective framework.
- Working within the limits of professional competence—avoiding the pitfalls of payer arrangements that may restrict access to specialty physicians and facilities, by clearly acknowledging when the symptoms or manifestations of a patient's illness require this higher degree of service, then working on behalf of the patient to seek access to them.
- Respecting different cultures and values—inherent in the support of the principle of autonomy is acceptance of values that may differ from one's own. As the United States becomes a more culturally heterogenous nation, health care providers are called upon to work within and respect the sociocultural framework of patients and their families;
- Seeking clarity on what constitutes marginal care—within a system of finite resources, physicians will be called upon to carefully and openly communicate with patients regarding access to marginal and/or futile treatments. Addressing the many needs of patients and families at the end of life will be an increasingly important challenge in both communications and delivery of appropriate, yet compassionate care.
- Exercising decision-making flexibility—treatment algorithms and clinical pathways are extremely useful tools when used within their scope, but physicians must follow the case-managed patient closely and have the authority to adjust the plan if clinical circumstances warrant.

FOSTERING A SOCIALLY RESPONSIBLE HEALTH CARE SYSTEM

The erosion of trust expressed by the public for the health care industry may only be reversed if those charged with working within or managing the system place community and patient interests ahead of their own. We must foster an ethical corporate culture within health care that rewards leaders with integrity and vision; leaders who encourage and expect ethical excellence from themselves and others and who recognize that ethics establishes the moral framework for all organizational decision making.

In a presentation to the Health Care Ethics Consortium of Georgia, Dr. Paul Hoffman, vice president of Provenance Health Partners, spoke of the importance of nurturing and sustaining an "ethical organizational culture" in which high standards of ethics and morality govern the behavior of all participants, from senior management and physicians, to nurses and technical staff. In such cultures, the ethical dimensions of decisions are weighed as heavily as the financial or operational factors, and actions are not taken if the outcome would conflict with the organization's stated values and mission. To assess the climate of an organization, Hoffman recommends conducting an "ethics audit" that would reveal real and perceived problems within the system; provide insights into ethical deficits that may exist; identify opportunities for education; and provide feedback from staff on their support for the organization's ethical culture.

Most important, Hoffman stressed that ethics must be integrated into every aspect of organizational work, calling for "a systems-oriented, proactive approach to improving an institution's health care practices, including both administrative and clinical practices." He went on to say that this "integrated ethics approach anticipates and responds to recurring ethical situations and applies an continuous quality improvement philosophy. This approach unites ethics activities throughout the organization." Whether your workplace is a 500-bed academic medical center or a small internal medicine practice, the purpose is the same—to foster and maintain an organization that is grounded in ethical behavior and dedicated to providing the highest quality of patient care.

In an article published in the Journal of the American Medicals Association, authors Ezekiel Emanual, MD, and Nancy Dubler, LLB, cited what they call the Six C's of the ideal physician-patient relationship: Choice, Competence, Communications, Compassion, Continuity, and [no] Conflict of interest. Physicians who accept a seventh "C"—the Challenge, and are imbued with the moral sensitivity embodied in their solemn oath, have an obligation to serve as the conscience of this new system dedicated toward caring for all Americans.

Writer and ethicist Emily Friedman said it best when she wrote,

> There are many communities in health care. But three to which I hope we all belong are the communities devoted to improving the health of all around us, to achieving access to care for all, and to providing our services at a price that society can afford. These interests are, of course, expressions of the deeper community of values that states that healing, justice, and equality must guide what we believe and do.

SELECTED REFERENCES

Dougherty, C. J. Back to reform: Values, markets, and the health care System. New York: Oxford University Press, 1989.

Hoffman, P. H. "Beyond ethics committees," presentation at the Annual Conference of the Health Care Ethics Consortium of Georgia, April 2, 2003.

Angell, M. (1993). The doctor as double agent. Kennedy Institute of Ethics Journal, Vol. 3, No. 3, September 1993.

"Ethical Issues in Managed Care." Report from the American Medical Association's Council on Ethical and Judicial Affairs. *Journal of the American Medical Association*, Vol. 273, No. 4, January 25, 1995.

Wicclair, M. R."Ethical Issues in Managed Care," Remarks at Fifth Annual Retreat of the Consortium Ethics Program, October 1995.

Philip, D. J. Ethics of managed care. *Medical Group Management Journal*, November–December 1997.

Pelligrino, E. D., Veatch, R. M., & Langan, J. P. Ethics, trust, and the professions: Philosophical and cultural aspects. Washington, DC: Georgetown University Press, 1991.

Brody, W. R. The end of health insurance—part II. In Crossroads: Essays on health care in America. Baltimore: Johns Hopkins University School of Medicine, June 5, 2002.

Kellerman, A. ER's cut back as patient loads rise. *The Atlanta Journal-Constitution*, June 5, 2003.

LaPuma, J. Managed care ethics: Essays on the impact of managed care on traditional medical ethics. New York: Hatherleigh Press, 1998.

"Managed health care: A brief glossary," Integrated Health care Association, Pleasonton, CA, 1997. Website: www.iha.org.

Carefoote, R. L. Medical Management Signature Series, Managed Care Resources, Inc. 1997. Website: www.mcres.com).

"Managed care and quality management," "Medical management: practice guidelines," "Medical management: oversight."

Konnor, M. Medicine at The crossroads. New York: Vintage Books, 1994.

Duffy, J. A. "Poll: Health advice ignored," *The Atlanta Journal-Constitution,* November 20, 1998.

Zwolak, J. Outside the box. *Tulane Medicine,* September 1995.

Emanual, E. J., & Dubler, N. N. Preserving the physician-patient relationship in the era of managed care. *Journal of the American Medical Association,* Vol. 273, No. 4, January 25, 1995.

Beauchamp, T. L., & Childress, J. F. Principles of biomedical ethics. New York: Oxford University Press,, 1989.

"Principles of Managed Health care," Integrated Health care Association, 1997. Website; www.iha.org.

Friedman, E. The right thing: Ten years of ethics columns from the health care forum journal. San Francisco: Jossey-Bass Publishers, 1996.

LaPuma, J. Understand guiding principles when mixing business, medicine. *Managed Care Magazine,* July 1998.

"What could have saved John Worthy?" The Hastings Center Report, Special Supplement, Vol. 28, No. 4, July–August 1998.

INTERVIEWS

Frank Brescia, MD, professor, Medical University of South Carolina, Charleston, SC.

Joseph DeGross, MD, professor, Mercer University School of Medicine, Macon, GA.

David DeRuyter, MD, pulmonologist, Atlanta, GA.

Daniel Russler, MD, vice president, HBOC, Inc., Atlanta, GA.

CHAPTER 26

Dissecting a Medical Malpractice Trial

Daniel J. Buba

> The scope of medical malpractice victims run the gamut from factory workers, electricians, laborers, carpenters, mechanics, shipyard workers, salesmen, merchant seaman, plumbers and maintenance workers to engineers, stay-at-home moms, doctors, attorneys, military dependents, clergy, and all the cubicle dwellers of the information technology age and beyond.
>
> —Dr. Jay S. Grife, MA, JD
> Medical Malpractice Consultants, Inc.

In the United States, a trial is thought to be the most common manner in which disputes are resolved. Contrary to what we see on television, however, very few cases actually make it to trial. The U.S. Department of Justice recently reported that only about 3% of all civil cases are resolved by a trial. The vast majority of civil lawsuits, and medical malpractice cases are settled or dismissed before any of the litigants see a courtroom.

TRIAL PARTICIPANTS

In every civil trial involving medical malpractice, there is a plaintiff (patient) and a defendant (doctor), collectively called the parties. The plaintiff is the party with the complaint, the accuser, and the defendant is the party against whom a complaint is brought, the accused. Some cases may involve multiple plaintiffs, multiple defendants, or both. Regardless of the numbers of parties, however, there are always two sides to a lawsuit. An attorney usually represents each side, though attorney representation is not always required.

Also participating in the trial are witnesses. Each party presents its case through the use of witnesses. Witnesses serve to tell the story of the parties. The plaintiff or defendant may also be a witness. The parties may also call a special kind of witness, called an expert witness, to testify on their behalf. An expert witness is simply a witness with experience in a particular field, whose testimony will aide the lay jury in understanding certain aspects of the case.

In most medical malpractice cases, the plaintiff must present expert testimony from a health care practitioner that the defendant fell below the standard of care required and caused injury to the patient. The reason for this requirement is that laypersons do not have the expertise to make an unaided determination that a doctor did or did not do anything wrong in treating a patient. The only time when expert medical testimony is not needed in a medical malpractice case is when the issue to be considered is within the realm of a layperson's knowledge. Leaving a surgical instrument in a patient's body or operating on the wrong limb need no expert testimony.

The judge and jury are the final participants in a trial. The judge presides over the trial and makes rulings regarding the law and its application to the case. The jury members are the fact finders. They listen to the evidence and determine the facts. For example, when two parties tell different versions of the same event, the jury decides which side is true. In cases where there is no jury, the judge decides both the law and the facts.

BURDEN OF PROOF

In all civil trials, the plaintiff, as the accuser, has the burden of proving his case. Much like a criminal defendant, a civil defendant has no burden and is presumed innocent of any claim by the plaintiff. As a result, if the plaintiff presents no evidence, or insufficient evidence to support his claim, the defendant wins without having to present his case. The burden the plaintiff carries is that he must prove his case by what is called a preponderance of the evidence. In other words, the plaintiff must prove it is more likely than not that he should win. The best way to visualize this burden is to imagine a set of scales. If the scales are even or tipped in favor of the defendant, then the plaintiff has not carried his burden, and loses. In order to prevail, the plaintiff must tip the scales in his favor.

To prove a case of medical malpractice, a plaintiff-patient must present evidence that the defendant-doctor was negligent, and the plaintiff does this by proving the treatment provided was below the applicable standard of care. The "standard of care" is the care and skill that a reasonably prudent practitioner would provide in treating a patient. It is established by the medical community at large and is constantly evolving. Care that violates the standard of care today may not necessarily violate the standard of care several years ago. This distinction is an important one, since most cases take several years to get to trial. The standard of care is never based on the outcome of the case; a bad result does not necessarily mean a violation of the standard of care.

Expert medical testimony is required to establish a violation of the standard of care in virtually all medical malpractice cases. A plaintiff who fails to present the required expert medical testimony in a medical malpractice case will lose. The plaintiff must also produce expert medical testimony that the alleged negligence caused the injury.

For example, suppose that a patient's widow brings a medical malpractice case against a surgeon who admitted the patient for removal of an AO plate embedded in bone. The plaintiff-widow alleges that the surgeon should have done something to prevent a pulmonary embolism, which occurred 3 days after the patient was dismissed from the hospital, killing him. The patient might have an expert who would testify that she or he would not have removed the AO plate, that she or he should have left it in place. Such testimony does not carry the burden of proving care below the standard required of the surgeon. Indeed, in most cases, the standard of care allows a practitioner to choose from a variety of treatment options within an acceptable range. Mere testimony by an expert witness that "I would have treated this patient differently" is insufficient to establish a breach of the standard of care. The bad result also is not itself proof of any negligence. Nor is there any evidence, in this example, that the doctor caused the patient's death (i.e., that the embolism would not have occurred without the alleged negligence of the surgeon). Therefore, doctor wins on all elements.

Trial Types

There are two types of trials: trial by jury and trial by judge. As noted above, in a trial by jury, the judge determines the law and the jury determines the facts. In a trial by judge—called a "bench" trial—the judge determines both the law and the facts. The U.S. Constitution guarantees a trial by jury. If a party does not request a jury trial, however, the right to a jury trial can be waived.

Most civil cases in the United States are tried by jury. Of the 3% of all cases that go to trial, the Department of Justice reports that about two thirds are jury trials and one third are bench trials.

Whether to try a case to the judge or to a jury is strictly a matter of choice by the litigants. If either party timely requests a jury trial, however, the case must be tried to a jury. Because of the constitutional implications, in most cases, both parties must waive their right to a jury trial in order for the case to be tried to a judge. In a few instances, such as trials for injunctions and family law matters, a jury trial is not an option and a judge must hear the case. However, the majority of civil issues offer the litigants a choice between bench or jury trials.

So why would anyone choose to have a case heard by a judge as opposed to a jury, or vice versa? The reasons are mainly based on preconceived notions about judge and juror biases. Generally, most litigants favor a jury over a judge because the decision is put into the hands of many rather than in the hands of one. Plaintiffs usually like juries because lay individuals are believed to be more sympathetic, and a plaintiff can appeal to the emotions of a jury. Conversely, defendants usually prefer bench trials because a judge is thought to be more objective in deciding a case. Requesting a bench trial can also result in a much quicker trial date. Since court dockets in most large cities are becoming increasingly congested, the time difference between a jury trial date and a bench trial date can be literally years.

None of the perceptions about the benefits of a jury trial or a bench trial apply to all situations—every case is different. There is at least some empirical evidence that some of the commonly held conceptions about bench and jury trials are actually misconceptions. For example, while it is almost universally believed that juries tend to favor plaintiffs and award much higher monetary amounts, a recent study by the Department of Justice[1] suggests that judges favor plaintiffs and return higher verdicts. Still, jury trials outnumber bench trials by about two to one.

---

[1] See Civil Jury Cases and Verdicts in Large Counties, Civil Justice Survey of State Courts at: www.usdoj.gov/bjs/abstract/cjcavilc.htm.

JURY SELECTION

The selection process for a jury begins with what is called the jury pool. A number of citizens are selected as potential jurors, usually several times the number of jurors needed for a trial. From this pool of potential jurors, the jury panel is selected.

The size of the jury panel varies by state and locale. Most juries consist of about 6 to 12 individuals on a panel. In addition, one or more alternate jurors may also be selected. Alternate jurors sit with the jury and hear evidence just as all the other jurors. In some states, they also sit in on jury deliberations, though they are not allowed to participate. If for some reason a member of the panel is unable to continue with the trial or deliberations, the alternate juror fills in. The number of alternate jurors varies, and determining the number is usually left to the discretion of the judge. Generally, the longer the trial, the more alternate jurors.

Before any potential juror appears at the courthouse for a trial, usually a questionnaire form is mailed for the individual to complete and return to the court. Such forms request information such as name, age, occupation, educational background, participation as a party or witness in previous litigation, previous jury service, and so on. Attorneys for the parties are able to obtain and review these questionnaires in advance of the trial date.

On the day of trial, when the potential jurors arrive at the courthouse, the judge typically asks some generic questions about their ability to serve. The judge may ask whether any potential juror has a problem staying for the duration of the trial or whether the potential jurors know any of the parties or their attorneys. The purpose of these questions is for the judge to determine which, if any, of the potential jurors will be excused immediately from service.

Many juries tend to be comprised of citizens with little or no college education. One of the possible reasons for this result is that many professionals, especially medical professionals, request to be excused from jury service, citing their professional commitments as justification. Ironically, professionals are usually the first to complain when juries who lack any representatives with advanced education hear their own cases. Once the judge is finished with the preliminary screening of the jury pool, voir dire begins.

A. Voir Dire: Questioning of the Jurors

Voir dire literally means, "to speak the truth." It is the term used to represent the preliminary questioning of potential jurors. The purpose of voir dire is to uncover any bias in potential jurors. Plaintiffs attorneys in medical malpractice cases will try to determine if the potential jurors have any strong connection to a health care provider, which might make the juror favor the defendant-doctor. Similarly, medical malpractice defense attorneys will try to uncover any bad experiences the potential jurors may have had with a health care practitioner, which might make the juror biased in favor of the patient. The judge, the attorneys, or both can conduct the questioning. Most jurisdictions allow the attorneys to conduct voir dire.

Beyond trying to eliminate bias against their clients, attorneys often use the voir dire process to try to "educate" the jury in their favor. They also use voir dire to begin placing before the potential jurors the theories of the complaint and defense thereto to try to gauge their reactions. Skillful attorneys will tacitly use the questioning process of voir dire to prepare the jury to find in favor of their clients.

B. Challenges of Jurors

When the attorneys and/or the judge have finished questioning the potential jurors, challenges may be made to remove potential jurors from serving on the jury panel. Attorneys use the challenge phase of jury selection to remove jurors who may favor the other side's case. To remove potential jurors, two types of challenges may be made to "strike" the individual from the jury.

The first type of challenge is a challenge for cause. A "for cause" challenge is one in which the attorneys are required to state a reason for removing the potential juror. The reason given is usually that the challenged juror cannot hear the case fairly for one reason or another. For example, a juror may have stated that he or she will not abide by a judge's instructions on the law because he or she does not think the instruction is fair. Such a situation is a clear case to have the juror removed for cause. The number of "for cause" challenges are unlimited, and the judge decides whether to excuse the challenged potential juror. Other challenges for cause may be based on a claim of juror bias. In practice, however, very few for cause challenges based on alleged bias are sustained.

The second type of challenge is a peremptory challenge (note the challenge is *per*emptory, meaning absolute, not *præ*emptory). Each party is given a certain number of peremptory challenges in which to remove any potential juror from the panel. In civil trials, each side generally has two or more peremptory challenges.

No reason is needed to strike a potential juror when using a peremptory challenge, and the individual is automatically excused. The only exception is the strike must be race and gender neutral. Where a pattern of strikes suggests peremptory challenges were used to remove potential jurors because of their race or gender, the entire process must be restarted. Volumes of law journal articles have been written about race- and gender-based peremptory challenges, and an extensive discussion is beyond the scope of this chapter. Suffice to say, objecting to peremptory challenges because they are race- or gender-based is the exception rather than the rule. In most cases, the number of challenges allowed is too small to show any pattern.

C. Jury Selection Logistics

Ordinarily, the jury box is filled with potential jury panel members by randomly selecting names from the pool of potential jurors. When a potential juror is removed by a challenge, that juror is replaced with another member of the jury pool. Each newly selected potential juror is questioned, and then, if appropriate, challenged. When each side has exhausted all of its challenges, the jury selection is complete.

The time to conduct jury selection varies. Supposedly, in the old days, jury questioning would take many days. In our current heavily congested court system, however, most judges limit the voir dire process to just a few hours.

D. Preliminary Instructions to the Jury

Once the jury is selected, the judge will give the jury preliminary instructions. These instructions usually involve statements of the law and the case such as the basic allegations in the lawsuit, which side carries the burden of proof, and the presentation of evidence. The judge will also instruct the jury regarding more general issues such as note taking, limitations on discussing the case, and breaks in the trial. Of course, in a bench trial, no preliminary instructions are necessary. After the judge gives the jury preliminary instructions, the formal presentation of the case begins with opening statements.

OPENING STATEMENTS

The opening statement phase of a civil trial is when the case really begins. Some lawyers very firmly believe that cases are won or lost during opening statements. In this phase, attorneys provide a road map of the trial by telling their client's side of the story, while at the same time trying to convince the jury to find in their client's favor.

Arguments are not allowed during opening statements. Rather, attorneys are only allowed to state what the evidence will show. Most attorneys find this to be a distinction without much of a difference. For example, the statement "Dr. Smith crippled Mrs. Jones by performing unnecessary surgery," could be considered an argument and not allowed during opening statements. Stating "the evidence will show that Dr. Smith crippled Mrs. Jones when he performed unnecessary surgery," however, is not considered an argument because the attorney is merely stating what he believes the evidence will show.

Depending on the complexity of the case, attorneys may use exhibits during opening statements. Such exhibits are not considered evidence but are only illustrative of what each side intends to prove. Some attorneys may even use very technical computerized presentations during opening statements. Any such "props" are fair game as long as the information presented can be described fairly as "what the evidence will show."

The time length for opening statements varies from jurisdiction to jurisdiction and from case to case. Cases that take several weeks to try may involve half-day long or longer opening statements. Cases that take a few days to try—which is probably most cases—involve an hour or so per side for opening statements.

PRESENTATION OF EVIDENCE

A. Witnesses

After the attorneys finish telling the jurors what the evidence will show, the presentation of evidence begins. Evidence is presented primarily by calling witnesses to testify on the client's behalf. The party calling the witness first asks questions during what is called direct examination, or "direct." The opposing party then gets an opportunity to ask questions of the witness during cross examination, or "cross."

Questions on cross must be limited in scope to the questions that were asked on direct. Issues not raised during the direct examination may not be raised. Cross-examination is not required. In some instances, an opposing party may have no questions at all for tactical reasons or because the witness testified to unimportant or uncontested issues.

Following cross-examination, the party calling the witness has an opportunity to conduct redirect examination, or "redirect," and following any redirect, recross examination may take place. Each subsequent examination, however, is limited in scope by the subject matter of the previous examination. The idea is that as each round of questioning is concluded, the focus gets narrower and narrower. Consequently, for example, if no questions were asked on cross, redirect is not allowed. After recross, the process is usually concluded, although on rare occasions a judge may allow further direct and cross if circumstances so warrant.

B. Exhibits

Exhibits are tangible pieces of evidence that are relevant to the case. Medical records, photographs, and objects are common examples of exhibits that may be used at a civil trial. Basically, any tangible object may be used as an exhibit if it will aid the finder of fact in the case.

The introduction of exhibits at trial is done primarily through witnesses. In order for an exhibit to be introduced into evidence, however, a witness must testify that the exhibit to be introduced is authentic, true, and accurate, and it must be relevant to an issue in the case. Such testimony is called foundation testimony. Before any exhibit can be introduced into evidence, a foundation must be laid.

Not all exhibits are introduced into evidence. For example, a skeletal model of the skull may be offered as an exhibit in a neurosurgery injury case because it might aid the jury in understanding the case. The skull model, however, may not be relevant to any issue in the case, and therefore cannot be introduced into evidence. Such an exhibit is called a demonstrative exhibit.

C. Objections

During the course of witness testimony or the attempted introduction of an exhibit into evidence, an attorney may state an objection. The main purpose of an objection is to prevent the presentation of certain information to a jury. Information that is not relevant or otherwise prohibited from being presented to a jury is objectionable. It is important to know that the conduct of a trial is not a wide-open search for the truth. Rather, it is a decision-making process in which the parties present their cases according to rules of evidence and procedure.

For routine objections, the attorneys will make brief statements in open court in support of or in opposition to an objection. The judge will then issue a ruling out loud from the bench. In some situations, however, an attorney may object to potentially damaging testimony that he or she wants to keep from the jury, in which case arguing the objection in open court may reveal the damaging information. In such an instance, the attorneys may ask to approach the bench for a "sidebar." Each attorney then approaches the judge's bench and will discreetly argue the objection out of the jury's earshot. If the objection involves a major issue that requires extensive argument, the judge will excuse the jury from the courtroom so the attorneys can present their arguments out loud and on the record.

If evidence is excluded and an attorney feels the judge's ruling was incorrect, the attorney may make what is called an offer of proof. In this instance, the excluded evidence is presented on the record but out of the presence of the jury. In this way, the evidence is preserved if the party decides to appeal the decision. An offer of proof is rare, but effective, if an appeal is contemplated.

D. Order of Evidence Presentation

Since the plaintiff has the burden of proof, the plaintiff presents his case first. The presentation of the plaintiff's case is called the plaintiff's case-in-chief. The plaintiff's case-in-chief includes what are called the essential elements of the complaint. A failure to present evidence on any one essential element produces a failure of the plaintiff to carry his burden. When the plaintiff finishes presenting his evidence, the defendant has the opportunity to make a motion for what is called a directed verdict.

When a defendant moves for a directed verdict, he is asking the judge to enter a judgment in his favor because the plaintiff failed to present evidence crucial to the plaintiff's case. If the plaintiff has in fact failed to present evidence on a crucial aspect of his case, the judge will enter a verdict in favor of the defense. The case is over, and the defendant need not present his case.

If, however, the plaintiff has presented at least some evidence, regardless of how weak that evidence may be, then a directed verdict motion will be denied. The judge will not substitute his judgment for that of the jury in determining whether evidence is strong enough for the plaintiff to win. In that situation, the defendant will have to present his case-in-chief.

Following the defendant's case-in-chief, the formal presentation of evidence is usually concluded, unless the plaintiff wants to present rebuttal evidence. Rebuttal evidence is evidence that may be presented to address any new issues raised by the defense that were not previously addressed by or disclosed to the plaintiff. The decision of whether to allow rebuttal evidence lies in the judge's discretion. In some cases, surrebuttal evidence, the defendant's "response" to rebuttal evidence, may even be allowed.

CLOSING ARGUMENTS

When each side has concluded its case, closing arguments begin. As with opening statements, the time length allowed varies from case to case and court to court. Unlike opening statements, however, just about anything goes during closing arguments. The parties are free to summarize and—as the name indicates—argue their case during closing in virtually whatever manner they see fit. All exhibits introduced into evidence are free game.

The only limitation during closing arguments is that the attorneys are supposed to confine their arguments to matters that are supported by the evidence. An objection that an attorney is misstating the evidence or arguing an issue not supported by the evidence, however, usually gets the following reply from the judge: "The jury heard the evidence, and knows what it is." In other words, the jury, as the official fact finder, knows whether a closing argument is or is not supported by the evidence. The parties are therefore given great latitude in presenting their closing arguments.

FINAL INSTRUCTIONS

Following closing arguments, the judge usually excuses the jury so that the attorneys can argue over final instructions. Final instructions are the instructions on the law the judge gives to the jury to guide them in reaching a decision. Only instructions of law that are supported by evidence in the case are given, and that is what the attorneys argue about. Each side will try to persuade the judge to read an instruction to the jury that is favorable to its case.

As noted above, the jury, as the fact finders, will determine what they believe to be the true version of the facts presented at the trial. The jury will then apply those facts to the law as provided in the final instructions. For example, a final instruction may read as follows:

> In order for the plaintiff to prevail, the plaintiff must prove that A, B, and C occurred. If you find the plaintiff has proven each of these elements, your verdict must be for the plaintiff. If you find the plaintiff patient has failed to prove even one of these elements, your verdict must be for the defendant doctor.

As with preliminary instructions, final instructions are omitted in a bench trial.

When the judge has decided which final instructions he or she is going to give, the jury is brought back into the courtroom and the final instructions are read. The judge also instructs the jury on the logistics of reaching a decision, such as choosing a foreman and taking breaks. The jury then retires to the jury room to deliberate.

JURY DELIBERATIONS

During jury deliberations, the jury is allowed to discuss the case amongst themselves. If the jury members have followed the judge's preliminary instructions, this will be the first time they discuss the case. Jury research shows that the process of reaching a decision varies widely from jury to jury, as does the time to reach a decision. Like many aspects of the trial process, a lot of conceptions exist about jury deliberations. If the jury deliberates for a relatively short period of time, it is believed they will return a verdict in favor of the defense. This conception comes from the belief that even if the jury quickly decided in favor of the plaintiff, it usually takes a long time to calculate damages. This conception, however, has proven to be a misconception in many cases.

While the jury is deliberating, the parties and their attorneys usually leave the courthouse and wait at a more comfortable location (usually a nearby restaurant, because, for some reason, most jury trials conclude at the end of the day). When the jury returns with a verdict, the parties are contacted to return to the courtroom.

If the jury is unable to reach a verdict, then the jury is hung. The remedy in the case of a hung jury is a new trial. Because most judges (and parties and attorneys) would rather crawl across a room full of broken glass than retry a case, judges will pressure the jury to keep deliberating until they are able to reach a decision. If that fails, the judge declares a mistrial, and a new trial is eventually scheduled.

THE VERDICT

When the jury returns to the courtroom to announce its verdict, the collective hearts of the parties and their attorneys can probably generate a registration on a Richter scale. It is the moment of truth, the climax of the entire trial process. After the verdict is read, either party may poll the jury to verify that each juror supports the decision, though a polling of the jury is always done, if at all, by the losing party.

Once the jury is polled, the losing party can also ask the judge to overturn the jury decision, called a "motion for judgment notwithstanding the verdict," or JNOV (judgment *non obstante veredicto*). A motion for JNOV is only granted if the judge, in hindsight, believes the case should not have been submitted to a jury because there was no evidence that a reasonable person would have credited on an essential element of the plaintiff's case. The judge has the discretion to enter a JNOV, but such discretion is rarely invoked. In most situations, judges are very hesitant to substitute their own judgment for that of the jurors. Once the judge enters a verdict, the trial is over.

A medical malpractice trial is nearly always a roller coaster ride of emotions. When the opposing side is putting on its case, you can feel as though you are being pummeled over the head with a baseball bat and that defeat is inevitable. Moments later, your attorney can perform a stunning cross-examination—and then, victory seems certain. Such is life in our adversarial system, where two parties present the case in a punch–counter-punch format. When the verdict is finally entered, regardless of the outcome, most parties are relieved that it is over. All have a more thorough understanding as to why 97% of civil cases never make it this far.

CHAPTER 27

Selecting Practice Management Advisors Wisely

Hope Rachel Hetico and Rachel Pentin-Maki

> Your representative owes you not his industry, but his judgment; and
> he betrays instead of serving you, if he sacrifices it to your opinion.
>
> —Sir Edmund Burke

There are many self-help publications and management gurus purporting to impart business information to their readers and to their physician clients. Within the current managed care climate, medical business advisors are currently all the rage. However, in the same vein, physician bankruptcies are mounting, medical student-loan delinquencies are increasing, and medical and ancillary practices are closing at record numbers. What gives?

Perhaps the answer lies in the lack of real business, accounting, and financial acumen by the average practitioner. This growing concern is prompting more and more MDs to seek the help of a financial or management consultant. But just what does a practice management consultant do, what credentials are needed to be in the business, and how can a financial advisor help you coordinate all aspects of your practice's life?

Examples of a Major Practice Management Fiasco

As the managed-care crisis exacerbates, there are too many examples of irrational practice-management behavior on the part of physicians, and no specialty is immune. Just reflect a moment on colleagues who were willing to securitize their practices a few years ago and cash out to Wall Street for riches that were not rightly deserved. Where are firms such as MedPartners, Phycor, FPA, and Coastal Health care now? A survey of the Cain Brothers Physician Practice Management Corporation Index of publicly traded PPMCs revealed a market capital loss of more than 95%, since inception.

Examples of a Major Financial Consulting Debacle

Recall the more recent tale of Dr. Debasis Kanjilal, a pediatrician from New York who put more than $500,000 into the dot.com company, InfoSpace, upon the advice of Merrill Lynch's star analyst Henry Bloget. Is it any wonder that when the company crashed, the analyst was sued, and Merrill settled out of court? Other analysts, such as Mary Meeker of Morgan Stanley and Dean Witter and Jack Grubman from Salomon Smith Barney are involved in similar fiascos.

Although sad, these stories are matters of public record. Hopefully, doctors now understand that the big brokerage houses that underwrite and recommend stocks may have credibility problems, and that physicians got burned with the adrenalin rush of "self-directed" portfolios, or relied too heavily on advice from low cost discounters.

More important, can the consultant you eventually hire on a smaller scale help you achieve your financial goals while still practicing medicine in an enjoyable and stress free manner? The answer to this and other questions follow, and the hallmarks of the myriad practitioners of medical management are explained in this chapter.

THE MEDICAL MANAGEMENT REVIEW PROCESS

Medical office management is very individualistic and focuses on the business factors that impact on your practice. Often, it is difficult to separate personal from professional business concerns. In short, management review provides a short-term and long-term strategy, taking into account every aspect of your office situation and how each affects your ability to achieve your objectives. Although constant vigilance is required in this rapidly changing field, the office management process can help you construct the foundation on which to build a secure and satisfying practice future. Accordingly, there are several distinct steps in the comprehensive management review process that should be considered by every business advisor

1. *Clarification of financial circumstances* by gathering all relevant financial data, such as a list of corporate and/or personal and financial assets and liabilities, tax returns, records of securities transactions (stocks, bonds, mutual funds, real estate and other partnerships), insurance policies, restrictive covenants, buy-out and partnership agreements, wills, trusts, IRAs and pension plans, and so on.
2. *Identifying practice goals and objectives* through a careful review of your personal attitudes and values. These may include more new patients to increase market share, increased or decreased frequency of existing patients, capital office improvements, new equipment or an ASC, more revenue per patient, spending more time with patients or for charity work, or just generating more gross revenues or profits. Some MDs may have overlapping or conflicting goals but there are some considerations, such as your net-worth statement, which may be important in determining your best management strategy.
3. *Identifying problems that may impede goals.* These might include too few paying patients or inappropriate payer mix, improper practice location or access, OSHA, the Health Insurance Portability and Accountability Act of 1996 (HIPAA), new or old partners, or inadequate cash flow or deflation. All must be identified before solutions can be explored.
4. *Constructing a written plan,* which can vary in length within the complexity of your current practice situation. It can be broad, like a general business or financial plan, or focused, like a marketing plan.

5. *Implementation,* since theoretical formulation is often easier than the actual execution of a plan. Why? Execution often delays current gratification in favor of future consumption. This may be hard to swallow in society's current attitude of immediate gratification and conspicuous consumption.

6. *Periodic review,* with the date used to create it. Just as health care is a rapidly changing environment, decreasing profits, marriage, death, divorce, eMR implementation, or poorly managed care contracting and negotiation strategies may signal a needed for the reformation of your plan.

CHARACTERISTICS OF GOOD PRACTICE MANAGEMENT REVIEW

Generally, although the presentation and style may vary, a well thought out and comprehensive management review should contain at least the following 10 elements. This should be obtained by completing a confidential business financial or data gathering questionnaire or by personal interview. Remember the adage, garbage in = garbage out, and recall that the review will only be as good as the information used to perform it.

1. *Goals and Objectives with Practice Data.* This means business data and a prioritization of your goals, with estimated time line and economic benchmarks for achieving them. For example, you may not expect to jump-start your practice over night, but it is not unreasonable to improve its efficiency and profitability over in a short time. Or, you may be able to decrease variable costs now, and slowly reduce fixed costs in the long run.

2. *Special Issues.* May include: illness, practice continuation, or buy/sell agreements. Especially noteworthy, according to Dr. Rex Huber, MBA, a professional practice management consultant in Minneapolis, Minnesota, "are the myriad new concerns involving practice mergers, acquisitions, antitrust, IPA, or regional network contracting issues."

3. *Business Economic Assumptions.* Will change over time but will usually include such items as medical specialty focus, payer and inflation factors and real rates of return, personal and corporate risk assumptions, geographic location and demographics, reimbursement rates, inflation, economic indicators, training, and age and sex, as well as personal risk tolerance or aversion.

4. *Consolidated Financial Statements.* Should include at least the last three annual corporate financial statements (balance sheet, net-income statement, and statement of cash flows) with tax returns.

   According to Dr. William P. Scherer, MS, who heads a computer-based testing firm in Ft. Lauderdale, "Initially, financial software such as Quicken-R made the creation of consolidated financial statements a pleasure, rather than a chore. But now, there are many application service providers (ASPs) to outsource this function."

5. *Net Worth Statement.* Net worth on the balance sheet represents practice equity levels obtained by subtracting short term and/or long term liabilities from assets at a particular point in time, as well as future estimates and projections. Practice net worth however, is not income—professional expenses are paid out of cash flows, not net worth. Nevertheless, more is usually better, except

when assets are overstated or liabilities are under reported. Physician practices are increasingly prone to show high gross incomes but low profit margins and net worth because of this problem.

6. *Income Taxation.* Should include, but may not be limited to, a review of corporate and personal income tax statements for all relevant years. This should include deductions, credits, and tax liability and rates, especially EGTRRA 2001 and the Bush Tax Act of May, 2003.

7. *Insurance and Risk Management.* This minimally should include an analysis of your personal and corporate financial exposure, relative to malpractice liability, morbidity, property-casualty, health, life, annuity, long-term care, buy-sell and key-person agreements, and disability insurance. It should also include an analysis of corporate buy/sell agreements and a review of all polices in force.

8. *Benefits and Retirement Planning.* Contains an evaluation of all traditional and Roth IRAs, SEPs, 401-Ks, 403-Bs, annuities, social security projected benefits, and personal pension and profit sharing plans of both the defined contribution and defined benefit types. A comparison should also be made of the taxable and tax-exempt rates of returns for these investment vehicles.

9. *Operational Audits.* Should generally include a review of most of the following processes: patient flow and controls, accounts receivable and cash management, fee schedule review with CPT and ICD-9 coding and compliance, IT and security, cost expense analysis, practice financial ratio creation and analysis, marketing and advertising plans, stationary, profit maximization and reimbursement issues, human resource issues and workplace violence, insurance and third-party payer processing and controls, personnel polices, administration, job structure, and benefits and productivity reviews; as well as any special concerns of the practice.

10. *Recommendations.* Implementation and follow-up: Oral and written communication between you and your consultant is important in order to understand, execute, and achieve your management goals and the costs associated with them, as well as the risks and benefits of each.

A prioritized schedule and action list is used to implement or reject recommendations for these 10 items.

In short, the practice management planning process denotes the method of how individuals can meet their business goals through proper management of resources. It is a broad-based approach that distinguishes the exceptional management consultant from other professions or nonintegrated advisors who typically focus on only a single area of the management picture.

ADVISOR CREDENTIALS AND CRITERIA

As you begin your search for a business advisor, call and ask for a short initial meeting with prospective advisors, which should be free of charge. Just as you would select your own physician or clergyman, you should base your decision on an advisor on comfort, credentials, experience, and, especially, education. Fee schedules are probably of least importance. By asking the following questions, you stand the best chance of finding an advisor that's right for your budget, practice, and personality.

Business Designations

What designation(s) should the advisor possess? Realize that the absolute terms *business advisor, practice management consultant,* and *business or financial planner* have no real meaning in terms of implying credentials, education, or standards! Anyone can use these terms and get into the advisory business—your brother, your neighbor, or the engineer down the street. Advisors of this nature are increasingly used by stockbrokers, bankers, and insurance agents and may or may not add value to your practice; also, keep in mind that they may be commissioned salespeople. Therefore, the following nomenclature is worthwhile to know:

CPE/CHE

The designations *Certified Physician Executive(CPE)* or *Certified Health Care Executive (CHE),* which are awarded by the Certifying Commission in Medical Management (CCMM: 4890 West Kennedy Blvd., #200, Tampa, Florida 33609-2575, phone: (813) 287-8944), may be earned by those physicians or lay professionals with the requisite requirements in education and demonstrated special competence and professional experience in the field of medical management. Specific requirements for certification include (1) current stature as a physician (MD/DO), or working lay professional; (2) completion of the American College of Physician Executive's *Graduate Program in Medical Management (GPPM), or,* completion of an accredited graduate management degree program (i.e., MBA, MHA, MPH, etc.), *or* completion of 200 hours of management education, with 120 hours of a core curriculum from the GPMM; (3) at least 1 year of medical management experience; or (4) completion of an approved week-long CPE tutorial program.

Upon receipt of the CPE designation, diplomate, fellowship, and distinguished fellowship status may be sought.

American College of Physician Executives (FACPE)

FACPE offers several educational programs over the entire field of medical management, such as certification curricula, master's degree programs at Tulane or Carnegie Mellon universities, CEUs, and other advanced standing or fellowship educational programs. A similar program for nonphysicians may lead to the designation Fellow of the American College of Hospital Executives (FACHE).

Certified Medical Planner (CMP©)

The certified medical planner (CMP©) mark is a rigorous new designation awarded to advisors who have successfully completed all requirements put forth by the Institute of Medical Business Advisors, Inc. (www.MedicalBusinessAdvisors.com). To obtain the CMP© certification, the following qualifications must be met:

- **Education.** An advisor must successfully complete a 20 course 12-month long intensive curriculum of accredited didactic material in order to sit for the MBA Board's Certification Examination. Medical practice management topics include: health care economics, managed-care reimbursement systems, setting up a medical office, physician unions, sexual harassment and workplace violence issues, insurance coding and billing, capitation econometrics, office expense models, marketing, advertising, sales and branding, cash-flow analysis, Medicare and Medicaid, HMOs, PPMCs, MSAs, IPAs, HIPAA, OSHA, ASCs, APCs, activity-based medical office costing, practice financial benchmarking, medical business decision making, fixed rate reimbursement, office compliance and medical credentialing, and others. Financial planning includes areas such as estate planning, retirement planning, investment management, tax planning, employee benefits, risk management, insurance, medical-practice valuation and sales, office-succession planning, and others (info@ MedicalBusinessAdvisors.com).
- **Examination.** An advisor must pass the MBA Board Certification Examination, which tests the knowledge of a multitude of integrated medical practice management and financial planning topics. Thereafter, a CMP© must obtain continuing education credit every two years, in the body of knowledge pertaining to core integrated principles.
- **Experience.** An advisor must acquire at least five years of management consulting and/or financial planning-related experience with physicians and medical professionals.
- **Ethics.** An advisor must voluntarily ascribe to the MBA Board's Code of Ethics and confidentiality, if also a CFP©. This voluntary decision empowers the MBA Board to take action if a CMP© holder should violate the code of ethics. Such violations could lead to disciplinary action, including the permanent revocation of the right to use the CMP© marks. http://www.fpanet.org/journal/Between TheIssues/Links/UsefulLinks/pracmgtlinks.cfm

CLU/ChFC/NAPFA

No one, especially doctors, likes to pay life and disability insurance premiums. Inadequate coverage, however, can completely devastate your family or medical practice, by quickly wiping out a lifetime of asset accumulation and business equity. Buying and maintaining the right amount and type of coverage from solid insurance companies at a reasonable price eliminates these risks in a very efficient manner. Unfortunately, an essential and relatively simple concept like this risk transfer has evolved into an area that makes many doctors downright queasy.

The easiest way to handle this issue is to get consensus agreement from the core team members as to the amount and types of coverage. Once that is accomplished, appropriate agents can be contacted. The agents could be captive agents with insurance companies with policies known to be good for the coverage in question. Otherwise, independent agents with access to a large number of companies and products can be contacted. Regardless, in addition to the usual questioning regarding competence and a background check, the agent should be aware that the core team will review all proposals. Proposals should include what is known as a ledger statement.

A chartered life underwriter (CLU), as granted by the American College, or chartered financial consultant (ChFC), are valid insurance designations demonstrating a focused expertise in the insurance business. But, these still are typically commission sales *agents* who work for their respective firms, or themselves, but not necessarily for you. The saying goes, "insurance is sold, not bought." They sell all sorts of personal and business insurance. Most recently, according to Beverly Brooks, president of the American Society of CLU and ChFC, in Bryn Mawr, Pennsylvania, the society has reconsidered its own strategy of insurance agents as the organization has changed its name to the Society of Financial Services Professionals to appeal to a broader base of financial practitioners beyond the insurance products it has traditionally provided. Finally, the National Association of Personal Financial Advisors (NAPFA) was formed in the 1980s, and the more than 800 NAPFA members are compensated on a fee-only basis.

Property and Casualty Insurance Agent

A good property and casualty (P&C) agent is needed to protect your home and business. The P&C agent should have an array of carriers with which the practice can be placed. One should not hesitate to place different types of coverage with different insurers. Most insurance companies will offer a discount if you place multiple coverage with them. However, this may not be as beneficial as insuring each need with a specialist.

Registered Representative

A retail or discount stock broker, regardless of compensation schedule, is also known as a registered representative. Other names include financial advisor, financial consultant, financial planner, vice president, and so on. Typically, the rigorous national test known as a Series #7 (General Securities License) examination, and state specific Series #63 license is needed, along with Securities Exchange Commission (SEC) registration through the National Association of Securities Dealers (NASD) to become a stockbroker. Since a commission may be involved and performance based incentives are allowed, be aware of costs.

Registered Investment Advisor

This securities license, obtained after passing the Series #65 examination, allows the designee to charge for giving unbiased securities advice on retirement plans and portfolio management, although not necessarily sell securities or insurance products. An RIA is also usually a fiduciary, while a RR, financial consultant, or stockbroker is not.

Certified Public Accountant (CPA)/Enrolled Agent (EA)/Certified Managerial Accountant (CMA)

A CPA, EA, CMA provides retroactive tax and financial accounting and proactive cost accounting information, respectively. Increasingly, in the medical managed care environment, the role of the CPA is yielding to the CMA or MBA, while EAs (usually former IRS agents with comprehensive knowledge of the tax code) can file your tax returns and are licensed to practice before the IRS. Do not expect EA fees to be necessarily lower than CPA tax rates.

However, for tax accounting, it seems that the higher the earnings the more complicated the tax code can become. Doctors in private practice, for instance, have an entirely different tax structure than do other business owners. In general, hiring an accountant to do your taxes is a smart financial decision. One gains expertise, leverages time, and obtains a higher level of accountability. Hiring an accountant for tax preparation, however, is only the tip of the iceberg.

Today's accounting firms provide a number of valuable services to physicians from bookkeeping to payroll to retirement plan administration and record keeping to business consulting.

The rules for selecting an accountant are the same as for selecting any other advisor. The search is for a specialist in the areas that require assistance. A CPA alone cannot provide all the services one may need. Each CPA being considered should be able to stand up to the scrutiny applied to any other role on the medical management team (www.aicpa.org). Ask lots of questions.

- How long have you been providing the services in question?
- Looking at my return from last year, how do I compare to your typical physician client?
- How do you get paid and what services do you provide outside of tax season?
- What would prompt you to refer me to another accountant?
- Will anyone else work on my return? (One should make sure that if part of the work is handed off to a support staff member, the accountant being interviewed will adequately supervise and review the work.)
- Do you provide tax planning services? If so, when do you prefer to render such? (If the accountant plans to give tax-planning advice only when doctors come in to get their return done, one must question whether a sufficient amount of time and attention will be available to render such advice.)
- How aggressive do you consider yourself with regard to deductions? (The accountant's disposition should match that of the client.)
- Are you conversant in the laws of the other states in which I am subject to tax?
- What percentage of the returns you have filed has been audited? (Some firms have quite a reputation with the IRS. An audit rate of over 2%–3% may warrant some concern.)
- Who will represent me in front of the IRS? (It does not have to be the accountant that prepares the return, but it should be someone with experience.)
- If you cause a problem with my return, will you cover the interest and penalties? This is a loaded question that may make the accountant a bit uncomfortable. If they get indignant or try to dismiss it out of hand as if they never make mistakes, look elsewhere.
- How do you resolve complaints, and how do I terminate the relationship?
- Are you willing to take a subordinate role to my other advisors?

Certification in Financial Planning (CFP©)

The premier personal financial planning designation of choice for the Financial Planning Association (FPA), located in Atlanta and founded in 1969, is board Certification in Financial Planning (CFP©).

This independent designation represents a professional who has completed a grueling 24-month course of study at an accredited institution and passed the exhausting two-day comprehensive Certified Financial Planner Board of Standards Examination. This test encompasses all aspects of the financial planning process, including insurance, economic principles, taxation, investments and retirement benefits planning. CFP©s may also work with JDs on estate planning or MBAs in business continuation issues. An ethics, continuing education and a confidentiality requirement is also mandated for this designation. (www.FPANet.org).

Chartered Financial Analysis© (CFA©)

A CFA© will usually work for a brokerage house and follow one or a few publicly traded companies. CFA© analysts may manage institutional money or run a mutual fund and have ethics requirements. Unfortunately, the previously unbiased nature of some Wall Street experts has been questioned lately with the collapse of such stocks as HealthSouth and others. Some authorities now feel that analysts have become merely promoters of the followed company, since sell recommendations are rarely made and non-CFAs may cozy up to insiders and corporate executives as they curry their favor. Contact the Association for Investment Management and Research (www.AIMR.org).

Health Care Quality Designations

ABQAURP

The American Board of Quality Assurance and Utilization Review Physicians (ABQAURP) (Professionals), certify diplomates who are MDs, DOs, DDSs, DMDs, DPMs, or other human service or health care professionals, such as RNs or PhDs. The ABQAURP board is accredited by the American Council for Continuing Medical Education (ACCME) to sponsor the program. Holders of the designation are distinguished by their knowledge of such diverse fields as case and risk management, managed care, credentialing and physician profiling, Workers' Compensation and medical ethics, ERISA, OBRA, CLIA, and Stark II antitrust laws, as well as NCQA, HEDIS, and Total Quality Assurance (TQA) principles and practices (48900 W. Kennedy Blvd., # 260, Tampa, Florida 33609 phone: (813)-286-4411).

CPHQ

The mission of the National Association for Health care Quality (NAHQ) is to improve health care by advancing the theory and practice of quality management in Health care organizations and by supporting the professional growth and development of Health care quality management professionals. The association has about 10,000 members and was established in 1976.

It has specialties in infection control, medical and staff records, nursing, risk management, utilization review and CQI/TQM. Annual educational conferences are available, along with integrated educational courses, the quarterly newsletter NAHQ News, and the bimonthly publication, *Journal for Health care Quality*. The NAHQ certification program, confers the designation Certified Professional in Health care Quality to members, and is accredited by the National Organization for Competency and National Commission for Health Certifying Agencies. It has certified more than 5,000 individuals. The NAHQ has liaison relationships with allied organizations, such as the American Hospital Association, JCAHO, National Health Council, and the National Association of Medical Staff Services. It has working relationships with the American Health Information Management Association, Health care Financial Management Association, and the U.S. Department of Health and Human Services. Corporate headquarters are at 5700 Old Orchard Road, first floor, Skokie, Illinois, 60077 (phone: (708) 966-9392).

Professional Education. What education and degree(s) does the planner possess, and in what field? The following nomenclature is worthwhile to know:

Masters of Business/Health Care/Hospital Administration (MBA/MHA)

An MBA or an MHA is probably the ideal complement to real-life experience, especially when combined with other insurance, investment advisory, and securities licenses. In fact, a subspecialty in finance, managerial or cost accounting, or health or hospital administration provides exceptional planning and investment-advisory credentials.

JD

Attorneys with a health and managed care background may provide valuable advice on such topics as: antitrust and corporate compliance, health care transactions, contracts and litigation, credentialing and peer review, federal and state fraud and abuse, elder care law, professional liability and malpractice defense, ERISA and welfare benefits, and third-party payments. They may also work with CFPs or MBAs on investment, retirement, and estate planning issues.

Beyond receiving a referral, contact your state bar association to obtain a list of qualified names. The search should be confined to attorneys specializing in the area of law that needs attention. The *Martindale-Hubbell Law Directory* is a complete listing of domestic and international lawyers by state and specialty. Questions to ask have a familiar ring:

- How long have you been practicing your specialty?
- Under what circumstances will you refer me to another lawyer or hand over my case?
- Will anyone else be working on this?
- How do you get paid, what is your background, and what other costs might I incur?
- How can I terminate this relationship?
- Have you ever had a complaint filed against you, or have you ever been sued for malpractice?
- Can you describe the general process for resolving my case?
- Are you willing to take a subordinate role to my other advisors?

Lawyers have a unique standard of advocacy and confidentiality in our society. The choice of a lawyer is accordingly a very important one. The ideal attorney is one that is pleasant to be around, though not a "yes" man, and who will also serve as a relentless advocate for you and your practice.

Expertise. Remember, there are only two types of experience, *good* and *bad*. Therefore, it may be worthwhile to recall that experience does matter, but only in the context of appropriate information and performance. After all, all physicians had to treat their first patient before a professional career was begun! For example, you may feel that an advisor that specializes in working with physicians represents a real value added service, or you may not think so. Admittedly, more and more advisors are beginning to understand the plight of modern physicians, so it might behoove you seek a consultant familiar with the risks and benefits of managed medical care.

Medical Management Education

The Center for Education in Medical Practice Management (CEMPM) is the source of all educational development and programming for the Medical Group Management Association (MGMA), American College of Medical Practice Executives and the Center for Research in Ambulatory Health care Administration (CRAHCA). The CEMPM comprises the knowledge base of all facets of the MGMA, ACMPE, and CRAHCA and is an experienced provider of education, focusing on the management and leadership of medical group practices and their strategic partners.

The Financial Management Society (FMS) was created by the MGMA in 1986 to meet the needs of managers/administrators involved in the financial aspects of a medical group practice

The Managed Care Assembly (MCA), of the MGMA, was previously known as the PrePaid Health care Assembly. The MCA was founded in 1981 to respond to the needs of MGMA members participating in capitated health care contracts.

Medical Business Advisors, Inc., was founded in 1995 as a resource center and referral exchange for physicians. It has recently launched its online CMP© educational certification program. The firm also produces textbooks, CD-ROMs and other medical-management tools for beleaguered physicians (www.MedicalBusinessAdvisors.com).

Bankers

Doctors carry notoriously heavy debt loads. Beyond the costs of a medical education are substantial costs for equipping and staffing a practice. Technology changes fast these days, and capital is required frequently.

Unfortunately, bankers are very conservative by nature. It may be increasingly difficult to borrow money, especially since modern bankers know that a medical degree is no longer the guarantee of a steady and high income that it once was. As more than one banker has often opined, "We don't usually loan money to doctors who really need it." They may also not have a clue about what the practitioner can do to better compete in the managed care arena. Bankers do have a good concept of local community politics, however, for those not familiar with a practice venue. They frequently can provide references to more focused advisors, and bankers generally do not charge a fee for their advice. The more business one does with a bank, the better the terms that can be obtained.

Real Estate Agents

Real estate agents come in all sorts of forms. A good one shortens the sales cycle immensely. The choice of agent should consider both the size of the real estate agency and the experience of the agent. The agent desired is not a part-timer, nor someone with only a couple of year's experience. Further, the agent should be focused on the price range and type of property in question. A good agent asks lots of questions in order to try to keep physician buyers or sellers from looking at properties that do not match what is wanted. When choosing a *listing agent,* the size and number of listings an agency maintains is an important consideration: the more the better. When interviewing an agent to sell a piece of property, ask about how they get and handle potential buyers. The essential question is, Would someone buy from this person?

Networks. A business advisor should work with a host of trusted and competent other professionals, such as those described above, for the best results. In the final analysis, the MD is considered captain of his or her the practice. It also goes without saying that your advisor should have errors and omissions (E&O) insurance, since he or she is creating and maintaining a chart on your case, just like the medical chart you create for your patients. In cases of dispute, items not documented in the chart likely do not exist.

Medical Management Resources. The following resources offer a variety of service consultants, information, and products to the economically harassed American health care provider. As always in these matters, *caveat emptor!*

Managed Care

- Apollo Managed Care Consultants www.apollomanagedcare.com
- InterStudy Publications www.hmodata.com
- Managed Care Information Center www.themcic.com
- Managed Care Marketplace.com is designed to provide information on companies that provide products and services to payors, purchasers, and providers. www.managedcaremarketplace.com
- Managed Care On-Line www.mcol.com
- MathMEDics www.mathemedics.com
- National Health Information www.nhionline.net
- Plexis Health care Systems www.plexisweb.com

Hospital & Health-System Management

- Cirdadian Information www.circadian.com/learning_center
- Joint Commission on Accreditation of Healthcare Organizations www.jcaho.org
- National Center for Health Statistics. Information on data and studies at www.cdc.gov/nchswww
- Opus Communications www.opuscomm.com
- National Institutes of Health. Information on grants and other resources at www.nih.gov

Health Law & Regulation

- Department of Health and Human Services. Information on the agency at www.os.dhhs.gov
- Health Care Financing Administration. Reports, data, and general information at www.hcfa.gov.
- Strafford Publications www.straffordpub.com.

Behavioral Health Care

- Manisses Communications: www.manisses.com.
- Therapistnet: www.therapistnet.org.

Clinical Care & Outcomes

- Agency for Health Care Policy and Research. Information on guidelines and outcomes at www.ahcpr.gov.
- Clinical Performance & Quality Health Care. Addresses the topics of clinical performance and quality health care at www.mcb.co.uk/cpqhc.htm.
- Healthweb. Lists medical libraries with topic-specific sites at www.health-web.org.
- Institute of Medicine. Information on studies and reports at www.nas.edu/iom.
- Medical Matrix. Ranks resources that are peer reviewed at www.medmatrix.com.
- National Library of Medicine. Information about publications and databases at www.nlm.nih.gov.
- PubMed. The National Library of Medicine's Web version of MedLine at www.ncbi.nlm.nih.gov/pubmed.

Health Care Information Technology

The Superior Consultant Company (SUPC-NASD) is a leader in health care IT consulting, IT outsourcing, and management consulting solutions for hospitals and health systems, integrated delivery networks, and other providers of care; payers; technology firms; health plans; and state and federal government agencies (www.SuperiorConsultant.com).

Health Care Industry

- AHA Central Office. ICD Medical Codes for Medical Transcription & Billing at www.ahacentraloffice.org.
- AHAData.com. www.ahadata.com.
- Alternative Link. www.alternativelink.com.
- CenterWatch. Information on clinical trials at www.centerwatch.com.
- Digital Health care Limited. Advanced digital systems for the health care market at http://www.digital-health care.com/
- Electronic Policy Network. www.epn.org.
- Pharmaceutical Information Network. Information on meetings, drug data, and resources at http://pharminfo.com.

- Pharmalicensing. Definitive resource for the pharmaceutical and biotech licensing executive. http://www.pharmalicensing.com.
- Psybermetrics. http://www.psybermetrics.com.

Health Care Associations

- Academy for International Health Studies www.AIHS.com
- American Academy of Managed Care Pharmacy www.amcp.org
- American Association of Health Plans www.aahp.org
- American College of Health Care Administrators www.achca.org
- American College of Health care Executives www.ache.org
- American College of Physician Executives www.acpe.org
- American Health Information Management Association www.ahima.org
- American Society for Health care Risk Management at www.ashrm.org
- College of Health care Information Management Executives www.cio-chime.org
- Health Care Compliance Association www.hcca-info.org
- Healthcare Financial Management Association www.hfma.org
- Healthcare Information and Management Systems Society www.himss.org
- Integrated Health care Association www.iha.org
- Institute of Medical Business Advisors, Inc. www.MedicalBusinessAdvisors.com
- Medical Association of Billers www.physicianswebsites.com
- Medical Group Management Association. Information on conferences and publications at www.mgma.com.
- National Association of Health care Access Management. http://www.naham.org.
- National Association of Physician Recruiters www.napr.org

THE ROLE OF TEAMWORK IN MEDICAL MANAGEMENT CONSULTING

The major practice management players have been assembled. Will the team function together well enough to assist your practice? Getting them on your advisory team to function well together may seem like a daunting task. In reality, it should be the easiest part of the process.

After taking the time to select the advisors, one should have a team comprised of competent ethical professionals who have shown that they communicate effectively. It is likely that, if these people are as good as they seem, they may already know each other and may have worked with each other. Moreover, good advisors want to learn more. They feed off good interaction with other advisors because it makes them better able to identify and address issues with their doctor clients.

This is not to say that merely hiring people adept in their particular field is all that is necessary for the development of good teamwork. There are steps that can be taken to help foster an appropriate level of teamwork.

- Designate the quarterback. Typically, the MBA, CFP©, CPA, or CMP© has the professional mandate to coordinate a doctor's business and financial affairs from the big picture perspective. Regardless, the quarterback must hand the ball off to the other players to get the job done properly.

- Make sure the players know about each other, and define everyone's role and communicate your wishes to all the advisors.
- Meet as a group on occasion, and tolerate no arguments. The advisors should not debate the issues at hand in the client's presence in a manner that is of a personal nature. This unprofessional behavior should force reconsideration of the advisor in question.
- Make the advisors clarify confusing issues. Sometimes a client, in a way that is not entirely accurate, may tell team member A what another team member B said regarding an issue. The inaccuracy might confuse A, who is now getting the information from the client. This happens frequently because the client is not an expert. A should call B directly to clarify. If instead A badmouths B, there may be a problem with team chemistry. Call team member C for an opinion. If a change is desired, elicit the help of the remaining team members to find a replacement, perhaps your second choice originally.
- Always remember, and remind people if necessary, the doctor client is the boss.

Once the core of the team is in place, other people will be needed from time to time—most commonly, attorneys, bankers, and real estate agents. To assemble these other players, one should get feedback from the core advisors. All other things being equal, an independent provider is usually better, the exception being the banker.

ADVISOR FEE SCHEDULES

Most management consultants charge for their services in one of three ways: (1) fee only, (2) commission only, or (3) a blended schedule. Typical hourly fees range from: $100–$350/hour; while insurance and broker commission rates vary from: 1%–7% and cost efficiency experts may garner one third of all cost savings the first year. Most clients prefer the blended approach so that they can pick and choose products and services depending or personal circumstances. An honest consultant will not only inform you of his fee schedule and scope of work, but empower you to produce the best outcome for the least cost. For example, a medical practice valuation may cost $5–$25 thousand dollars but return 5–10 times that amount. Remember, it is perfectly reasonable to compensate a business consultant who works with you to achieve your practice's business goals.

CONTEMPORANEOUS HEALTH CARE CONSULTING FIELDS FOR PHYSICIANS AND GROUP PRACTICE MANAGERS

On the other hand, if you, as a medical practitioner with specific expertise in a particular administrative area, are interested in working as a management consultant, the following health care facilitators and fields are on the upswing, according to Susan A. Cejka, president, Cejka & Co., a national health care search firm for physician executives. Usually, real world experience is as important as advanced degrees or designations:

- *Assemblers.* Organize physicians and physician organizations in a single or multi-specialty group-practice setting.
- *Care Managers.* Triage leaders for fields such as nursing, physical therapy, oncology, and electronic-data interchange.
- *Financial/Capitation Analysts.* Reviews financial ratios and crunch capitation numbers, utilization rates, and other economic numerics on a large scale.
- *Integrators.* Serve to decouple the recent wave of practice mergers and acquisitions, since some have failed and experts are needed to undo the damage—especially in the hospital or PHO setting. Efficiency and capacity utilization expertise and reengineering are included in this employment model.
- *Insurance Experts.* Require large-scale capitation contracting experience and negotiating skills to integrate the myriad of existing networked managed medical care products of the future.

Moreover, you must have the flexible mindset to bridge the gap between the clinical world of medicine and the administrative world of business. According to the MGMA, the following chart modification represents a descriptive contract between physician/clinicians and physician/administrators.

Clinicians vs. Administrators

PHYSICIAN/CLINICIAN	PHYSICIAN/ADMINISTRATOR
*Physiologic and anatomic disorders	*Health organization with finite budgets
*Defined specialty and scope	*Generalists in business knowledge
*Individuals and patients	*Trends and cohorts
*Science and medicine	*Finance, accounting and business
*Slow change with flexibility	*Rapid change with flexibility
*Short term goals	*Long-term strategic plans
*One-on-one interactions	*Group dynamics/organizational structure
*Independent	*Dependent
*Performer (action)	*Delegator (assignor)

Contemporaneously, the just released Management Compensation Survey (2002) of MGMA reported that compensation was essentially unchanged for many key medical group-practice manager positions. For example, compensation rose about $2,500 for CEOs and administrators of groups with 7 or more FTE physicians, and about $1,000 for administrators with 6 or fewer FTE physicians. Compensation for other core management positions marginally increased, from about 1%–5%, such as chief operating officer (COO), $82,000; chief financial officer (CFO), $73,000; business office manager, $41,000; and medical office manager, $37,000. Moreover, according to Jerome T. Henry, MBA, MSHA, of the MGMA, "With more physicians participating in MSOs, PPMCs or other outside management entities, there is a significant demand for qualified managers. When an MSO or PPMC wants to hire proven talent, they appear willing to pay a top salary." Accordingly, compensation for physician executives, who spend at least 50% of their time in administrative duties, saw minor pay increases last year. CEOs made about $255,000, and medical directors made $187,000, up 5% and 4.3%, respectively. But, turnover and burnout, may be rapid in these fields.

For those physicians serious about developing a consulting career, a variety of insurance products may be required for your own protection. These might include the following policies, as offered by Executive Risk (phone: (860) 408-2000, or www.execrisk.com).

- Health care consultants professional liability insurance.
- Medical directors and officers liability insurance (private and public companies) for health care and managed care organizations.
- Employment practices liability insurance for health care organizations.
- Managed care errors and omissions liability coverage.
- Employment practices, crime, and fiduciary liability insurance.
- Antitrust, staff privilege discrimination, and restraint of trade conspiracy insurance.
- Credentialing, peer review, and miscellaneous professional liability insurance.
- Diversified errors and omission insurance.

In addition, be aware that several states (Maryland, Mississippi, New Jersey, and Ohio) are now considering legislature to make certain decision making/denying medical directors/consultants responsible for care. In effect, such bills make physician executives/consultants as responsible as attending physicians when action, or lack of it, causes patient harm. Therefore, malpractice liability riders are important in this regard.

CONCLUSION

Despite the fact that some physicians and lay professionals believe that they can employ all aspects of the practice management planning process without professional guidance, history seems to suggest otherwise. In fact, the competitive health care marketplace of today mandates not only credible practice management advice, but experienced skills, as well. Savvy advice, if executed properly, is often worth its weight in gold, and it is a shame that more doctors do not recognize this fact, even as their incomes are plummeting.

Remember, just because you are a very good doctor doesn't mean that you are a business management or financial guru. Arrange to have a qualified management consultant, Certified Financial Planner©, and/or Certified Medical Planner© on retainer before its too late.

AGENCIES FOR PRACTICE MANAGEMENT ASSISTANCE

- Atwater Consulting and Recruiting: (888) 227-1118 or www.healthjobs.com
- American College of Physician Executives: (813)-287-2000

- Doctor's Advisory Network (MA): Attorneys and consultants.
- American Academy of Family Physicians: Network of Consultants.
- Consumer Credit Counsel (CCC): (800)-388-2227
- ICON (Interactive Career Opportunity Network: 1-877-877-MGMA
- Tax Assistance: (800)-829-1040
- National Fraud Exchange: (800) 822-0416 Ext.: 33
- CFP Board of Standards: (303)-830-7543
- Institute for Investment Management Consultants: (800) 449-4462
- Investment Management Consultants Association: (303) 770-3377
- International Association for Financial Planning (IAFP): 800-945-IAFP
- Institute of Medical Business Advisors, Inc.: (770) 448-0769
- Medical Group Management Association: (303)-799-1111
- Securities Exchange Commission (SEC): (202)-272-3100
- National Association of Securities Dealers (NASD): (800)-289-9999

Physician-Practice Management Systems

Physician-Practice Management Systems—*These organizations provide medical-practice management services, including financial, administrative, and clinical services. Many include consulting services, billing components, accounting/finance, electronic medical records, and other related services for physician practices. Several include physician data-system design and engineering.*

CPU Medical Management Systems
(An ASP medical practice management system)
9235 Activity Road
Suite 104
San Diego, CA 92126
www.CPUmms.com

IDX Systems Corporation
(An integrated clinical, financial, administrative, scheduling, billing, and managed care Internet based practice management solution)
401 IDX Drive
Burlington, VT 05402
www.IDX.com

Data Solutions and Services, Inc.
(Data processing design and implementation solutions)
1807 Britton Lane
Montgomery, AL 36106
www.Datasolutions1.com

Vital Works, Inc.
(A management software solution to include financial, clinical, billing, prescription writing, registration, automated data entry and PDA integration)
Ridgefield, CT
www.Vitalworks.com

Medisoft
(Insurance billing software with electronic submission, AR tracking, billing, accounting and practice management)

916 E. Baseline Road
Mesa, AZ 85204
www.Medisoft.com

McKesson HBOC, Inc.
Physician Office Manager
(Includes software for patient information at point of contact, practice management,
eligibility, registration and scheduling, and managed care contracts)
One Post Street
San Francisco, CA 30005
www.HBOC.com

Medic Computer Systems
(Physician practice management system to include financial, administrative, clinical,
and managed care)
8529 Six Forks Road
Raleigh, NC 27615
www.Medic.com

Advanced MD, formerly Perfect Practice MD
(Web-based practice management software for physicians including billing, scheduling, accounts receivable tracking, document scanning, and other services)
2795 Cottonwood Parkway
Suite 120
Salt Lake City, UT 84121
www.amdsoftware.com

Sure Claim 2000
(Physician billing software solution linked to PDA applications)
www.Sureclaim.com

EdgeMed Solutions, Inc.
(Medical practice management software)
1650 S. Powerline Road, Suite F
Deerfield Beach, FL 33442
www.Edgemed.com

Healthpac Medical Billing Systems
(Patient billing, electronic claims filing, electronic remittance posting, and insurance claim scrubber)
5105 Paulsen Street
Suite 225-D
Savannah, GA 31405
www.healthpac.com

Doc-tor.net
(Web enabled practice management software)
9 Post Road
Oakland, NJ 07436

Alta Point Data Systems
(Physician software package including billing, inventory, scheduling, clinical records, speech recognition, electronic claims, and PDA application)
1100 East South Union Avenue
Midvale, VT 84047
www.altapoint.com

Microsys Computing, Inc. (MicroMD)
(Practice management software and system configurations)
790 Boardman-Canfield Road
Youngstown, OH 44512
www.Microsys-computing.com

Smart Move Software
(Medical office management software to include scheduling, billing, ledger, and reports)
1151 Sheldon Drive
Westbury, NY 11590
www.smartmoveinc.com

E Claims, Inc.
(Electronic processing of claims)
9393 Second Avenue
Kearney, NE 68847
www.eclaims.com

Companion Technologies
(Comprehensive practice management system and electronic medical record)
6975 Union Park Center
Suite 500
Midvale, UT 84047
www.megawest.com

Physician Computer Network (PCN), Inc.
(Develops and supports information systems for physician practices)
180 Passaic Avenue
Fairfield, NJ 07950
www.pcn.com

NextGen Healthcare Information Systems
(ASP Medical Management Package)
Horsham, PA
www.nextgen.com

EZ Claim Medical Billing Software
124 W. University
Suite 206
Rochester, MI 48307
www.ezclaim.com

Soft Aid Inc.
16291 N.W. 57th Avenue
Miami, FL 33014
www.soft-aid.com

A4Health Systems
(Electronic medical record and practice management system)
3501 Dillard Drive
Cary, NC 27511
www.a4healthsys.com

Physician Micro Systems, Inc.
2033 6th Avenue
Seattle, WA 98121
www.pmsi.com

Athena Health
(ASP practice management system for offices)
One Moody Street
Waltham, MA 02453
www.athenahealth.com

Medical Electronic Billing
(Outsourced billing firm)
2121 Andrea Lane
Ft. Myers, FL 33912
www.m-e-b.com

Info-X, Inc.
(Claim check, medical necessity and coding compliance firm)
20 Charles Street
Northvale, NJ 07647
www.info-x-inc.com

Voice Recognition Software—*Dictation and transcription service via voice activation*

Speech Technology
www.speechtechnology.com

Dragon Systems, Inc.
www.Dragonsys.com

ViaVoice
www.IBM.com

21st Century Eloquence
www.voicerecognition.com

Digital Dictation Solutions, United Kingdom
main@src.co.uk

iDigital
(ASP digital dictation/transcription service)
www.idigital.com

Voice Network Systems
2201-2205 Maryland Avenue
Baltimore, Maryland 21218
www.vnsi.net

Medical Diagnosis Software—*Links symptoms or test results with associated conditions*

Diagnosis Pro
www.Medtech.com

Mioti—medical reference information
www.Mioti.com

www.Medicalsoftwareforpdas.com

5GL-Doctor
Australia
lisadev@uzemail.com.au

Electronic Medical Record Software Programs—*Depending on the package, average electronic medical record software can range from $6,000 to $15,000. Some of the packages include entering data, others include predetermined templates that the physician checks, and others include the ability to dictate your clinical medical record creating your own template.*

6520 N. Irwindale Avenue
Suite 215
Irwindale, CA 91702
www.Medicware.com

Medscape
(digital medical record capabilities with PDA)
20500 NW Parkway
Hillsboro, OR 97124
www.Medscape, Inc.

SOAPware Electronic Medical Record
www.Docs.com

IknowMEd
1608 Fourth Street
Third Floor
Berkley, CA 94710
www.Iknowmed.com

PowerMed Corporation
50 Monument Square

Portland, ME 04101
www.powermed.com

Blue Heron Software Development Ltd.
PO Box 59
Gananoque., On., Canada K7G2T6
www.Smartchartsmd.com

Berdy Medical Systems
(Smart Clinic and MD Trends)
www.berdymedical.com

Ergo Partners L.C.
Emritus—electronic medical record product
202 Hillcrest West
Lake Quivira, KS 66217
www.ergoparnters.com

Fax Software

Win Fax Pro 10.0
www.symantec.com/winfax

eFax
(receives and sends secure faxes)
www.efax.com

GFI Software USA Inc.
GFI Faxmaker
201 Towerview Court
Cary, NC 27513
www.gfisoftware.com

Clinical Websites for personal digital assistants (PDAs)

http://www.acponline.org/pda/ All sorts of medical books, programs, etc. Check Clinical References for documents on calories, ICD-9 codes, normal lab values, vaccination information, and ADA guidelines.

http://www.pdacortex.com/ More medical reference documents, patient tracking, databases, etc.

http://cgwebermd.tripod.com/Clinical-med/ Clinical medical textbook series.

http://www.handheldmed.com 5-Minute Consult Guides, Taber's Cyclopedic Medical Dictionary, Patient Tracker Desktop, the Merck Manual, Patient Tracker 5.11 for Palm OS, a to Z Drug Facts from Facts and Comparisons, etc.

http://www.emedicine.com Click PDA for a list of e-books.

http://www.medscape.com/viewarticle/442736 Although written for primary care providers, there is information on PDA's, programs, and more links to related PDA sites.

Medical-Practice Management Service Agreement

MPMSA Template: *Some key provisions of a medical practice management service agreement* (Institute of Medical Business Advisors, Inc.):

Definitions;
Relationship of the Parties;
Services to Be Provided By Administrator;
Overall Function;
General Administrative Services;
Facilities;
Premises;
Personal Property;
Expenses;
Disposition;
Acquisition and Assistance;
Financial Planning and Budgeting;
Inventory and Supplies;
Marketing, Advertising and Public Relations;
Personnel;
Provider and Payer Relationships;
Quality Assurance;
Other Consulting and Advisory Services;
Events Excusing Performance;
Obligations of the Group Practice;
Employment of Physician Employees;
Distributions to Physicians Stockholders;
Professional Services;
Medical Practices;
Group Practice's Internal Matters;
Group Practice Board Meetings;
Name;
Compliance With Laws;

Ancillary Operations;
Premises and Personal Property;
Group Practice Employee Benefit Plans;
Joint Planning Board;
Restrictive Covenants and Liquidated Damages;
Restrictive Covenants of the Group Practice;
Noncompetition;
Acknowledgment of Proprietary Interest;
Covenant Not-to-Divulge Confidential and Proprietary Information;
Return of Materials to Administrator;
Return of Materials to the Group Practice;
Restrictive Covenants and Liquidated Damages Provisions;
Enforcement of Physician Agreements;
Enforceability of Liquidated Damages Provisions;
Enforcement of Restrictive Covenants and Other Provisions;
Remedies;
Financial and Security Arrangements;
Service Fees;
Payments;
Repayment;
Security Agreement;
Performance Incentive/Reduction;
Records;
Insurance and Indemnity;
Insurance To Be Maintained By the Group Practice;
Insurance to Be Maintained By Administrator;
Continuing Liability Insurance Coverage;
Additional Insured;
Indemnification;
Guaranty;
Term and Termination;
Term of Agreement;
Extended Term;
Termination By the Group Practice;
Termination By Administrator;
Effective Date of Termination;
Effect Upon Termination;
General Provisions;
Assignment;
Amendments;
Waiver of Provisions;
Additional Documents;
Attorneys' Fees;
Contract Modifications for Prospective Legal Events;
Parties In Interest; No Third Party Beneficiaries;
Entire Agreement;
Severability;
Governing Law;

No Waiver;
Remedies Cumulative;
Arbitration and Mediation;
Mediation;
Initiation of Procedure;
Selection of Mediator;
Time and Place for Meditation;
Parties Represented;
Conduct of Mediation;
Fees of Mediator;
Disqualification;
Confidentiality;
Binding Arbitration;
Communications;
Captions;
Gender and Number;
Reference to Agreement;
Notice;
Counterparts.

Medical Unions, Public Sympathy, and Physician Salaries

Medical Unions and Public Sympathy: a recent issue of *Fortune* magazine carried the headline, "When Six Figured Incomes Aren't Enough. Now Doctors Want a Union."[1] Rightly or wrongly, the public has no sympathy for affluent doctors, and public support, as was seen in last year's UPS strike, is not in favor of organizing physicians. the doctors, on the other hand, want to unionize not for the purpose of getting more money but to get MCOs to return to them the power to practice as they see fit. But recall that perception is often reality, as the physician salary table below might suggest.

Specialty	Average	Lowest	Highest
Primary Care			
Family Practice	147,516	111,894	197,025
Internal Medicine	160,318	117,984	205,096
Pediatrics	149,754	111,113	201,086
Primary Care Surgical			
OB-GYN	238,224	184,045	350,455
Ophthalmology	246,823	161,763	417,000
Otolaryngology	254,978	180,084	392,890
Internal Medicine Specialties			
Endocrinology	160,085	123,984	221,633
Neurology	196,563	130,872	252,765
Hematology/Oncology	269,298	155,475	473,000
Pulmonary	198,956	143,229	280,278
Rheumatology	165,218	119,076	218,113
Nephrology	233,824	161,039	405,142

(continued)

---

[1]www.fortune.com and www.lib.usf.edu

(*continued*)

Specialty	Average	Lowest	Highest
Gastroenterology	282,133	179,000	381,340
Cardiology	300,500	186,667	434,607
Surgical Specialties			
General Surgery	261,276	175,314	364,279
Cardiovascular Surgery	558,719	351,108	852,717
Colon/Rectal Surgery	291,199	186,000	420,175
Neuro Surgery	438,426	279,655	713,961
Oral & Maxillofacial	208,340	157,404	352,879
Orthopedic Surgery	346,224	237,731	540,524
Plastic Surgery	306,047	196,711	411,500
Urology	273,326	180,808	375,000
Vascular Surgery	359,339	237,525	636,995
Miscellaneous Specialties			
Dermatology	232,000	168,988	407,000
Psychiatry	150,610	121,000	189,499
Hospital Based			
Anesthesiology	265,753	219,850	392,960
Radiology	309,361	225,181	429,716
Emergency Medicine	210,830	160,000	250,000

Source: Physician's Search: 2003

Major Doctor Unions[2]

National Doctors Alliance [affiliated with the Salaried Employees International Union (SEIU)] an umbrella group for:

Committee of Interns and Residents
Membership: > 11,000
Growth: 1,000
Dues: 1.375%–1.5000% of salary

Doctors Council
Membership: > 3,500
Growth: 1,000
Dues: $720/year

United Salaried Physicians and Dentists
Membership: 1,200
Growth: 300
Dues: .85% salary with $650 annual ceiling

[2]Membership may include: physicians, dentists, podiatrists, or veterinarians. May also include independent as well as employed doctors.

Federation of Physicians and Dentists
Membership: 8,500
Growth: 250
Dues: $672/year

Physicians for Responsible Negotiations (MD/DO only)
AMA sponsored Union: Mark Fox, MD
Membership: N/A
Growth: N/A
Dues: $300–$720/year

Union of American Physicians and Dentists
Membership: 6,000
Growth: 15–17% annually
Dues: $465 initial fee, plus $400/year, plus $100 annual IPA surcharge

Useful Healthcare Web Sites and Resources on CRM

HIPAA

- *HIPAA:* http://www.hcfa.gov/hipaa/hipaahm.htm
- *American Hospital Association:* www.aha.org

Privacy

- www.privacyrightsnow.com
- Online Privacy Alliance—www.privacyalliance.org
- Electronic Privacy Information Center—www.epic.org
- The Direct Marketing Association (DMA)—www.the-dma.org
- State or local chapters of the Better Business Bureau www.bbbonline.org

Data Mining

- www.kdnuggets.com
- www.dmg.org the Data Mining Group, a consortium of industry and academics formed to create standards for defining and sharing predictive models
- Data warehouse info center www.dwinfocenter.com has a list of tools available in the market.

Research

- www.gartner.com
- www.forrester.com
- www.aberdeen.com
- www.metagroup.com

CRM destination sites:

- www.crm_forum.com
- www.crmguide.com
- www.crmcommunity.com
- www.crmguru.com

CRM Healthcare Software Providers (in alphabetical order)

Act!—*www.act.com*
Aspect Communications—*www.aspect.com*
ASTEA communications—*www.astea.com*
Avaya Communications—*www.avaya.com*
Chordiant—*www.chordiant.com*
Commence—*www.commence.com*
Concerto—*www.concerto.com*
Convergys—*www.convergys.com*
Data Distilleries—
Delano Technologies—*www.delanotech.com*
Epiphany—*www.epiphany.com*
Front Range Solutions—*www.frontrange.com*
Magma Solutions—*www.magmasolutions.com*
Maximizer—*www.maximizer.com*
Microsoft—*www.microsoft.com*
NCR—*www.ncr.com*
Onyx—*www.onyx.com*
Peoplesoft—*www.peoplesoft.com*
Pivotal—*www.pivotal.com*
Protagona—*www.protagona.com*
Quadstone—*www.quadstone.com*
Salesforce—*www.salesforce.com*
SalesLogix—*www.saleslogix.com*
SAP—*www.sap.com*
SAS—*www.sas.com*
Serviceware—*www.serviceware.com*
Siebel—*www.Siebel.com*
Talisma—*www.talisma.com*
Upshot—*www.upshot.com*
Unica—*www.unica.com*
Viryanet—*www.viryanet.com*
White Pajamas—*www.whitepajamas.com*

Afterword

In his dictionary, Webster defines the word visionary as "one who is able to see into the future." Unlike some pundits, prescience is not a quality we claim to possess. To the purveyors of health care gloom and doom, however, the future for physicians is a bleak fait accompli. If you were of this same philosophical ilk prior to reading this book, we hope that you now realize the bulk of medical-management activity for physicians, payers, and patients may take place at the physician/executive level, as doctors take back their place as maestro of the medical-care symphony.

In the future, this doctor/manager dichotomy will blur as physicians control their professional and economic lives, leave tightly controlled HMOs, and form medical provider service networks or other delivery models, to obviate the need for broker-middlemen-agents sucking huge profits out of the system at the expense of all concerned. By other delivery model, we mean a medical-care organization run by physician executives who contract directly with employers, rather than managed-care intermediaries.

For this physician driven health care migration to occur, providers will need to consider the example of our contributing authors and graduate from business school and law school; or take management or technology courses to reengineer their practices with the needed organizational tools of this Millennium. Hopefully, *The Business of Medical Practice: Advanced Profit Maximization Techniques for Savvy Doctors* will prove useful in this regard and serve as a valuable resource for every medical, business, and graduate-school library in the country.

Do not be complacent, for, as onerous as it seems, we may not survive autonomously as a profession without utilizing this sort of information, because the bar to a new level of medical care has been raised in this decade. Although we still need actuarial and accounting data, working capital, marketing techniques, and correct product pricing, we believe that all physicians will look back on the Year 2005–2006 and recognize it as the turning point in the current health care imbroglio. Already, there are growing signs of this sea change as indicated by recent settlements of class-action lawsuits against giants Cigna and Aetna Health Care.

And, the growth of new health care technology and distribution models bodes well for future practitioners and patients through the following:

- e-health care technology, connectivity, eMRs, and computer physician order entry (CPOE) systems
- medical practice outsourcing
- global managed health care
- biotechnology, human genomics, and prospective health care

Therefore, as medical professionals, please realize that the experts of *iMBA* all face the same managed care issues as you do. And although the multidegreed experts of this textbook may have a particular business expertise, we should never lose sight of the fact that, *above all else*, medical care should be delivered in a personal and humane manner, with patient interest, rather than self-interest, as our guiding standard. *Omnia pro aegroto* (All for the patient).

Good medicine, Good business, Good day!

Fraternally,

David Edward Marcinko,
Hope Rachel Hetico, and
Contributing Authors

Index

Springer Publishing Company

Telemedicine and Telehealth
Principles, Policies, Performance, and Pitfalls

Adam William Darkins, MD, MPH, FRCS
Margaret Ann Cary, MD, MBA, MPH

"Darkins and Cary maintain a singular voice that is informative, providing a reasoned perspective that is devoid of cliches that typically are offered as insight about telemedicine and telehealth...This is a book that I can recommend to my colleagues to gain a balanced perspective on the implications of the Internet on modern healthcare."

—Telemedicine Journal

Contents:

- Introduction
- Definitions of Telemedicine and Telehealth and a History of the Remote Management of Disease
- Telehealth: A Patient Perspective
- Telehealth and Relationships with Physicians
- Using Telehealth to Make Health Care Transactions
- Telehealth Services
- Regulatory, Legislative and Political Considerations in Telehealth
- The Market for Telehealth Services
- Contracting for Telehealth Services
- The Business of Telehealth
- The Management of Telehealth Services
- Choosing the Right Technology for Telehealth
- Other Important Influences on Health Care that Affect the Future of Telehealth
- References
- Glossary of Terms and Abbreviations

2000   328pp   0-8261-1302-8   hard

---

11 West 42nd Street, New York, NY 10036
Order Toll-Free: 877-687-7476 • Order On-line: www.springerpub.com

Springer Publishing Company

Distinguishing Psychological from Organic Disorders, *2nd Edition*
Screening for Psychological Masquerade
Robert L. Taylor, MD

This volume is designed to help clinicians assess medical conditions which are "masquerading" as psychological ones. The author provides essential clues to our understanding of organic disease and shows us how to look for these clues during the clinical interview process. Common clinical pitfalls, simple assessment tests, and over 100 case studies are included. An annotated bibliography to this practical guide makes this an essential resource for mental health practitioners.

New to this edition: obsessive / compulsive disorders; the "love delusion"; postictal psychosis; an update on AIDS dementia complex; addition of atypical neuroleptics; SSRI's and newer general medications; an alternative medicine section; multiple sclerosis; ADHD; Lyme's disease; and an updated bibliography and references.

Contents:
- Appearances Can Be Deceiving
- Design of the Nervous System
- Clinical Traps
- A First Step: Recognition of Brain Syndrome
- More Clues to Psychological Masquerade
- Looking for Psychological Masquerade in the Clinical Setting
- Four Masqueraders
  (Brain Tumors, Epilepsy, Endocrine Disorders, AIDS)
- Drug-Induced Organic Mental Disorders
- Somatization: The Other Side of Things
- The Old and the Young
- Putting It To the Test: A Summary and 15 Test Cases
- Annotated Bibiography

2000   280pp   0-8261-1329-X   hardcover

11 West 42nd Street, New York, NY 10036
Order Toll-Free: 877-687-7476 • Order On-line: www.springerpub.com